Community Health Nursing

For Baillière Tindall:

Senior Commissioning Editor: Ninette Premdas
Project Development Manager: Dinah Thom
Project Manager: Samantha Ross
Designer: Judith Wright

Community Health Nursing

Frameworks for Practice

Edited by

Dianne Watkins MSc PGCE RN RM HV RNT

Director of Educational Development, School of Nursing and Midwifery Studies, University of Wales College of Medicine;
Formerly Director of Primary Care and Community Nursing, University of Wales College of Medicine, Cardiff, UK

Judy Edwards OBE BSc(Econ) PGCE

Formerly Director of Community Nursing Studies, University of Wales College of Medicine, Cardiff, UK

Pam Gastrell BA MPhil

Formerly Director of Studies, Primary Health Care, University of Southampton, Southampton, UK

Foreword by

Joan Higgins

Professor of Health Policy, University of Manchester, Manchester, UK

SECOND EDITION

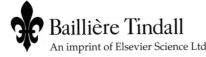
Baillière Tindall
An imprint of Elsevier Science Ltd

EDINBURGH LONDON NEW YORK OXFORD PHILADELPHIA ST LOUIS SYDNEY TORONTO 2003

BAILLIÈRE TINDALL

An imprint of Elsevier Limited

First edition 1996
Second edition 2003

ISBN 07020 2659X

British Library Cataloguing in Publication Data
A catalogue record for this book is available from the British Library

Library of Congress Cataloging in Publication Data
A catalog record for this book is available from the Library of Congress

Notice
Medical knowledge is constantly changing. Standard safety
precautions must be followed, but as new research and clinical
experience broaden our knowledge, changes in treatment and drug
therapy may become necessary or appropriate. Readers are advised to
check the most current product information provided by the
manufacturer of each drug to be administered to verify the
recommended dose, the method and duration of administration, and
contraindications. It is the responsibility of the practitioner, relying on
experience and knowledge of the patient, to determine dosages and
the best treatment for each individual patient. Neither the Publisher
nor the editors assume any liability for any injury and/or damage to
persons or property arising from this publication.

Contents

Contributors

Graham Allan BA MA PhD
Professor of Social Relations, School of
Social Relations, Keele University, Keele, UK

Carol Alstrom BSc(Hons) RGN DN CPT
Acting Deputy Director of Nursing,
St Mary's Hospital, Newport, Isle of Wight, UK

Michael L Burr MD DSc(MED) FFPHM
Reader in Epidemiology, Centre for Applied
Public Health Medicine, University of Wales
College of Medicine, Cardiff, UK

Lynda Carey BA(Hons) MSc(Nursing) RGN
Professional Lead, Practice Nursing, Blackburn
with Darwen Primary Care Trust, UK

David Cohen BCom MPhil
Professor of Health Economics, University of
Glamorgan School of Care Science,
Pontypridd, UK

Carole Crocker BSc(Hons) PGCE RGN DipProfPrac (spec)
Senior Nurse – Community Child Health,
Risca Health Centre, Newport, Gwent, UK

Graham Crow BA MA PhD
Reader in Sociology, Department of
Sociology and Social Policy, University of
Southampton, UK

Bridgit Dimond MA LLB DSA AHSM Barrister at Law
Emeritus Professor, University of Glamorgan,
Pontypridd, UK

David Fone MB BS MRCGP MFPHM
Consultant in Public Health Medicine,
Gwent Health Authority, Pontypool,
Gwent, UK

Neil Frude MPhil PHD CPsychol FBPsS
Clinical Research Tutor, Clinical
Psychology Training, Whitchurch Hospital,
Cardiff, UK

Elizabeth Gould BA(Hons) RGN RHV MPH
Development Manager, Gwent Health
Authority, Pontypool, Gwent, UK

Ben Hannigan BA(Hons) MA PGCE RMN RGN DPSN
CertCounsSkills
Lecturer, School of Nursing and Midwifery
Studies, University of Wales College of
Medicine, Cardiff, UK

Michael Hardey BA MA
Lecturer in Sociology, School of Nursing and
Midwifery, University of Southampton,
Southampton, UK

Harriet Jefferson BA(Hons) MSc RGN RHV PGDHPE RNT
Lecturer, School of Nursing and
Midwifery, University of Southampton,
Southampton, UK

Mark Jones BSc(Hons) MSc RN RHV
Director, Community Practitioners' and Health
Visitors' Association, London, UK

Gordon Macdonald PhD MPhil MA BSc(Econ) PGCE PGDipHEd
Head of Public Health and Health Promotion, School of Care Sciences, University of Glamorgan, Pontypridd, UK

Julia Muir BSc MSc RGN RSCN
Formerly Principal Lecturer, Faculty of Health and Social Care, University of the West of England, Bristol, UK

Elizabeth J Muir MSc(Econ) PhD CertEd
Project Director – Enterprise Education, Welsh Enterprise Institute, University of Glamorgan, Pontypridd, UK

Stephen Peckham BSc(Hons) MA(Econ)
Head of Department of Sociology and Social Policy, Reader in Health Policy, Oxford Brookes University, Oxford, UK

Brenda C Poulton BA MSc PhD RGN RHV
Professor of Community Health Nursing, School of Nursing, University of Ulster at Jordanstown, Newtownabbey, Co. Antrim, UK

Lisa Rhead BSc(Hons) RNMH
Community Nurse Learning Disability, Llanfrechfa Grange Hospital, Llanfrechfa, Cwmbran, Gwent, Wales

Graham C Rumbold BA MSc RGN NDNCert CHNT RNT
Coordinator, International Affairs and CPD, Centre for Healthcare Education, University College Northampton, Northampton, UK

Anna Sidey RSCN RGN DNCert
Independent Adviser in Community Children's Nursing, Church Stretton, Shropshire, UK

Eileen Thomas MA PhD RGN RHV MA
Nursing Director/Honorary Reader in Healthcare Practice, Portsmouth Health Care NHS Trust, Portsmouth, UK

Wendy Warren BSc(Hons) BSc(OU) Dip(HE)NursingStudies DN DipSS CertED CertHP
Head of Organisational Development St Mary's Hospital, Newport, Isle of Wight, UK

Ruth Wyn Williams BN(Hons) RNMH
Lecturer, School of Nursing and Midwifery Studies, University of Wales College of Medicine, Cardiff, UK

Foreword

In reviewing the period of health and social policy covered by this book two contrasting themes – continuity and change – emerge clearly. For many community nurses the nature of the clinical relationship, one to one with patients, may have remained relatively unchanged. As the different chapters of the book demonstrate, the factors influencing their working environment – patterns of ill health and health inequalities, the nature of family life and the legislative framework – have undergone change, but essentially at the margins. On the other hand the organizational superstructure, governing primary and community care, has experienced seismic shifts. If 'primary carers' were the forgotten partners in health care after the creation of the NHS in 1948, they suddenly came into their own in the 1990s. The notion of a 'primary care led NHS', which seemed like a 1990s catch phrase, is becoming a reality and the rest of the NHS has discovered the vital role which community nurses and their colleagues can play. In England, Primary Care Trusts now control the majority of NHS resources and community nurses are discovering new opportunities to make and influence policy as they take up roles as members of the management structure of primary care organizations. In other countries of the UK a similar prominence is being given to the contribution of primary and community care, even though organizational structures vary slightly.

Despite a degree of continuity, the relationship between professional and client is beginning to change. The younger generation, with whom community nurses work, have a different concept of 'service' from those who grew up with the NHS and who may have been uncritically grateful for the help it provided. The new users of healthcare services are more instrumental and expect a relationship of equals as well as collaboration and partnership in their care. They are less sentimental about the benefits of the 'welfare state' and more knowledgeable about their options. Different chapters of this book demonstrate how changing social and economic circumstances can have an impact upon need and demand and upon families' expectations of the services they receive. In periods of social change the immediate effects are often felt first by community staff and only later by those working in institutional settings. In this sense, community nurses are always on the 'front line,' both shaping and responding to the new environment. In these changing circumstances there are new pressures upon community nurses, but also new opportunities as the nature of nursing roles begins to change. The serious shortage of skilled individuals in advanced healthcare systems has led to a re-evaluation of the clinical workforce, with the result that traditional boundaries are being breached and ways of working are becoming more flexible. These trends present both new challenges and new opportunities to professional staff in community health nursing.

As the editors of this book have observed, community nurses occupy one of the most sensitive positions in the whole healthcare system. They are welcomed into people's homes, when clients are often at their most vulnerable. This places enormous pressure on community nurses, who work with a high degree of autonomy, to deliver the highest quality of care in often demanding circumstances. They may not have a wide range of colleagues upon whom to draw when they are delivering care, and a great deal rests upon their own knowledge and personal integrity. It is crucial that they have a broad understanding of a very wide range of issues, which can affect the care they give, and this book provides a thorough grounding in these areas.

This new edition of the book adds a great deal to our understanding of the context in which community nursing takes place. It illustrates the complexity and challenge of the task but the centrality of the community nurse's position in the NHS today and in the future.

Joan M Higgins

Editors' introduction

The political context has changed the face of primary health care over the last decade, hence the need for revising the content of this book, ensuring it is as up-to-date as any textbook can be. The NHS is witnessing radical reforms in an attempt to redress the balance in health across social groups in society (DoH 1999a, 1999b, 2001a). Inequalities in health influenced by structural and environmental issues, beyond the control of the individual, are guiding public health practice, whilst the organization of primary health care is again under review (Audit Commission 2002, British Medical Association 2002). Different models of primary care organizations are emerging across the four countries of the United Kingdom, with devolution playing a major part in determining the differences. A new General Practice Contract is on the horizon, and NHS Frameworks are directing practice in an effort to promote the delivery of clinically effective care (DoH 1999c, 2000a, 2000b, 2001b, 2001c). Professional regulation and protection of the public are major drivers for change, merging with a more informed general public.

This second edition of *Community Health Nursing – Frameworks for Practice* brings these issues to the forefront and considers the implications for community nursing. It not only updates each chapter, but also responds to a range of critical comments for improvement received from reviewers. Recommendations suggested an increased emphasis on quality improvement, inclusion of a chapter on the prevention of child physical abuse, community mental health nursing, community learning disability nursing and school

nursing, and the greater significance of public health as a framework for practice. This second edition has included these suggestions in its text.

The text remains broad based and is designed to support students undertaking graduate programmes, at a pre-registration and post-registration level. Students studying for first registration in the fields of mental health, learning disability and adult and children's nursing would benefit from using elements of this book as an accompaniment to their community modules and associated clinical placements. It would help them to understand the broad nature of primary health care and the roles of various nursing professionals working within the field, as well as guiding them through those factors that adversely affect health and well-being.

Qualified nurses studying for a specialist community nursing qualification in district nursing, health visiting (public health nursing), community mental health nursing, community learning disability nursing, practice nursing, school nursing or community children's nursing will find this book invaluable to their studies. This new edition has incorporated chapters specifically relating to community mental health nursing, community learning disability nursing and school nursing, in turn increasing its acceptability to these groups of specialist community nurses. It aims to provide a stimulating resource for both community nursing students and educators in clinical practice and higher education institutions. The book poses questions and issues for reflection, seminars and debate, as well as offering referenced and recommended reading to promote depth and breadth of study.

As editors we made a decision to continue with a 'framework' approach to education and professional development that links social and health policy with innovation and community nursing practice. There is a deliberate overlap in some parts of the book to guide the reader through a multitude of subject areas that interlink, thus reinforcing important messages. Each chapter is cross-referenced with other chapters, which allows the reader to gain an in-depth knowledge of particular areas and assists with building the 'picture of nursing in a community and primary care environment'.

STRUCTURE AND ORGANIZATION OF THE BOOK

The book is organized into six sections, each using a different perspective to explore the issues relevant to community nursing practice. Section one focuses on the pressures for change, highlighting relevant health and social policy developments and their consequent effects on the organization and management of primary care. The section proceeds with a vision of the modern public health movement and emphasizes the use of a social model of health. The final chapter in this section draws the reader's attention to the clinical governance framework and the implications of this policy development on clinical practice and professional regulation. The provision of a quality service to clients and patients, delivered through a collaborative approach, where the client/patient is an equal partner in care, is an important message that arises throughout this chapter.

Section two uses public health as a framework for practice, with chapters that explore the use of epidemiology as an evidence base for disease prevention and structural issues related to poverty and its influence on health. The emphasis in this section is on those factors that adversely affect health and the associated issues for preventative work. The final chapter outlines opportunities for the community nurse to work in a proactive manner to contribute to the achievement of health

gain, using the resource of the local community to improve health status.

Section three reviews the family as a framework for community nursing practice, outlining sociological and psychological perspectives. Society's view of what constitutes a family changes in its structure over time, and the perceived functions of a family all impact upon the way in which nurses deliver care in the home environment. Violence and abuse in families is a major health-related problem and one which community nurses need to be aware of when undertaking the assessment process in a home environment. Protecting children from abuse is of importance to all community nurses, and an ecological framework for prevention of violence to children by their parents is presented in this chapter. In the final chapter in this section the family is discussed as a provider of health care, as well as the unit for nursing assessment. It presents a way of working with families that would suit all community nurses, regardless of the specialism being studied.

The fourth section is concerned with professional frameworks based around legal and ethical issues, team working and leadership. The emergence of new nursing roles associated with greater autonomy are rapidly developing in primary care settings, leading to new issues associated with accountability and legal frameworks for practice. These concerns are addressed in the first chapter of this section, closely followed in the second chapter, by the ethical issues encountered in community nursing practice. Primary healthcare provision is closely aligned with effective team working, which is addressed in the chapter on team working and team development in health and social care. The final chapter in this section discusses leadership in community nursing and presents the qualities of effective leaders. It outlines the importance of leadership in leading and managing change in nursing practice.

Section five contains chapters pertaining to each of the specialist areas of community nursing previously mentioned. Each chapter outlines the historical development of that area of nursing, highlights issues relevant to current practice, and discusses the future development in relation to health and social policies. The section, read in its totality, will serve to provide an overview of nursing in a community and primary healthcare setting, accurately describing how each diverse discipline contributes to the delivery of care through collaboration and team working.

The final section of the book is based around challenges for the future of community nursing. It is unique in its attempt to offer future aspirations for practice, which provide a springboard for debate and discussion. It presents an overview of innovation and developments in nursing and questions whether the National Health Service provides value for money. Information technology is presented as both a challenge and an opportunity for community nurses, and the section ends with a chapter on the shift from health promotion to the 'modern' public health movement, outlining opportunities for community nurses to make an active contribution to the public health agenda.

This book is by no means inclusive of all issues influencing the specialist community nurse. It does, however, provide an overview of the complexities influencing and shaping the current and future practice of community health nursing. An important message for community nurses based on our personal beliefs is that, although we play a critical part in the lives of many people on their pathway to recovery or death, our role will only be valued if we value others. Each person's

experience of illness or health is unique, shaped by personal life experience, and this must be respected. As community nurses we are privileged to share people's homes and families and we must never abuse our position. This philosophy underpins each page of this new edition of *Community Health Nursing – Frameworks for Practice*.

REFERENCES

Audit Commission 2002 A focus on general practice in England. Audit Commission, London

British Medical Association, General Practitioner Committee 2002 Improving general practitioners' working lives. BMA, London

Department of Health (DoH) 1999a Saving lives: our healthier nation. HMSO, London

Department of Health (DoH) 1999b Making a difference: strengthening the nursing, midwifery and health visiting contribution to health and health care. HMSO, London

Department of Health (DoH) 1999c Mental health: National Health Service Frameworks. HMSO, London

Department of Health (DoH) 2000a National Service Framework: coronary heart disease. HMSO, London

Department of Health (DoH) 2000b The national cancer plan. HMSO, London

Department of Health (DoH) 2001a Investment and reform for NHS staff – Taking forward the NHS plan. HMSO, London

Department of Health (DoH) 2001b National Service Framework for older people. HMSO, London

Department of Health (DoH) 2001c National Service Framework for diabetes. HMSO, London

Pressures for change

The material contained in this introductory section seeks to set the scene for the reader. The pressures for change in primary care relate to the political agenda, inclusive of devolution and emerging primary care organizations. The emphasis on professional regulation, risk management and protection of the public are major developments influencing healthcare provision in the 21st century, all of which are alluded to in this first section.

The first chapter opens with a review of recent health and social policy developments, their background, introduction and likely impact. Against this backdrop the second chapter examines the growth of primary care in the United Kingdom and explores some of the reasons why primary care is seen as having an increasingly important role within the National Health Service. It examines some of the key policy issues and their effect on patient care and current community nursing practice. Readers are reminded the landscape of primary care is changing across the United Kingdom, leading to diversification of primary care organizations. The chapter concludes by urging nurses to consider the impact of the changes outlined, on primary healthcare services and the development of community nursing.

Chapter three follows with a discussion on innovation and change in public health. It commences with an overview of the function and historical development of public health practice and draws attention to the pressures for change. It explores the need to incorporate a social model of health in the drive to reduce the impact of poverty and key health issues are discussed from a public health perspective. The author concludes with examples, drawn from a case study of health and social needs assessment carried out in Caerphilly

County Borough, south Wales, which illustrates a social model of health in action.

The final chapter in this section is concerned with issues relating to quality assurance and clinical governance. It begins with a discussion of policy development in the face of media coverage of scandals, pointing to (among other things) the failure of the professions in self-regulation and the rising costs of claims for negligence. Implications for nurses working in primary care and community settings are explored and readers are asked to consider the critical significance of continuous professional development and life-long learning. The importance of evidence-based practice and patient safety is emphasized, in conjunction with working in partnership with clients, improving clinical outcomes and promoting equity in service provision.

1

Recent health and social policy developments

S. Peckham

INTRODUCTION

The last 15 years have seen some fundamental changes in healthcare policy in the UK which have had important implications for community nursing. At the time of writing, the NHS is going through yet another major organizational change and the NHS continues to retain its position as one of the key topics of political debate and media interest. The election of a Labour government in 1997 had important consequences for the development of healthcare policy and a new organizational pattern has been set out for the 21st century. Continued change is now planned for the next few years as the proposals contained in the Labour government's *The NHS Plan* (DoH 2000) unfold and develop. This chapter discusses the broad sweep of these healthcare policy changes as they relate to the NHS and, more specifically, to community nursing. The aim of the chapter is to set out broad themes relating to NHS policy developments and particularly the extent to which such changes represent a break from, or continuity with, the past. It is, though, becoming increasingly difficult to talk about health care in the UK as a unitary system due to devolution and the increasing number of differences between England, Northern Ireland, Scotland and Wales. These differences are addressed in this chapter, as is devolution in relation to health policy; however, the main emphasis is on the English policy framework. Many changes relate specifically to primary care and these are dealt with in more detail in Chapter 2.

POLICY HISTORY

While this chapter focuses on the period since 1997 it is important to understand these policy changes within the overall context of health policy in the UK over the last 150 years. Much of the shape of the NHS and key problems to which policy is addressed, are the result of professional and policy developments in the 19th century, at the birth of the NHS in 1947 and organizational changes in the 1970s, 1980s and 1990s. This history has been amply dealt with elsewhere (Klein 1998, Ottewill & Wall 1990). In fact, many of the policy developments since 1947 have been to address key tensions which continue to haunt the delivery of health care in the UK today:

- The tension between central or local control and management
- The tension between medical and management power
- The tension between treating individuals and providing a population-based service within a capped budget
- The tension between treatment and prevention of ill health.

Furthermore, current policy developments can be seen as part of the continuing response to developments in health and welfare which have been termed as the 'crisis in health' (Ham 1992). In the 1970s there was an increasing recognition of a growing number of problems and issues facing healthcare systems in developed countries. While labelled as a 'crisis', this was not a single incident but the coming together of a range of factors. Many of the features of the 'crisis in health' were visible in all industrialized countries and had their roots in concerns about the rapidly escalating costs of health care (Saltman & Von Otter 1992), although the 'crisis' reflects concern about a range of issues of which those given in Box 1.1 are seen to be the most significant.

Part of the response to the 'crisis' was the recognition that changes in the epidemiology and demographics of disease required a different approach from one that focused on the delivery of acute care. Thus in dealing with chronic illness and supporting older people the role of general

Box 1.1 Factors in the 'Crisis in Health'
◆ Demographic changes – the UK has an ageing population while at the same time a reduction in the proportion of the population of working age, leading to an increasing demand for health care at a time when health systems will be limited in their ability to respond to this demand.   ◆ Epidemiological transition – a move from a major preoccupation with infectious diseases to one concerned with chronic conditions.   ◆ Changing relationships between patients and healthcare professionals.   ◆ Concern with social factors – the biomedical or curative approach to health is being questioned, with a search for a broader approach which takes into account social factors, recognizes the harmful effects of the environment and shifts the emphasis on to prevention of ill health.   ◆ Continuing concerns about inequalities of health and the recognition that these are deep seated.   ◆ The ever-widening gap between demands made on healthcare services and the resources which the Government is prepared to make available.

practice and community health services became more central. In the UK the response was to develop general practice and primary healthcare teams and led to an increasing engagement of government and the NHS in developing the quality and role of primary care (DHSS 1986, 1987, Ottewill & Wall 1990). There was also a retrenchment with an initial focus on high-spending hospitals but a recognition that control also needed to be exercised over the gatekeepers to the NHS. The last 20 years have also seen an increasing overlap between primary and community care services. The issue of collaboration between health and social care agencies is not a new one (Exworthy & Peckham 1998) but there has been an increasing emphasis on health and social care partnerships during the 1990s and the Labour government has placed partnership at the centre of its proposals and developments for the NHS and Social Services (Glendinning et al 2001).

THE CONTEXT OF NHS REFORMS AT THE TURN OF THE CENTURY

Since coming in to office the Labour government placed priority on three policy areas which have impacted on health and health care in the UK:

1. *political devolution* to Scotland, Wales and Northern Ireland
2. *modernization* of the NHS including organizational reform and an emphasis on standards
3. an ideology of the *third way*, a more pragmatic approach to policy formulation and implementation.

Tensions exist within this policy direction. On the one hand, Labour stresses 'one nation' policies and stresses greater uniformity through new institutions such as the National Institute for Clinical Excellence (NICE; England and Wales only). On the other, it emphasizes local targets and local responses to particular circumstances, for example through developments in primary care. Political devolution may increase diversity as it allows greater policy experimentation but it may also facilitate uniformity through 'policy transfer' – the sharing of policy developments in one country with another (Dolowitz et al 1999).

The reforms pursued by the Labour government post 1997 were further focused around a modernization agenda for the NHS in a new approach to healthcare organization. There were a number of strands to this which sought to make a break with the Conservative government's internal market approach of the early 1990s. However, the new Labour government was also constrained by developments in the 1990s and hence NHS policy changes in the period after 1997 must be seen in the context of previous policy developments.

One prime consideration was the level of agreement about the focus on primary care and there was also some hesitation about launching into major NHS reform so soon after the major reforms of 1991 and consolidation of health authorities in 1996. The new Labour government was also faced with a number of high-profile incidents which heightened public anxiety about medical practice including the Alder Hay case regarding the removal of tissue and organs during post mortems, Harold Shipman and the Bristol child heart surgery cases.

These incidents raised questions about medical competence and the robustness of the machinery established to monitor medical competence within the NHS and through the General Medical Council.

It was these factors which led to an increased emphasis on accreditation and performance management and an emphasis on national standards. (See Chapter 4 for a more detailed discussion of quality improvement and the implications for community nursing.)

Labour policy has been developed in two White Papers; *The New NHS* (DoH 1997) on NHS organization and *Saving Lives: Our Healthier Nation* (DoH 1999) on public health. These were followed up in 2000 with *The NHS Plan* and the development of a modernization strategy for the NHS which built on the White Papers. One key change was a shift away from competition within an internal market, introduced in 1991, to an approach based on partnership between agencies, although retaining the essential distinction between purchasers (health authorities and primary care organizations) and providers (hospitals and community health services). The other major change has been the increasing impact devolution has made to the shape of the NHS, with distinctive differences in policy development in Scotland and Wales. Nevertheless there were important continuities of policy across the home nations, which focused on the development of primary care organizations, improved management performance, an emphasis on increasing quality through improved management systems and accreditation, together with a focus on a national service with national standards brought about in England through the instigation of National Service Frameworks (NSFs), the NICE and the Commission for Health Improvement (CHI) (now to become the Commission for Healthcare Audit and Inspection (CHAI)).

NEW LABOUR AND THE NHS

The publication of *The New NHS* White Paper in the autumn of 1997 set out the foundations of the new government's approach to the NHS in England which was also reflected in developments in Scotland, Northern Ireland and Wales (Secretaries of State for NI, Scotland and Wales). The Labour government set out six key principles for the NHS (see Box 1.2) underpinned by values for delivering care:

◆ at home: easier and faster advice and information for people about health, illness and the

NHS so that they are better able to care for themselves and their families;

♦ in the community: swift advice and treatment in local surgeries and health centres with
family doctors and community nurses working
alongside other health and social care staff to provide a wide range of services on the spot;

♦ in hospital: prompt access to specialist services linked to local surgeries and health centres
so that entry, treatment and care are seamless and
quick (DoH 1997).

The New NHS (DoH 1997) proposed to renew
the NHS and to tackle the 'unfairness', 'unacceptable variations' and 'two-tierism' of the Conservative internal market (Powell & Exworthy 2000). To
this end the White Paper included proposals for
NICE and CHI to promote such equity.

These proposals also suggested a more bureaucratic approach to ensuring national standards and
alongside the development of National Service
Frameworks, establish national criteria for standards and quality of care and approaches to clinical practice. The Government also promised to
shift £1 billion of NHS funding from red tape into

patient care, the establishment of NHS Direct (a 24-
hour nurse helpline), an NHS information super-
highway and to develop guaranteed fast-track
cancer services. *The New NHS* provided a framework for a range of changes in the organization of
primary care with the introduction of Primary Care
Groups/Local Health Groups – building on earlier
models of Total Purchasing projects. (See Chapter
24 for further discussion on NHS Direct).

Public health was also identified as a key area
for government action with a clear recognition of
the problems of health inequalities. Since 1997, the
Labour government has taken various steps associated with tackling health inequalities. One of its
first actions was to commission an Independent
Inquiry into Inequalities in Health, chaired by Sir
Donald Acheson, the former Chief Medical Officer.
The inquiry reported in November 1998 (Acheson
1998). The inquiry reviewed the research evidence
related to health inequalities and made 39 recommendations. Only three of the recommendations
were directed to the NHS, thereby underlining
the relative contribution of healthcare services to
tacking health inequality compared to poverty,
education, employment, housing, transport and
nutrition. (See Chapter 6 for information on structural issues related to poverty and health.)

The planned policies for the NHS and for the
improvement of public health in England were
set out in *The New NHS* (DoH 1997) and then in a
Green Paper the following year (DoH 1998). The
Green Paper *Our Healthier Nation* (DoH 1998) was
seen as a follow-up to the *Health of the Nation* (DoH
1992). The strategy aimed to improve the health
of the population as a whole and to improve the
health of the worst off in society, as a means to
narrow the 'health gap'. It proposed four targets
related to heart disease and stroke, accidents, cancer and mental health. The subsequent White
Paper *Saving Lives: Our Healthier Nation* was published in 1999. It reaffirmed the proposed targets
but did not set national health inequality targets
and it did not allocate specific monies to the task.
Instead, local areas were to set their own targets.
These aims have also been reflected in the policy
developments for Northern Ireland, Scotland and
Wales. However, there are important distinctions
in relation to the role of the elected assemblies in

these countries as well as to the exact nature and responsibilities of their primary care organizations. One key weakness of national policy is the seeming lack of co-ordination between NHS organizational policy and public health, although government policy and guidance have been very clear about the central role of primary care in public health.

Partnership was a central theme of *The New NHS* and the Government was keen to support the development of partnership as an alternative to the internal market. This approach was emphasized as a 'third way'; neither central planning (hierarchy) nor the internal market. It includes developing local health economies and long-term service agreements between purchasers – which would increasingly be primary care organizations (Primary Care Trusts and new Care Trusts) – and providers – hospital and specialist service trusts, other primary care trusts and provider Care Trusts. Community Health Trusts would, by and large, be merged into the new Primary Care Trusts. The Government also signalled a major investment plan in the NHS and stated its intention to modernize and to improve standards and the quality of care. The framework for these developments was established in *The NHS Plan* (DoH 2000). This set out ten core principles for the NHS (see Box 1.3).

The NHS Plan states that health care is a basic human right and that the NHS will not exclude people because of their health status or ability to pay. Access to the NHS will continue to depend upon clinical need and not the ability to pay. It will also continue to provide access to a comprehensive range of services throughout primary and community health care, intermediate care and hospital-based care. In addition the NHS will also provide information services and support to individuals in relation to health promotion, disease prevention, self-care, rehabilitation and after care with new specific services such as NHS Direct (see Chapter 24), and by supporting increased patient information and support. In order to improve patient responsiveness, the Plan provides for structures to give patients and citizens a greater say in the NHS, and promises that the provision of services will be centred on patients' needs.

Box 1.3 NHS plan: principles for the NHS

1. The NHS will provide a universal service for all based on clinical need, not ability to pay.
2. The NHS will provide a comprehensive range of services.
3. The NHS will shape its services around the needs and preferences of individual patients, their families and their carers.
4. The NHS will respond to different needs of different populations.
5. The NHS will work continuously to improve quality of services and to minimize errors.
6. The NHS will support and value its staff.
7. Public funds for health care will be devoted solely to NHS patients.
8. The NHS will work together with others to ensure a seamless service for patients.
9. The NHS will help keep people healthy and work to reduce health inequalities.
10. The NHS will respect the confidentiality of individual patients and provide open access to information about services, treatment and performance.

The Plan reiterates that patient confidentiality will be respected throughout the process of care and that the NHS will be more open about information concerning health and healthcare services. The Government is committed to the continuing use of information to improve the quality of services for all and to generate new knowledge about future medical benefits. Developments in science such as the new genetics, offer important possibilities for disease prevention and treatment in the future (see Chapter 12 for further discussion on the implications for family nursing). As a national service, the NHS is well-placed to take advantage of the opportunities offered by scientific developments, and will ensure that new technologies are harnessed and developed in the interests of society as a whole and available to all on the basis of need.

There is a strong emphasis on the quality of services and proposals outlined in the Plan include new national standards, greater performance management, improved clinical governance and new national organizations to support high-quality care (NICE) and to ensure standards are maintained by service providers (CHI). The Government has also signalled its intent to support staff through additional education and training and to expand the numbers of doctors and nurses. At the same time the Plan identifies professional and organizational protectionism within the healthcare system which needs to be addressed in order for the NHS to develop. The Modernisation Agency, together with local modernization committees, has been established to lead change throughout the service and much of its work is based on using examples of 'good practice' within the NHS such as NHS Beacons, although the use of pioneers, whose anticipated success will be rolled out to the rest of the NHS, is also evident in the Booked Admissions Programme, the Collaboratives in cancer, orthopaedics, primary care and other services, and the 'Action On' initiatives for cataracts, ENT, dermatology and orthopaedics. In addition, numerous Department of Health documents now use brief 'case studies' to illustrate desired behaviour. Perhaps aligned to this approach there has also been the drawing in of leaders to focus on areas of clinical care (e.g. cancer and CHD) and also on services such as food (Lloyd Grossman) and buildings (Prince Charles).

Central to the development of a quality service are proposals for substantive changes to the regulatory machinery for healthcare professionals which are set out in *Modernising Regulation in the Health Care Professions* (DoH 2001) and specific consultation documents for a new Health Care Professions Regulatory Board and a new Nursing and Midwifery Council – the proposals for which are incorporated in the Health Services Reform Bill 2001. These developments involve a complete overhaul of the regulatory bodies and are set alongside changes to the General Medical Council and how complaints are dealt with. For nursing the English National Board and UKCC have been abolished and are to be replaced by a new Nursing and Midwifery Council which incorporate separate arrangements for health visitors. In addition there will be a new Health Professions Council for the regulation of healthcare professionals previously covered by the Council for Professions Supplementary to Medicine and there are proposals for a Council for the Regulation of Healthcare Professionals to oversee the activities of the various regulatory bodies (see Chapter 13 for discussion of related legal issues).

Drawing on the partnership theme (of central importance to the NHS) would be the development of a 'seamless' service. The health and social care system will be shaped around the needs of the patient, not the other way round. There will be an increased emphasis on developing partnerships and co-operation at all levels of care – between patients, their carers and families and NHS staff; between the health and social care sector; between different government departments; between the public sector, voluntary organizations and private providers in the provision of NHS services. The aim will be to ensure a patient-centred service. Proposals include new approaches to partnerships to provide improved care for older people especially by supporting intermediate care, developing 'one-stop shops' (integrated health and social care services) and developing new care trusts – combined health and social care organizations. Specific proposals include:

◆ rapid response teams: made up of nurses, care workers, social workers, therapists and GPs working to provide emergency care for people at home and helping to prevent unnecessary hospital admissions;

◆ arrangements at GP practice or social work level to ensure that older people receive a one-stop service: this might involve employing or designating the sort of key workers or link workers used in Somerset, or basing case managers in GP surgeries;

◆ integrated home care teams: so that people receive the care they need when they are discharged from hospital to help them live independently at home.

There is little in the Plan about public health issues although it set out a commitment that the NHS will focus efforts on preventing, as well as treating, ill health. There is a clear recognition of the wider determinants of health, such as deprivation, housing, education and nutrition, with a commitment that the NHS will work with other public services to intervene, not just after, but before ill health occurs. Of key importance is the commitment to reduce health inequalities and a promise to introduce health inequality targets which was honoured and lengthy consultation was undertaken on targets to:

◆ reduce by at least 10% the gap in mortality for children under 1 year between manual groups and the population as a whole by 2010

◆ reduce by at least 10% the gap between the fifth of health authority areas with the lowest life expectancy at birth and the population as a whole by 2010.

DEVOLUTION

Since the beginning of the NHS there have always been important differences in the organization and delivery of healthcare services between England, Northern Ireland, Scotland and Wales. Essentially England and Wales operated the same structure and organization with Scotland having a similar structure, but with health boards rather than authorities, and Northern Ireland having combined health and social care departments. Many elements of the system were, however, the same, including the general practitioner system, the role and location of public health, delivery of community services, etc. Since the Labour government came to power in 1997 much has changed, with political devolution to the Scottish Parliament and Welsh Assembly and with political change now occurring in Northern Ireland.

The Labour government's political devolution to a Scottish Parliament, and to Welsh and N. Ireland Assemblies, has created the capacity for further spatial differences. Moreover, other policies support greater diversity. The proposed NHS reforms, published in 1997 and 1998, incorporated different territorial policies. Although the capacity for policy diversity post-devolution will vary in each territory, some policy uniformity might be expected; the UK operates as a unitary state with a parliamentary system (based at Westminster). However, whilst the impact of policy proposals upon existing systems is only emergent, devolution is likely to unleash a dynamic whose longer-term impacts are currently unknown.

Currently the Department of Health (DoH) (for England) is the responsibility of the Secretary of State for Health whereas, elsewhere, responsibility lies with the Secretary of State for each territory. The DoH (in London) takes responsibility for UK-wide issues and for international health policy issues (such as liaison with the European Union) (Hunter 1998a, Jervis & Plowden 2000). This division of responsibilities is liable to change as devolved territories renegotiate their relationships within and outwith the UK.

Scotland already enjoys considerable administrative devolution which is complemented by political devolution to the Scottish Parliament (Hazell & Jervis 1998, p. 31). The White Paper envisaged 'greater flexibility … over the pace and detail of the primary care changes' (Hunter 1998b, p. 11). Parliament can alter income tax for Scottish residents by three percentage points and vire between and within their total budgets. Hazell and Jervis (1998, p. 42) foresaw the possibility that the Parliament could introduce radical changes such as adding greater democratic input into healthcare commissioning, or ending the independent contractor status of GPs. Recent measures proposed in Scotland (e.g. long-term care charges and student grants) have demonstrated that the Scottish Parliament is determined to set its own political course. In particular, the decision to provide long-term care free of charge, is beginning to have political and service ramifications across the whole of the UK, not just in Scotland.

The Welsh Assembly is responsible for allocating £2.5 billion of NHS expenditure in Wales but has no law-making powers. However, it can introduce structural changes – such as transferring powers to the Assembly itself (Hazell & Jervis 1998, p. 34). It will also be able to abolish or reform HAs and NHS Trusts – a reform it wishes to invoke with regard to the former (NAW, press release, WO1123, 2 February 2001). The Assembly cannot pass primary legislation and will have no tax raising powers. However, by passing secondary legislation, it will 'dictate the **detail** of health policy' (Whitfield 1998, p. 15; emphasis added). The NHS in Wales underwent revision before the Assembly was established by reducing the number of Trusts in Wales from 26 to 16 in April 1999 (Garside 1999). The Assembly was given a central role in health policy, for example HAs are held to account by the Assembly. The White Paper (*A voice for Wales*, 1997) defined its health remit as monitoring the health of the population, determining the scale of financial resources for health and the identification and promotion of good practice (para. 2.1). (This complements earlier innovations in, for example, health promotion services.) In February 2001, the NHS Plan for Wales was published which proposed the abolition of HAs in Wales by April 2003. The National Assembly will take 'direct democratic control, its responsibilities providing leadership, direction and oversight through a newly created Health and Well-being Partnership Council which will be chaired by the Minister' (NAW Press Release, WO1123, 2 February 2001).

CURRENT CHANGES

As we begin the 21st century we continue to see governments grappling with what are somewhat traditional concerns of healthcare policy – the funding and organization of healthcare systems (e.g. The Wanless Report (2002) and review for the Treasury), trying to improve quality, tackling issues of accountability and addressing the roles and regulation of healthcare professionals. Certainly the changes being made are new in the sense that the organizational focus of the NHS is shifting through devolution and the focus on primary care but many key policy issues remain to be addressed in terms of accountability structures, how to improve efficiency, provide high-quality universal care and balance the demands of clinical care and public health.

The Government is pursuing change at every level of the NHS with proposals for changes to organization (nationally, regionally and locally), professional regulation, patient and public involvement – although these are being pursued to different degrees within England, Northern Ireland, Scotland and Wales. For example in Wales there will be 22 local health boards, local commissioning partnerships and public health will be led by the Welsh Chief Medical Officer,

centrally under the direction of the Assembly. In England, since *The NHS Plan* (2000) there has been a continuing debate about the structure and organization of the NHS in England given the proposals for moving quickly to comprehensive PCT coverage, the development of Care Trusts and the abolition of Health Authorities and Regions and the establishment of 28 Strategic Health Authorities (StHAs). The details for these developments are contained in a Department of Health consultation paper *Shifting the Balance of Power: Next Steps* (DoH 2002a). In addition to those proposals which had been outlined in *The NHS Plan*, the Government proposes re-merging the NHS Executive and the Department of Health. Emphasis is also placed on the need to pursue the changes quickly (at odds with the developmental approach outlined in the White Paper *The New NHS*), to use the Modernisation Agency and Leadership Centre to develop new ways of working, to develop a new and more patient-centred service and to make organizational changes to support longer-term cultural change. (See Chapter 4 for further discussion of the link between quality improvement and culture.)

While there are clear similarities in policy proposals across the UK, emphasizing a focus on primary care organizations as key organizations in the NHS, drawing clinicians into management and policy development, emphasizing partnership and developing national standards, there are still some very distinct and interesting differences. Welsh organizational structures have resulted in Local Health Boards (LHB) matching local authority boundaries with broader LHB membership than in either England or Scotland. In Scotland partnership arrangements are being developed through interorganizational arrangements rather than by unifying health and social care as in the English Care Trusts (see Chapter 3). Of perhaps most interest, in relation to community health services, are the different arrangements for structuring and delivering community services – where England is moving towards incorporation in primary care organizations (Peckham & Exworthy 2002). Key differences are emerging over public health where the Welsh Assembly and Scottish Parliament have placed more emphasis on this area of work with the Welsh Assembly, in particular, taking a stronger role in addressing public health issues (see Chapter 3 for more detailed discussion of public health issues). Essentially devolution has created a stronger divergence and thus rather than one modernization programme being driven from London there are a number of organizational and policy experiments being developed within the UK healthcare system.

Conversely, proposals for changes to the professional regulatory machinery will apply across the whole of the UK and represent both a more structured role for professional regulatory bodies and one in which the regulatory mechanisms themselves are more centrally regulated. The new Nursing and Midwifery Council will be smaller than the UKCC and be made up of directly elected practitioners and a strong lay input, which will be charged with strategic responsibility for setting and monitoring standards of professional training, performance and conduct. The Council will maintain a new streamlined professional register. They are to be given wider powers to deal effectively with individuals who present unacceptable risks to patients. Health visitors will continue to have separate registration and representation within the new Council. The new Health Professions Council will oversee the 12 regulatory boards for professions allied to health care and will have similar powers to the Nursing and Midwifery Council. These changes are currently being implemented. At the same time there have been changes to the General Medical Council to strengthen its powers through a scheme of regular revalidation of the fitness to practice of doctors on its Register, and it is now consulting on new governance arrangements, revalidation and improved fitness to practice procedures. The Government is also consulting on the establishment of a new Council for the Regulation of Healthcare Professionals to which all professional regulatory councils would be accountable. These changes apply to the whole of the UK and represent a significant change to healthcare professional regulation with greater government involvement in establishing and prescribing the functions of regulatory bodies and by establishing clearer links between regulation, accreditation and continuing professional development and re-accreditation.

There are also new proposals for dealing with complaints, lay scrutiny of the NHS and the development of new structures and mechanisms for patient and public involvement. These proposals vary in England, Scotland and Wales. However, there is generally an increased emphasis on lay involvement, alongside increased healthcare professional involvement in the management and organization of healthcare services. Central to these developments is an attempt to open up healthcare services to greater public scrutiny. So while Community Health Councils (CHCs) are to be abolished in England, they are to be retained in Wales, and Scotland is retaining the Community Health Boards. However, in all areas there is a strengthening of such lay agencies. England is to replace CHCs with a range of new organizations and structures, the Government proposing to establish new elements for patient and public participation, Trust-based patient 'advisory services' (PALS) and new scrutiny powers for local authorities (DoH 2001). To support patient and public involvement the proposals include Patient Forums (PFs) for each PCT and NHS Trust. A new independent complaints advocacy service (ICAS) will also be established to support patients making complaints. Locally these new arrangements for patient and public involvement will have to link into existing networks of voluntary organizations and arrangements at practice level for patient participation. It is not clear how these relationships will develop.

At the same time the Government is establishing a national Commission for Patient and Public Involvement in Health (CPPIH) to advise the Government on arrangements for patient advice and advocacy services, to support local patient forums, set standards, facilitate training and monitor PALS, Patients' Forums and ICASs. The CPPIH will have regional outposts based on the 28 strategic Health Authority areas. Staff will be employed by CPPIH and work with a local reference panel. Their role will be to facilitate capacity building and to assist patients' forums, providing the glue that binds local arrangements together and which links them to the national body. Members of the Commission will be drawn from patients' forums, local strategic partnership lay members and others, in particular the voluntary sector. CPPIH local outposts will commission independent complaints advocacy services and the CPPIH will conduct the appointment process for patients' forum members. The Chief Medical Officer is also reviewing the procedures and systems for clinical complaints and further developments in professional regulation and the operation of complaints machinery are likely in the near future. However, a key issue is whether sufficient resources will be made available to support this new structure of patient/public involvement as it is more costly than the CHCs which it is replacing and on the whole CHCs have not been generously funded in the past – perhaps contributing to some of their identified weaknesses.

Alongside these changes there is a wider emphasis on developing standards of care within the health service. Increasingly government policy is setting national standards and the National Service Frameworks – covering CHD, mental health and older people in 2001 with children's services early in 2002 – provide a framework for healthcare providers. Coupled with guidance from NICE and the inspection approach of CHI a new quality framework is being established governing patient care. This fits with the Government's intentions set out in *The New NHS* to establish a national health service delivering high standards of care.

CONCLUSION

NHS policy is currently at a time of rapid development with a strong central drive towards a new, although not always clear, modernization programme. Two things would appear to be happening at the moment, which at first glance would seem to be diametrically opposed. The first is the emphasis on decentralization and devolution pushing responsibility for the NHS away from central government to the elected assemblies in Scotland and Wales and to frontline clinicians/ managers within primary care organizations. At the same time central government and the Scottish and Welsh NHS are applying more central control on standards and quality. Thus we may see increasing diversity in organizational structure in

the future but clearer goals regarding standards and quality of care with nationally driven guidelines and national inspection, all emphasizing a national health service. This tension will become increasingly difficult as the Government increases expenditure on the NHS over the next few years. The publication of the Wanless Report (2001) has led to an increasing Treasury presence in health policy and it is not clear to what extent this exercise of control will be increased over the next year or so. How far such centralized control can sit alongside a more decentralized and fragmented service is not clear.

The other main area of increasing policy interest relates to professional practice. An interest in quality and standards of care immediately overlaps issues of regulation and accreditation of professionals who work within the NHS. In 2000, the Prime Minister attacked professional practice in the public service as being a conservative force not amenable to change as seen by the Government. Hence much effort has been placed in trying to change professional practice and involve professionals in pioneering and supporting change in the NHS. In any large organization there will be disagreements about the nature and rate of change. Clearly, increasing patient and public involvement can only further ratchet up the pressure on professionals in the service. Yet it is important to view such changes as an opportunity for reflection, listening and reviewing practice – key components of any high-quality public service. Professionals will need to be aware that their practice will in future be more open to scrutiny. The recent agreement on agenda for change will provide flexibilities in the NHS workforce upon which to base new professional roles (DoH 2002b).

Finally, it is important to consider what role public health will have in this new modernized NHS. There is a danger of insufficient attention being paid to developing an adequate performance management structure for public health. Public health professionals in England are being absorbed into primary care organizations. At the same time there is an emphasis on developing public health skills across all professional groups. Such moves may dilute public health activity or they might increase it. Two dangers are present.

The first is that there is insufficient development of the notion of a multidisciplinary public health force. In Scotland there is an emphasis on the role of health visitors but this is missing from England where the emphasis remains on a medicalized workforce. Secondly, the preoccupation with service delivery (standards, quality, commissioning, professional regulation, etc.) tends to overshadow public health policy and activity. The new patient/public involvement structures are focused on service delivery as well. Thus it is not clear whether the potential for developing a broader public health approach – particularly for community nurses – will be fulfilled.

SUMMARY

◆ This chapter focuses on the UK National Health Service since 1997, with a summary of the period before then.

◆ Major organizational changes to the structure of the NHS since 1997, introduced by the Labour government, including legislation are covered.

◆ The introduction of the devolved electoral assemblies in Northern Ireland, Scotland and Wales and the impact on each other and on the NHS in England are discussed.

◆ The three policy areas of priority to the Labour government are political devolution, modernization of the NHS and the ideology of the third way.

DISCUSSION POINTS

1. The extent to which devolution in Scotland, Wales and N. Ireland will create new tensions within the NHS and health policy more generally.

2. The Government is pursuing a modernization agenda in the NHS but whose view of modernization is being carried forward?

3. In what ways could increased accreditation, regulation and patient/public scrutiny ensure higher quality care.

4. The importance of developing a public health role for community nursing.

REFERENCES

Acheson D (chair) 1998 Independent inquiry into inequalities in health. HMSO, London

DHSS 1986 Primary health care: An agenda for discussion. Cmnd. 9771. HMSO, London

DHSS 1987 Promoting better health: The Government's programme for improving primary health care. Cmnd. 249. HMSO, London

Department of Health 1992 The health of the nation: a strategy for health in England, Cm 1986. HMSO, London

Department of Health 1997 The new NHS. HMSO, London

Department of Health 1998 Our healthier nation, Green Paper, Cn 3852. HMSO, London

Department of Health 1999 Saving lives: Our healthier nation. HMSO, London

Department of Health 2000 The NHS plan. HMSO, London

Department of Health 2001 Shifting the balance of power. DoH, London

Department of Health 2002a Shifting the balance of power: Next steps. DoH, London

Department of Health 2002b Human resource framework: Next steps. DoH, London

Davies HTO, Nutley SM, Smith PC (eds) 2000 What works? Evidence-based policy and practice in the public services. Policy Press, Bristol

Dolowitz DP, Hulme R, Nellis M, O'Neil F 1999 Policy transfer and British social policy. Open University Press, Buckingham

Exworthy M, Peckham S 1998 The contribution of coterminosity to joint purchasing in health and social care. Health and Place 4(3): 233–243

Exworthy M, Powell M 2000 Variations on a theme: new Labour, health inequalities and policy failure. In: Hann A (ed) Analysing health policy, Chapter 4, pp. 45–62. Ashgate, Aldershot

Garside P 1999 Evidence based mergers. British Medical Journal 318: 345–346

Glendinning C, Coleman A, Shipman C, Malbon G 2001 Primary care groups: Progress in partnerships. British Medical Journal 323: 28–31.

Ham C 1992 Health policy in Britian. MacMillan, Basingstoke

Hazell R, Jervis P 1998 Devolution and health. Nuffield Trust series 3. University College London and the Nuffield Trust, London

Hunter DJ 1998a The NHS: looking to the future. British Journal of Health Care Management 4(5): 226–228

Hunter DJ 1998b A disunited kingdom? Health Management October: 10–12

Jervis P, Plowden W (eds) 2000 Devolution and health: first annual report. The Constitution Unit, UCL, London

Klein R 1998 The new politics of the NHS. Longman, London

Ottewill R, Wall A 1990 The growth and development of the Community Health Services. Business Education Publishers Ltd, Sunderland

Peckham S, Exworthy M 2002 Primary care in the UK: Policy, organisation and management. Palgrave/Macmillan, Basingstoke

Saltman R, Von Otter C 1992 Planned markets in health care. Open University Press, Buckingham

Secretary of State for Northern Ireland 1998 Fit for the future: a consultation document on the government's proposals for the future of Health and Personal Social Services in Northern Ireland. The Stationery Office, Belfast

Secretary of State for Scotland 1997 Designed to care: renewing the National Health Service in Scotland. Cmd. 3811. The Stationery Office, Edinburgh

Secretary of State for Wales 1997 A voice for Wales. Cmd. 3718. The Stationery Office, Cardiff

Secretary of State for Wales 1998 NHS Wales: putting patients first. Cmd. 3841. The Stationery Office, Cardiff

Wanless D 2002 Securing our future health: taking a long term view. HM Treasury, London

Whitfield L 1998 Assembling ideas. Health Service Journal 108(5630): 14–15

FURTHER READING

Baggott R 2000 The politics of public health. MacMillan, Basingstoke

Hennessey D, Spurgeon P (eds) 2000 Health policy and nursing: Influence, development and impact. MacMillan, Basingstoke

Klein R 1998 The new politics of the NHS. Longman, London

Ottewill R, Wall A 1990 The growth and development of the Community Health Services. Business Education Publishers, Sunderland

2

Developments in primary care

S. Peckham

KEY ISSUES

◆ Primary care is central to developments in the NHS and health policy in the UK.

◆ There is a lack of clarity over the exact definition of primary care.

◆ There is an increasing emphasis on multidisciplinary and multiagency partnerships within primary care.

◆ Primary care nursing is becoming an increasingly important element of primary care.

INTRODUCTION

Primary care is now recognized as playing a central role in the UK National Health Service and has become a major focus of health policy (DoH 2002). The changes introduced by the Labour government from 1997 have significantly shifted healthcare policy from an emphasis on secondary care – which has dominated health policy since before the Second World War – to placing primary care at the centre of healthcare development, commissioning and public health. These changes to the healthcare system came at the end of a sustained period of healthcare reform in the 1990s, not only in the UK but also in many other developed countries. As we enter the 21st century it is perhaps timely to review this movement towards primary care and to examine why the role of primary care in healthcare systems has become so important.

The 20th century saw the emergence of primary care as a specific area of health care, albeit dominated for the most part by general practice. However, this process was accompanied by a separation of the generalist model of primary care from the specialist approach of secondary care services. This separation was evident for the first third of the century and was formalized by the creation of GPs as independent contractors within the NHS, even though GPs' gatekeeping role was considered vital to the functioning of the NHS. In many ways, other primary care professions (especially community nursing) experienced a similar separation from the rest of the healthcare system by virtue of their distinctive professional developments in local authorities. The integration of GPs and community nursing became most apparent with the effective development of primary care teams from the 1960s onwards.

While the managerialism of the 1980s, and the internal market in the 1990s, has been seen as inimical to primary care teamwork, these two developments were instrumental in placing primary care at the centre of health policy and in a pivotal role in the organization and management of health care. It is no surprise therefore that the 1990s witnessed the most concerted attempt to shape primary care through policy reform, in part because of the pressures and needs elsewhere in the NHS. Though autonomy has been valued by all professions throughout, and the legacy of the generalist/specialist separation and of the 1948 settlement persist, the Government has become less deferential to the professions. For much of the century, the Government was wary about upsetting the professions (primarily medicine) given their status within society and the power which they wielded. However, with the rise of managerialism, policies have made fundamental advances in shaping the organization and management of primary care. This is resulting in a wider and more inclusive definition of primary care, a greater managerial role in what had been a professional enclave, and a more central role in meeting NHS objectives. There are also changes in the organization of primary care and in the roles of healthcare practitioners such as GPs and nurses, and though an increasingly inquisitive and sceptical public is placing more demands on practitioners, primary care has thus moved from the margins to the mainstream of health policy in the UK. This chapter examines the growth of primary care in the UK and explores some of the reasons why primary care is seen as having an increasingly important role within the NHS. It then goes on to examine some of the key policy issues and the effect these have on current practice mainly as these relate to England.

THE GROWTH OF PRIMARY CARE IN THE UK

Central to the organization of primary care services in the UK are general practice and community health services and since the Second World War there has been an enormous expansion of these services. From the 1960s there has been a steady increase in the workload and, consequently, the numbers of staff. Today primary care is a major employer with, in England, Scotland and Wales, over 100 000 people now working in general practice with over 40 000 additional members of the primary healthcare team (PHCT) who also work in, or with, practices (see Table 2.1).

A simple review of the history of UK health policy demonstrates little interest in general practice and community health services. As Moon and North (2000) argue:

… the current status that general practice enjoys as a speciality within medicine and the influence that GPs wield are in sharp contrast with its origins and much of its history, during which general practice was overshadowed by the more prestigious branches of medicine (p. 13).

Traditionally, the sidelining of general practice and community health in the UK is seen as a by-product of the establishment of the National Health Service in 1948. The settlement achieved ensured that the focus of government was on the secondary and tertiary sectors given the dominance of hospital-based services (Klein 1998). Two consequences of the establishment of the NHS were the independent practice status of general practice, outside of the mainstream NHS administration, and the retention of community and public health services within local authorities (Klein 1998, Ottewill & Wall 1990, Timmins 1995). For the UK this tended to push policy interest in these areas to the sidelines. This is not to say that these areas were ignored as there has been a continuing debate within the UK about the relationship between community health and hospital services (Ottewill & Wall 1990) and since the 1950s an interest in the development, quality and role of the general practitioner services (Moon & North 2000). However, the interest of government in primary care services rapidly escalated from the mid 1980s. This interest grew for a number of reasons but can be seen as arising from the coincidence of a number of trends as shown in Box 2.1 (Peckham & Exworthy 2002).

While identified as separate contributors to policy and organizational changes, there are clear

Table 2.1   Practice staff in England and Wales, 1992 & 1997, and Scotland 1998

Job title	E&W 1992 WTE	E&W 1997		Scotland 1998[1] WTE
		WTE	Number	
Fund manager	–	1677	2559	–
Management & admin	6409	–	–	834[2]
Practice manager	–	7094	8715	–
Secretarial & clerical	13 300	–	–	3685[3]
Secretarial	–	6157	9622	–
Receptionist	20 717	–	–	–
Receptionist/clerical	–	30 899	50 507	–
Computer operator	1195	2287	3805	190
Other admin	–	3396	5713	–
Practice nurse	9450	10 724	19 455	968
Dispenser	1065	1213	2155	26
Physiotherapist	77	94	358	–
Chiropodist	10	27	176	–
Interpreter/link worker	24	58	112	–
Counsellor	174	253	1184	–
Comp. therapist	–	10	62	–
Other duties	661	710	1568	801
Total number of staff	53 082	64 599	105 991	6504

[1] Figures for Scotland provisional as at 1 April 1998; [2] Category in Scotland is 'Management'; [3] Category in Scotland is 'Secretary/clerk/receptionist'.

Box 2.1   Trends affecting the development of primary care

◆ Broader changes in the delivery of healthcare services associated with the 'crisis in health care' and the 'crisis of the welfare state';

◆ An interest in the organizational relationship of general practice to the NHS as the key to managing activity;

◆ A desire to extend managerial control over primary care and, following the failure of earlier cost-control measures, to engage general practitioners in financial management;

◆ The growth of the 'new public management' and consequent changes in approaches to the management and organization of public services particularly to curb expenditure, contain demands and increase efficiency and effectiveness;

◆ Changes in patients' expectations about being treated more promptly and closer to home;

◆ A fragmenting medical profession with changing professional expectations – especially for GPs – towards more flexibility in their working arrangements and career choices;

◆ The rise of professionals as managers and a desire to control the gatekeepers to the NHS as general practice was seen as the last untouched bastion of clinical and medical autonomy;

◆ An increasing emphasis on localization and community-based services.

---

inter-relationships between these areas. In the UK, general practitioners have traditionally adopted a managed care approach being both first point of contact for health care for the majority of the population, providing immediate health care to individuals and families and making referrals to secondary care (Fry & Hodder 1994, Starfield 1998). As Starfield notes, the UK system of general practice is the most universal and comprehensive system in the world. Thus they have a critical role to play in dealing with long-term chronic illness. Similarly, the UK has one of the most comprehensively developed community health services which has increasingly become integrated with general practice. Interestingly this integration combines both primary *medical* care and, to a certain extent, primary *health* care. Thus the need to address changes in disease management from mainly acute episodes to the management of chronic disease places a greater burden on primary care and has perhaps led to the 'rediscovery' of the GP's role. At the same time there have been significant changes in demand by patients leading to pressure on consultation times, length of time waiting for an appointment and particularly out of hours work. It is not clear however, the varying contribution of providers and patients in this upturn in demand, nor is there any simple answer to dealing with these problems (Rogers et al 2000). All these issues are explored in more depth by Peckham and Exworthy (2002) but it is important to recognize the complex background that lies behind current developments in policy and practice.

This discovery of the important role of primary care within the UK NHS has occurred at a time when there has also been a re-examination of the role of the GP and developments in primary care nursing. It is perhaps the convergence of these factors which has provided an impetus to the exploration of new models of primary care organization. These developments have also led to a re-evaluation of the nature of primary care.

RE-EVALUATING PRIMARY CARE

Primary care has long been acknowledged as one of the major strengths of British health and social care arrangements, with its focus on universality of access, emphasis on continuity of family and individual care, and its role as a gateway to other services (Starfield 1998). However, the theory and practice of primary care has been undergoing re-evaluation and change (Macdonald 1992, Starfield 1998, WHO/UNICEF 1979) a situation reflected in the re-examination of primary care in the UK (Fry & Hodder 1994, Meads 1995, Peckham 1999).

This re-evaluation from within primary care services has been accompanied by impetus for change coming from national policy (DHSS 1986, 1987, DoH 1996, 1997, 2000). Initially, the main thrust for change was on quality and then, with the introduction of the internal market and fundholding, on the purchasing role of primary care, which was intended to lead to greater efficiency and responsiveness (Le Grand et al 1998). At the same time, there has been a re-assessment of the role of general practice and latterly, more radical solutions have been sought, with a range of new developments, from the mid 1990s onwards. These included Primary Care Act Pilots (PCAPs) which are exploring new organizational arrangements for general practice, Total Purchasing – where groups of practices held the whole purchasing budget for

their population, and GP Commissioning which brought together GPs and health authorities on commissioning. These latter two were the forerunners of the Primary Care Groups (PCGs), Primary Care Trusts (PCTs) and Care Trusts – in England (and imminently in Northern Ireland), Scottish Primary Care Trusts (SPCTs) and Local Health Boards (LHBs) in Wales. Current government policy emphasizes the promotion of primary and community care, with the intention of ensuring a more efficient response to the needs of vulnerable groups, by managing the care of these groups as much as possible in the community and by developing interagency work. The emphasis on developing services and commissioning health care is, however, secondary to promoting the health of the local community creating a new, key emphasis, on public health and the role of PCOs (DoH 1997, 1999, NHSE 1998).

THE CURRENT CONTEXT OF PRIMARY CARE IN THE UK

Primary care became seen as both an issue ('problem') to be tackled and also as a solution to 'difficulties' elsewhere in the NHS during the 1980s and especially the 1990s. As the contribution of primary care to the wider NHS became increasingly recognized, there was a greater need to incorporate it into the NHS's organization and management. Perhaps the most significant trigger for this was a process of managerialization which took place right across the public sector – the rise of New Public Management (NPM). It established new patterns of policy, organization and management. Although it initially had a marginal effect on primary care, NPM began to permeate primary care through the introduction of managerialism in community health services and other providers, the shift in focus from FPCs to FHSAs and the more managerial approaches (often associated with IT) within individual general practices.

This process of incorporation continued into the 1990s with a series of reforms which were both an attempt to re-organize primary care and to act as an additional lever upon secondary care. This was most clearly evident in the GP fundholding scheme and Trust status but also through a series of policy statements. Although the internal market had profound inter- and intraprofessional consequences, the policy direction continued to move towards further integration with the introduction of PCGs and PCTs (and LHGs and SPCTs), not least because these were not voluntary schemes. Once community health services had been reorganized into PCGs and PCTs, primary care was effectively incorporated into the NHS. A process which had begun some 30 years earlier, had finally been realised.

However, such incorporation has not been absolute and nor is it complete. Primary care has always been noted for its diversity, in terms of service provision and quality. Despite many initiatives oriented around quality improvement (often associated with NPM) in the 1980s and 1990s, the linkage between management and quality only formally became established with the introduction of clinical governance in 1997. In 1998, Alan Milburn, then Minister of Health, said 'It is important to understand that the variations in quality in secondary care are as nothing compared to variations in quality in primary care' (Evidence to Health Select Committee, 12 November 1998, qu. 32). (See Chapter 5, for further discussion of clinical governance.)

As mentioned previously, primary care is also becoming increasingly characterized by diversity in its organizational form. Incorporation has not been, and is unlikely to be, a uniform process, applying to all areas and to all services, equally. Devolution has created further complexities and diversity in primary care (Exworthy 2001) but there are common themes in policy across the UK which demonstrate a new emphasis on developing primary care services. In England, for example *The NHS Plan* (DoH 2000) provides for an expansion in primary care. It also provides a framework for developing primary care services based on the following five principles.

ACCESS

Improved access to primary care is based upon setting standards for accessing a primary care practitioner (24 hours for any practitioner and 48 hours for a GP), an expansion of practitioners (2000 more GPs and 450 more GPs in training by 2004), new organizational structures and services (such as walk-in clinics and NHS Direct), investment in premises (up to 3000 family doctors' premises including 500 new primary care centres will benefit from a £1 billion investment programme by 2004) and new organizational structures (PCTs and Care Trusts). It is likely that the Government's goals of increased access will not be possible based on the traditional general practice model of GP as the first contact for patients. The development of primary care nursing is an important element of a new approach to the provision of primary care through walk-in clinics and NHS Direct where nursing input is central to service delivery such as telephone advice, triage and face-to-face care (see Chapter 24).

INFORMED PATIENTS

The Government is placing an increased emphasis on patient information and patient and public involvement. As discussed in Chapter 1 there is a growing movement for changing both professional practice and organizational structures to deliver such policies in practice. This will not only involve a change in the way services need to be delivered – something primary care professionals are already engaged in – but also substantial changes to the way patients input into both their own care, and the organization and delivery of primary care services.

EXTENDED HIGH-QUALITY SERVICES

The next few years will continue to see a change in the organization of primary care. The aim is to create a bigger role for GPs and other primary care professionals in shaping local services. Professionals will also take on different roles with more specialist GPs, nurse practitioners, the incorporation of social services as well as community health services and an expansion in the range of services offered in practices and primary care centres (different therapists, complementary health professionals, etc.). There is also a greater emphasis on clinical governance within primary care with a stronger quality framework through new national standards (for example National Service Frameworks for Coronary Heart Disease and the Care of Older People), national guidance from the National Institute for Clinical Excellence, performance measurement frameworks and inspection (Commission for Health Improvement) and internal audit and governance mechanisms. There is also a new wider governance framework through changed board structures, patient and public involvement frameworks and new procedures for professional accreditation, regulation and complaints.

MODERN PRIMARY CARE SETTINGS

New approaches to primary care are being developed based on both widening access and integrating services (especially health and social care). Proposals include one-stop health and social care services, additional investment in new intermediate care services and new Care Trusts (similar joint management organizations are proposed for Scotland). The development of Care Trusts was a key proposal of *The NHS Plan* and was seen as one approach to addressing problems of partnership. Initially the proposals related to areas where developing partnerships between primary care organizations and social care agencies were not progressing. However, the first real proposals for developing Care Trusts have been in Wiltshire – a county with a strong tradition of interagency partnerships with Care Trusts being seen as a positive move to restructure both health and social care. There are also 15 other pilot sites which focus on specific patient groups and one which includes housing. It is too early to know whether such moves will be successful in creating clearer and more effective partnerships and the first few will start in 2003.

TRAINING AND EDUCATION

There is an increased emphasis on continuing education programmes and the training of new practitioners. GPs will be helped with their continuing professional development through earmarked funds. Perhaps one of the key changes to primary care practitioners will be the development in accreditation and regulation and changes in dealing with complaints. These stem from high-profile medical mishaps such as that of the Bristol children's heart surgery case where a number of children died unnecessarily, and from the imprisonment of Harold Shipman, a GP convicted of murdering large numbers of his (primarily) older patients. There has also been a general increase in scepticism of medical practitioners and general public mistrust. Of particular concern has been the self-regulatory arrangements of healthcare professions with a view that bodies such as the General Medical Council and UKCC were more sympathetic to the practitioners than to patients who have made complaints. The upshot is likely to be more government intervention in regulatory frameworks such as those currently being developed (discussed in Chapter 1).

PUBLIC HEALTH

Another key area of development which is having an increasing impact on primary care is that of public health. From an international perspective public health is seen as central to primary health care (Macdonald 1992). However, developments in the UK highlight the tensions between the different models of health which underpin approaches to health and health care – namely the medical and social models. The dominance of the medical model in UK primary care practice must, therefore, raise important questions about the potential of primary care to take on key public health roles – to transform itself from primary *medical* to primary *health* care (Macdonald 1992). It is also pertinent to ask whether such a public health role is new in terms of wider definitions of primary care (e.g. WHO 1978, 1991) which recognize different models and practice of primary care and public health. For example what has been the contribution of 'Health for All', the community health movement and, with specific relevance to the UK, community health services (Ottewill & Wall 1990, Turton et al 2000)?

Since the early 1990s, with the publication of *The Health of the Nation* (DoH 1992) there has been a growing debate about the role of primary care nurses in public health activity (Lindsay & Craig 2000). This was particularly stimulated by the report of the Standing Nursing and Midwifery Advisory Committee *Making it Happen* (DoH 1995). In England, primary care organizations were given three main functions which remain central to guidance for Primary Care Trusts:

◆ to improve the health of, and address health inequalities in, their community
◆ to develop primary care and community health services across their area (including improved integration of services)
◆ to advise or take on the commissioning of hospital services for patients within their area to appropriately meet patients' needs (DoH 2002, NHSE 1998).

NHSE guidance also identified the need for primary care organizations to work with other local partners including local authorities and housing agencies, to adopt community development approaches to reach local people, to develop more one-to-one health promotion interventions and work with all local stakeholders to address local health issues (NHSE 1998). While the overall lead for public health remains with Health Authority Directors of Public Health, PCGs '… should … assess the public health capacity and capability available locally, to agree the best organisational arrangements, whilst ensuring clear lines of responsibility and accountability …' (NHSE 1998, para. 18). In *Saving Lives: Our Healthier Nation* White Paper, government policy is very clear about the centrality of the Health Improvement Programme (HImP) and the important role to be played in the development of local HImPs by PCGs: '… Over time they will forge powerful local partnerships with local bodies … to deliver shared health goals. They will help shape the health improvement programme and draw up their own plans for implementing it and for hitting the targets in it.' (DoH 1999, para. 10.11). This suggests that the Government saw PCOs as being

key local actors within public health, taking both a responsibility for addressing the local communities' health needs but also collaborating with other local agencies on public health activities. While the links between public health and primary care are widely accepted (Popay 1999) this indicates a significant change in the nature of primary care, and more specifically general practice. Yet the seeds of such a change were already sown before the Labour government policy initiatives of the late 1990s and it is worth examining the development of the relationship between public health and primary care.

Subsequent policy documents have further emphasized the Government's commitment to public health and tackling health inequality. Whilst there is some sense in charging such organizations with this responsibility, there are currently doubts about their capacity to fulfil this task and also the relative priority accorded to it, compared with commissioning and primary care development. This issue was identified by the Health Committee's inquiry into public health (2001).

The NHS National Plan was published in July 2000. Although it focused primarily on the structure and organization of the NHS, it recognized that 'the wider inability to forge effective partnerships with local government, business and community organizations has inhibited the NHS's ability to prevent ill-health and tackle health inequalities' (p. 29). The effectiveness of these (and other) strategies to tackle health inequality is not yet known since many of the mechanisms proposed in these documents have only been established within the last couple of years. Empirical evidence (at the local level) suggests that there is widespread support for such policies but their implementation is being hampered by competing priorities from central government and local partnership difficulties (Exworthy et al 2000).

The importance of the role of PCTs in England is likely to be further emphasized by the changes to health authorities and the abolition of the NHSE Regions (DoH 2002). Larger health authorities will lead to more devolved public health functions with Directors of Public Health taking a more strategic role through the development of regional public health networks that draw together NHS and local authorities. Such developments see an expansion of multiprofessional public health practice with new public health specialists including those with nursing and community backgrounds (Chief Medical Officer 2001). (It is at the regional level of interorganizational collaboration that the shape of public health will be formed in England, taking on the role that the assemblies in Northern Ireland, Scotland and Wales are beginning to perform.) Gillam et al (2001) argue that the development of PCOs provides an opportunity to develop partnerships and take a population approach which was not possible from an individual practice approach. This will require dealing with substantial complexity and involve developing new skills. Considering the tendency of general practice not to become involved in such activities in the past and, notwithstanding the experience of community health services which are now being integrated into PCOs (in England at least), developing public health within primary care will require a cultural as well as organizational shift. As PCTs in England absorb public health specialists from the dismantled health authorities we may see an increased emphasis on medical approaches which may be at odds with the need to develop a multidisciplinary public health workforce (HDA 2001) which works with local communities rather than delivers public health to them. There may also be opportunities for drawing on the wider primary care workforce, particularly the experience of community nurses (Lindsay & Craig 2000). In Scotland, the Executive has proposed extending the role of public health nurses (Scottish Executive 2001) – also envisaged in England and Wales with SNMAC (1995) but yet to be fulfilled.

However, it is worth sounding a note of caution. Professor Jennie Popay in her evidence to the House of Commons Health Committee referred to the 'awesome' expectations now laid upon primary care to deliver the public health agenda and to address inequalities in health and that 'there is little if any evidence from research or practice that past primary care organisations or primary care medical professions have the capacity or the inclination to do this' (Popay 2001).

CHANGING PATTERN OF PROFESSIONAL WORK IN PRIMARY CARE

Current changes in organization and practice in primary care will provide challenges and new opportunities for professional practice. However, the pattern of professional work in primary care has rarely been static, reflecting fluctuations in the balance between and within professions as well as the myriad of changes in the organization and management of primary care. However, the medical profession has remained largely dominant in various incarnations of interprofessional working. Nonetheless, the degree of interprofessional working has grown in the latter part of the 20th century such that it is now a well-established feature of primary care in the UK.

Nursing has undergone the most distinctive and significant professionalization in recent years. Moreover, nurses represent a significant and varied professional group within primary care. The professionalization of nursing has largely been shaped by its relations with medicine, perhaps the most significant demonstration of which concerns nurse education and training. Nursing's curriculum used to be prescribed by doctors (Parkin 1995); indeed, women were excluded from medicine in the 19th century (Green & Thorogood 1998, p. 141). For many, the inter-relationship between medicine and nursing reflected the distinction between curing and caring (Witz 1994, p. 33, Wilson 2000, p. 50), a differentiation as much about gender as about professions. Parkin (1995) argues that nursing continues to be seen as essentially a female occupation which carries social perceptions of it as low-status work, involving menial tasks, uninteresting/routinized work and domestic duties. One of the most significant attempts in primary care to enhance nursing's professionalization was the Cumberlege Report on neighbourhood nursing (1986) (Exworthy 1994, Parkin 1995, Wilson 2000, p. 50). The report proposed that community nursing should be based on neighbourhoods of 10 000 to 25 000 population and managed by a neighbourhood nurse manager, drawn from any nursing background and responsible for all community nurses in that patch. This report advocated nurse practitioners who could work independently, run certain clinics, refer, diagnose and prescribe certain medications (Parkin 1995). It also made recommendations about the PHCT liaison and nurse training. The report sought to re-define the role of community nursing within primary care but in ways that were complementary or parallel to general practice. This led to much criticism by doctors and pharmacists. The report's almost exclusive focus on community nursing and its failure to integrate with the wider primary care, helped to shape the report's relatively small impact. Although about 30% of community health services had implemented Cumberlege's proposals after 2 years (King's Fund 1988), the internal market reforms of 1991 overtook the concept of neighbourhood nursing, and the dominance of GP Fund Holding effectively put pay to this professionalization strategy (Exworthy 1994).

The 1990s was a period of huge change for primary care nursing/community nursing as a result of the rise in the number of practice nurses and the development of nurse practitioners. The growth in the number of practice nurses was aided by subsidies to practices who employed practice nurses. Their numbers rose spectacularly from 1920 in 1984 to 9100 in 1994 (Green & Thorogood 1998, p. 100). Though working with the practice population and for the practice, practice nurses also experienced a huge rise in, and expansion of, their workload (associated with the 1990 GP Contract). Richards et al (2000) estimate this rise to be 75% (p. 187) as practice nurse roles were extended especially into chronic disease management (e.g. asthma), health promotion, smoking cessation, family planning and treatment of minor illnesses. This was despite some delegation of practice nurse tasks to healthcare assistants. Although the number of therapy staff such as osteopaths, counsellors and physiotherapists also rose in the early 1990s (Green & Thorogood 1998), the number of new entrants to health visiting declined (Richards et al 2000, p. 186).

In the late 1990s, there was an equivocal reaction to the introduction of PCGs among primary care nurses. On the one hand, nursing was guaranteed a role in decision-making but, on the other, it was only allotted two places on a committee dominated by up to seven GPs. Only two nurses were appointed chairs in 481 PCGs in April 1999 (Richards et al 2000) and only one was chair of the Executive Committee in the first two waves of (40) PCTs (from April 2000) (Robinson & Exworthy 2001). The recruitment of nurses and their quasimanagerial position on PCGs have, to some extent, been part of recent attempts to revive health visiting in a wider public health role (Acheson 1998, DoH 2000, Turton et al 2000).

The rise in number of practice nurses was initially thought to be at the expense of nurse practitioners. Such practitioners are distinguished from their nurse colleagues by virtue of their additional knowledge and skills which facilitate first-level assessment and treatment. Nurse practitioners are those with 'a level of education, clinical activity and responsibility higher than that of other nurses, but different from that of a GP' (RCGP 1998). Their tasks involve diagnosis, prescribing, telephone advice and home visits. Some see the nurse practitioner as shifting nursing towards a medical orientation and hence a diminished nursing role whereas others see them as an alternative or complementary rather than subservient to doctors. The growth of nurse development units, nurse-led units and minor injuries clinics (often led by nurses), often part of walk-in clinics and healthy living centres, illustrate how nurse practitioners are extending nursing into new clinical and organizational areas. However, many such developments have coincided with nursing's professionalization rather than having been initiated by nursing. These developments should be viewed cautiously within the wider context of policy changes in primary care, in which GPs remain mostly in control of resources. Witz (1994) has argued that this 'points to the limited expansion of the nurse's role, as [they] simply take on routine tasks performed by GPs, without necessarily expanding her decision-making or forging new partnerships with patients' (p. 37). As a result, she argued, the localized power of doctors and managers will remain crucial in influencing the direction of nursing and the roles that nurses undertake. (See Chapter 17 for a more detailed discussion of practice nursing.)

But the role of the GP is also changing – although it would be wrong to say that their role will be substantially different in the short term as a result of current policy developments. One key change over the last ten years has been the feminization of general practice. More women than men now enter general practice training. This has led to pressures on working patterns and has particularly fed pressures to change out-of-hours support. Working practice has also been changed through the Primary Care Act pilot schemes which have introduced changes to the General Medical Services contracts, with an increase in the number of salaried GPs. Clearly the context of practice will change. Increased accreditation, changes in organization and increases in medical knowledge will directly affect practice. However, it is likely that the daily routine of general medical practice will change little – the frontline is where continuity will be retained. The central role of general practice is to manage patient care and make appropriate referrals for further care or investigation. This is central to both medical practice and the way the NHS operates.

Conversely we may expect to see greater changes in the roles of primary care nurses. Gillam argues that 'In many respects, nurses are the future of primary care ...' (2001, p. 123). Certainly the reforms following 1997 have placed nurses in a stronger position both in terms of practice and involvement in management and policy. One immediate consequence of the 1997 reforms has been the inclusion of community nurses within the local management and policy process through their position on primary care organization boards. This has led to the development of more cohesive local nurse networks which have drawn together community nurses and practice nurses. Interestingly the development of networked practices has re-introduced ideas of area-based working into community nursing – echoes of Cumberlege from the 1980s. Community nurses are more likely to draw boundaries within the defined limits of their employing primary care organization. While there will continue to be overlaps between PCOs due to the differences between the resident (those people living within the PCO boundary) and registered (those registered with GPs within a PCO) populations there will be an increasing emphasis on area-based work.

The second major influence of the development of PCOs has been the bringing together of practice nurses and community nurses. How far this will continue is still open for discussion. There are calls for more generic approaches to primary care nursing but there are still major differences between practice, school, and community nurses and health visitors. There is likely to be some blurring of roles as time goes on but it is likely that there will be a fierce debate between ideas for generalist versus specialist primary care nurses.

Two other factors complicate the development of primary care nursing in the future but which provide welcome opportunities for many nurses. The first is the extension of nurse prescribing and the second is the nurse practitioner. The development of walk-in centres and changes to local contracts through the Primary Medical Care Services projects are providing new ways of working and new organizational structures within primary care for nurses to take on more responsibility. New opportunities are also provided through developments such as NHS Direct, which uses nurses to staff 24-hour patient helplines (see Chapter 24).

Finally, we are also likely to continue seeing an increasing complexity of community nurse tasks. More and more people are being cared for in their own home, or within a community setting. At the same time it is increasingly true that people with a dependence on an increasingly complex medical technology, are also being cared for at home. Specialist tasks, which used to be undertaken in hospital, are now routinely carried out in the home and requiring more specialist skills from community nurses. There is also a growing number of specialist community-based nurses, and hospital-based nurses who have a community workload, in the areas of cancer, paediatrics and HIV/AIDS.

CONCLUSION

The landscape of primary care is changing fast. While general practice will remain the cornerstone for the immediate future, policies across the UK will lead to a greater diversification of primary care organization. In particular, we can expect community nurses to take on additional responsibilities both in terms of clinical practice and organizational management. There is also an increased level of technicality in the provision of primary care. This creates a challenge to the notion of primary care as being holistic with the practitioner dealing with the whole person. The changing nature of professional, patient and lay-carer roles also challenges the notion of practitioner as expert. Thus, in the future we can expect to see an increasing blurring of roles such as that which is already happening in nursing and social care for people with learning difficulties, where integrated professional training already exists. This may in future lead to a blurring of roles between carers and nursing professionals in particular.

Organizationally we will be seeing community nurses integrated into primary care structures bringing together a range of primary care nurses offering opportunities for changes to nursing organization and practice. With nurses providing much of the new developing agenda within primary care (NHS Direct and walk-in centres) and being engaged within the new management structures of primary care organizations it is likely that the future will bring greater management of primary care nursing within primary care but also a greater involvement of primary care nurses in the management of primary care. Primary care in the future may also offer greater diversity for nurses with the range and level of roles expanding providing new career paths – especially for practice nurses who have traditionally been constrained by their general practice location. There is also a danger that there will be a push for greater generalization in nursing (from medics) with their main role as supporting primary medical practice. This may downgrade nursing responsibilities and tasks and open up the development of low-grade nursing auxiliary functions instead of more developed and central roles for primary care nurses.

SUMMARY

◆ Primary care is now recognized as playing a central role in the NHS.

◆ There has been a huge growth in the number of primary care workers since the 1960s and the trends which have affected this are discussed.

◆ The re-evaluation of primary care over the past 20 years and the current context within the UK NHS, particularly since the coming to power of the Labour government, are aimed at access, informing patients, extending high-quality care, providing modern primary care settings and the training and education of staff.

◆ Public health has an increasing impact on primary care.

◆ The latter part of the 20th century saw a 'professionalization' of the UK NHS workers in primary care, which has had an impact on the roles of all involved particularly the lines between medical and nursing staff becoming blurred.

DISCUSSION POINTS

1. How important are organizational changes in primary care to shaping clinical practice and patient care?

2. To what extent will local practitioners be able to shape local healthcare services?

3. How will newer developments such as walk-in centres and NHS Direct affect nurse roles in the future and traditional general practice?

4. How will nurse roles expand in the future? To what extent will specialisms in nursing remain, or will there be a move towards more generalist nurses?

5. How will multidisciplinary working and increasing carer and patient self-care affect nurses' roles?

REFERENCES

Acheson D (chair) 1998 Independent inquiry into inequalities in health. HMSO, London

CMO 2001 The report of the Chief Medical Officer's project to strengthen the public health function. DoH, London

DHSS 1986a Primary health care: An agenda for discussion. Cmnd. 9771. HMSO, London

DHSS 1986b Neighbourhood nursing: A focus for care [The Cumberlege Report]. HMSO, London

DHSS 1987 Promoting better health: The Government's programme for improving primary health care. Cmnd. 249. HMSO, London

Department of Health 1995 Making it happen: public health – the contribution, role and development of nurses, midwives and health visitors. Report of the Standing Nursing and Midwifery Advisory Committee. DoH, London

Department of Health 1996 Primary care: Delivering the future. HMSO, London

Department of Health 1997 The new NHS: Modern, dependable. HMSO, London

Department of Health 2000 The NHS plan. HMSO, London

Department of Health 2001 Shifting the balance of power. DoH, London

Department of Health 2002 Shifting the balance of power: Next steps. DoH, London

Exworthy M 1994 The contest for control in community health services: professionals and managers dispute decentralisation. Policy and Politics 22: 1, 17–29

Exworthy M, Powell M 2000 Variations on a theme: new Labour, health inequalities and policy failure. In: Hann A (ed) Analysing health policy, Chapter 4, pp. 45–62. Ashgate, Aldershot

Exworthy M 2001 Primary care in the UK: understanding the dynamics of devolution. Health and Social Care in the Community 9(5): 266–278

Fry J, Hodder JP 1994 Primary health care in an international context. Nuffield Provincial Hospitals Trust, London

Gillam S, Abbott S, Banks-Smith J 2001 Can primary care groups and trusts improve health? British Medical Journal 323: 89–92

Green J, Thorogood N 1998 Analysing health policy: a sociological approach. Longman, London

Klein R 1998 The new politics of the NHS. Longman, London

Le Grand J, Mays N, Mulligan J-A (eds) 1998 Learning from the NHS internal market: a review of evidence. King's Fund, London

Lindsay J, Craig P 2000 Nursing for public health: Population-based care. Churchill Livingstone, Edinburgh

Macdonald J 1992 Primary health care: medicine in its place. Earthscan, London

Meads G (ed) 1996 A primary care-led NHS: Putting it into practice. Churchill Livingstone, London

Milburn A 1999 Evidence to the House of Commons Select Committee on Health, Report on Primary Care Groups, Hc 153. TSO, London

Moon G, North N 2000 Policy and place: General medical practice in the UK. MacMillan, Basingstoke

Ottewill R, Wall A 1992 The growth and development of the Community Health Services. Business Education Publishers Ltd, Sunderland

Parkin PAC 1995 Nursing the future: a re-examination of the professionalization thesis in the light of some recent developments. Journal of Advanced Nursing 21: 561–567

Peckham S 1999 Primary care purchasing: Are integrated primary care providers/purchasers the way forward? PharmacoEconomics 15(3): 209–216

Peckham S, Exworthy M (2002) Primary care in the UK: Policy, organisation and management. Palgrave/Macmillan, Basingstoke

RCGP 1998 The primary health care team RCGP information sheet number 21. RCGP, London

Robinson R, Exworthy M 2000 Three at the top: preliminary report on chief executive and boards chairs at first wave primary care trusts. LSE, London

Rogers A, Hassell K, Nicolaas G 1999 Demanding patients? Analysing the use of primary care. Open University Press, Buckingham

Starfield B 1998 Primary care: Balancing health needs, services and technology. Oxford University Press, New York

Summerton 1999 Accrediting research practices. British Journal of General Practice 49(438): 63–64

Taylor P, Peckham S, Turton P 1998 A public health model of primary care: from concept to reality. Public Health Alliance, Birmingham

Timmins N 1995 The five giants. Fontana, London

Turton P, Peckham S, Taylor P 2000 Integrating primary care and public health. In: Lindsay J, Craig P (eds) Nursing for public health: Population-based care, Chapter 11, pp. 195–218. Churchill Livingstone, Edinburgh

Walsh JA, Warren KS 1979 Selective primary health care: an interim strategy for disease control in developing countries. New England Journal of Medicine 301(18): 967–974

WHO/UNICEF 1978 Primary health care: The Alma Ata Conference. WHO, Geneva

WHO 1991 Community involvement in health development. Report of a WHO study group. WHO Technical Report Series No. 809. WHO, Geneva

Wilson AE 2000 The changing nature of primary health care teams and interprofessional relationships In: Tovey P (ed) Contemporary primary care: the challenge of care, Chapter 3, pp. 43–60. Open University Press, Buckingham

Witz A 1994 The challenge of nursing. In: Gabe J, Kelleher D, Williams G (eds) Challenging medicine, Chapter 2, pp. 23–45. Routledge, London

FURTHER READING

Moon G, North N 2000 Policy and place: General medical practice in the UK. MacMillan, Basingstoke

Ottewill R, Wall A 1992 The growth and development of the Community Health Services. Business Education Publishers Ltd, Sunderland

Peckham S, Exworthy M 2002 Primary care in the UK: Policy, organisation and management. Palgrave/Macmillan, Basingstoke

Starfield B 1998 Primary care: Balancing health needs, services and technology. Oxford University Press, New York

3

Innovation and change in public health

D. Fone

INTRODUCTION

This chapter provides a framework for understanding recent innovations and change in public health practice. It explores the history of public health from the pioneering days in Victorian times to the pressures for change that have led to the redefinition of the functions of public health and the development of modern public health practice.

A case study of innovation in local collaborative public health practice highlights how modern public health can work to improve community health and reduce health inequality.

WHAT IS PUBLIC HEALTH?

Public health is about understanding and improving the health of populations or communities, rather than the health of individuals. The key feature is of a geographically defined population, such as a country, region or health authority, or at smaller levels, a local authority, electoral ward, enumeration district or smaller postcode-defined areas. Within these, public health practitioners may focus on people with a particular illness, such as coronary heart disease, or a client group such as children or the elderly.

Population measures to improve health include population screening programmes, such as breast or cervical cancer screening to identify disease at an early stage for treatment, health promotion activities aimed at the underlying determinants of poor health, such as smoking cessation programmes, and health protection in which, for example, environmental safety is enhanced to reduce dangers from unfenced ponds or traffic-calming measures.

The scientific basis of public health practice is the discipline of epidemiology, which is often described as the study of the distribution of diseases in populations. In fact, the science of epidemiology is broad ranging and of fundamental importance to everybody who is working towards improving the health of the population. Epidemiological methods can help us understand the aetiology and natural history of disease, they can measure the size of health problems to inform planning and then evaluate the effectiveness and cost-effectiveness of interventions to improve health.

One of the fundamental principles of epidemiology and public health is that the subject of interest must be defined. The most commonly used definition of public health was suggested in the Acheson Report (1988) which reviewed the public health function: 'the science and art of preventing disease, prolonging life, and promoting health through the organised efforts of society'.

This definition makes it clear that public health is not the responsibility of one professional group or organization, but involves the whole of society/ is a societal process. But how can it be achieved? In a report on strengthening the public function, the Chief Medical Officer for England (DoH 2001a) considered that 'this definition is still widely used because it reflects the essential elements of modern public health' (Beaglehole & Bonita 1997):

◆ a population perspective
◆ an emphasis on collective responsibility for health
◆ an emphasis on prevention
◆ the key role of the state linked to a concern for the underlying socioeconomic determinants of health as well as disease
◆ a multidisciplinary basis
◆ an emphasis on partnership with the populations served.

See Chapter 6 where Harriett Jefferson explores structural issues related to poverty and health.

WHAT ARE THE PUBLIC HEALTH FUNCTIONS?

Much consideration has been given to defining the public health functions required to move towards a better understanding of how to improve population health through public health practice. Ten public health functions have been defined by the UK Faculty of Public Health Medicine. They are shown in Box 3.1.

These broad definitions of the functions of public health show that everyone, both public and professionals, has responsibilities for improving public health. Public health is clearly not just one activity but requires a broad multidisciplinary team to implement the defined public health functions. The functions will be discharged by many people working for a variety of different organizations in different settings, but all with the same aim of improving the health of the population.

WHO PRACTISES PUBLIC HEALTH?

In his report on strengthening the public health function (DoH 2001a), the Chief Medical Officer

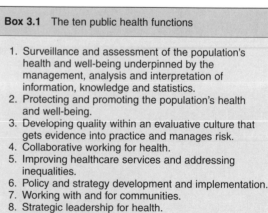

Box 3.1   The ten public health functions

1. Surveillance and assessment of the population's health and well-being underpinned by the management, analysis and interpretation of information, knowledge and statistics.
2. Protecting and promoting the population's health and well-being.
3. Developing quality within an evaluative culture that gets evidence into practice and manages risk.
4. Collaborative working for health.
5. Improving healthcare services and addressing inequalities.
6. Policy and strategy development and implementation.
7. Working with and for communities.
8. Strategic leadership for health.
9. Research, development and education.
10. Managing self, people and resources.

Source: Faculty of Public Health Medicine. See online: http://www.fphm.org.uk

for England defined three broad categories of people who work to improve public health:

1. Those whose primary role is public health: these are the public health 'specialists' whose primary role is maintaining and improving the public's health. They come from a variety of professional backgrounds and experience including social science, public health science, environmental health, public health medicine, pharmacy, nursing, health promotion and dentistry.

2. Those for whom public health is part of their role: these public health practitioners include people whose role includes (but not exclusively) furthering health by working with communities or groups. They include health visitors, health promotion specialists, community development workers and environmental health officers.

3. Those whose role would benefit from an awareness of public health issues: these could include managers in the NHS and local authorities, teachers and employers in local organizations.

Public health practitioners may be located in a wide range of organizations, including Strategic Health Authorities, Primary Care Organizations, NHS Trusts, local government departments, and the business and voluntary sectors.

So how have we arrived at the current state of public health practice? The next section considers a brief history of public health from Victorian times and the recent pressures for change that have led to the present day.

HISTORY OF PUBLIC HEALTH

As medical science developed in the 19th century, a growing awareness that the major causes of epidemic infectious diseases, such as cholera, were preventable through ensuring a clean water supply and safe disposal of sewage led to growth of the Public Health Movement. Edwin Chadwick, a lawyer and engineer and secretary to the Poor Law Commission was one of the pioneers of the day and the architect of the first Public Health Act of 1848. This was a defining moment in the history of public health. It established a General Board of Health and local boards were set up which became the forerunners of local government. The 1848 Act

gave the Boards of Health permissive powers to monitor and enforce control of the environment, through activities such as inspecting drains. It recommended the appointment of Medical Officers of Health to advise on matters relating to the health of the community. These appointments were not obligatory until the next major Public Health Act of 1875, which obliged local health boards to improve a range of sanitary and environmental provisions.

But what was the role of the Medical Officer of Health? One of the most perceptive comments on this subject was made by PH Holland Esq., the General Board of Health inspector sent to assess the condition of Merthyr in 1853. In a letter to C Macauley Esq, the secretary of the General Board of Health, dated 15 December 1853, he recommended the appointment of a Medical Officer of Health and believed that:

the labour of such officer will do much to **remove the ignorance** which has permitted such evils to arise, to **arouse the apathy** which allows their continuance, and to overcome the opposition which impedes their removal. Such officers would **show** the fearful amount of suffering disease and death produced for want of means for bringing pure water into the town, and for taking foul water out of it. They would **prove** that the losses occasioned by avoidable sickness and its consequences reduce a well paid population to poverty.

A sequence of four public health activities was envisaged to carry out these duties. These are shown in Box 3.2.

As a result of the Public Health Acts of the 19th century, public health practice was based in local authorities. Environmental health departments employed environmental health officers whose

---

Box 3.2

1. Epidemiological investigation of disease prevalence and incidence (**to show**).
2. Evidence-based assessment of the socioeconomic impact of the disease burden (**to prove**).
3. Dissemination of knowledge about disease and their causes (**to remove ignorance**).
4. Advocacy for changing environmental conditions (**arouse the apathy**).

role was to investigate and control outbreaks of communicable disease, and be responsible for enforcing standards relating to food, water supplies and sewage disposal, housing and air quality. The responsibilities of the Medical Officer of Health widened to include responsibility for community health services, such as maternity and child welfare, and responsibility for the new municipal hospitals.

Local authorities continued to provide these public health services until the 1974 NHS reorganization. After 1974, the Medical Officer for Health role became the responsibility of health authorities and the medical speciality was renamed Community Medicine. This fragmented the public health service and removed the focus for public health doctors away from public health and their colleagues in nursing and environmental health to a more medical administrative role. This 'new' specialty of Community Medicine further lost its way in successive NHS reorganizations and in 1988 the Acheson Report (1988), taking stock of the 'crisis' in public health, suggested renaming the specialty back to public health medicine. He recommended the appointment of Directors of Public Health as an executive director and member of the board to health authorities. The professional role of the Director of Public Health was to assess the health needs of the health authority resident population, to publish an annual independent report on the health of the population and play a key role in organizing the necessary multisectoral and multidisciplinary links to implement change to improve the health of the population.

However, despite this role, the speciality of public health medicine in health authorities became increasingly isolated in the 1990s from the wider practice of public health. Public health physicians were increasingly drawn into the commissioning of secondary and tertiary hospital services within the NHS purchaser/provider split. The health service reforms of 1990 brought in by the NHS and Community Care Act 1990 established an 'internal market' healthcare system in which health authorities and some GP fundholding practices acted as *purchasers* of health care, setting up contracts for provision of services with hospitals, the *providers* of health care. Despite

the rhetoric that services should be commissioned on the basis of healthcare need and interesting theoretical frameworks for healthcare needs assessment (Stevens & Raftery 1994), there was little evidence that assessment of health need actually drove the process, contracting for health care within the internal market was essentially a financial accounting process, with small marginal shifts in provision over time.

This was the situation up until as recently as 1997. What then were the pressures for change that led to the refocusing and ongoing development of modern, multidisciplinary public health practice?

PRESSURES FOR CHANGE

The fundamental pressure for change has been the refocusing of the public health agenda back to its core purpose of improving the health of the population and reducing health inequalities through action on the wider societal determinants of health. An understanding of social exclusion, which refers to individuals living in communities on the margins of society as a result of a cycle of problems such as low educational achievement, unemployment, poor health, crumbling community infrastructure and the need for action, was made possible through societal change which included an increasing awareness of these issues and a greater individual and community involvement in solutions. All those practising public health realized the need to move away from the traditional medical model of public health practice to a multiprofessional approach in order to rise to the challenges posed by health inequalities. The newly elected Labour government in 1997 provided the necessary policy frameworks for change.

INEQUALITIES IN HEALTH

The fundamental pressure for change has been the awareness of increasing evidence for health inequalities within the UK and the need for action to address them. Although absolute levels of health have improved in the UK over the last 20 years, the effect has been simultaneously to widen the health divide between affluent and deprived populations (Shaw et al 1999).

The story starts with the Labour government of the late 1970s which established the Black Committee on Inequalities in Health, chaired by Sir Douglas Black. Their report published in 1980, The Black Report, has since become a landmark in the history of understanding inequalities in health (Department of Health and Social Security 1980, Townsend & Davidson 1988). The Report highlighted the substantial variations in health that existed in the UK, arguing that these inequalities were caused by inequality in material well-being and poverty. However the report was rejected by the Conservative government of the day on the grounds that implementation of the recommendations was considered financially unrealistic. The Report was effectively suppressed as the Government restricted the number of copies published to a few hundred and there was no official publicity.

Although increasing evidence on health inequalities was published during the 1980s (Whitehead 1987), it was not government policy to explicitly address them. Eventually the overwhelming research evidence that was being published did lead the Conservative government to establish a Health Variations Group in 1994 (the word 'inequalities' was never used), chaired by the Chief Medical Officer for England. Their comprehensive and enlightened report (DoH 1995) identified that although some activity within the NHS was addressing the so-called 'variations' in health, it was taking place at the margins of health authority business. The report reinforced the need for 'alliances' with local government, voluntary and community organizations to make progress, and made a series of recommendations that paved the way for change later in the decade.

Following the election of the new Labour government in 1997, an Independent Inquiry into Inequalities in Health was commissioned, chaired by Sir Donald Acheson. Their report (DoH 1998) made 39 recommendations for action. A detailed examination of the evidence presented to the Inquiry was published a year later (Gordon et al

---

Box 3.3

1. All policies likely to have an impact on health should be evaluated in terms of their impact on health inequalities.
2. A high priority should be given to the health of families with children.
3. Further steps should be taken to reduce income inequalities and improve the living standards of poor households.

Source: Department of Health (1998b).

1999), summarizing the evidence base for each recommendation.

The three areas considered by the Independent Inquiry to be crucial to reducing inequalities in health are shown in Box 3.3.

WHAT INNOVATIONS AND CHANGE ARE HAPPENING?

MEETING THE HEALTH INEQUALITIES AGENDA

It became increasingly apparent that in order to respond to the health inequalities agenda, new modes of multidisciplinary collaborative teamwork were required. A broader view of the different roles and scope of public health practitioners necessitated a careful consideration of training and professional standards of public health practice. An important debate on the need for appropriately trained and accredited public health specialists who are not medically qualified developed and the question of leadership in public health has more recently been aired in the *British Medical Journal* (McPherson et al 2001).

A national tripartite project between the Faculty of Public Health Medicine, the Multidisciplinary Public Health Forum and the Royal Institute of Public Health and Hygiene has redefined the three levels of public health practice as Generalists, Practitioners and Specialists. This project is managed by Healthworks UK, the National Training Organization for Healthcare.

Generalists include all those whose roles have an influence on the wider socioeconomic and environmental determinants of health. This may be either at a strategic or policy level, such as government officials or those working with communities or individuals, such as voluntary workers, teachers or housing officers. Public health practitioners have a more direct professional role in public practice, such as health visitors or environmental health officers. As well as their core professional training and qualification, public health practitioners may have had more specific training in the public health sciences and practice, for example taking a Masters in Public Health degree. Public health specialists may come from a variety of professional backgrounds and will have completed specialist training in public health. Specialists will lead public health programmes across organizational boundaries to manage change at strategic and operational levels.

The tripartite project mentioned above has adopted the Faculty of Public Health Medicine's ten public health functions as the basis for standards of specialist practice. Work on developing standards for public health generalists is now underway.

Specialist training schemes, to the standards required to achieve the defined core competencies within the Faculty's ten public health functions, required by public health medicine and higher specialist training for doctors, are now available. Membership of the Faculty of Public Health Medicine is available through examination to non-medically qualified candidates, and the specification and appointment of public health specialists with equivalent status to medical public health specialists (consultants in public health medicine) is now starting to happen.

Appointees to these posts will have demonstrated achievement of the Faculty of Public Health Medicine core competencies and the national standards for practice in public health. Local job descriptions within the ten public health functions will vary, but the key principle of the role of public health specialists is to take a local leadership role, facilitating and leading partnership working between the statutory organizations with a public health remit, such as Primary Care Organizations and the Local Authority, with links into wider public health networks. A new cadre of well-trained and enthusiastic public health specialists will be the key with which the door to modern public health practice can be opened.

SURVEILLANCE AND ASSESSMENT OF THE POPULATION'S HEALTH AND WELL-BEING

Growing acknowledgement of the need for a greater understanding of inequalities in health at a local level, for local planning, has given a new focus to public health practitioners in the surveillance and assessment of the population's health and well-being. This focus has moved away from large population areas to geographically defined small areas (such as administrative local government units of the electoral ward or division, population of around 5000 people). At this small area level, information on disease and health status is usefully displayed in maps. Maps of disease will highlight areas of greatest risk and reveal patterns of local geographical variation that may not be suspected from inspection of the same data as numbers in tables. Maps are an important source of information for local planners, as well as generating hypotheses on causal mechanisms that can be tested in further research studies.

There is a long history of geographical public health and the use of maps of disease to highlight health inequality. The first example is that of John Snow and the Broad Street pump in Soho, London in 1854 (Donaldson & Donaldson 2000). The increasing availability of information at a small spatial level, coupled with the growth in computer technology and Geographical Information Systems (GIS), small area statistical methods and advances in disease-mapping techniques, has led to a much wider use of geographical information in health needs assessment. These techniques have greatly enhanced the presentation and analysis of information as a basis for strategic planning to address health inequality.

New Internet-based interactive GIS technology has resulted in the wider availability of small area data for planning. For example the Office for National Statistics Neighbourhood Statistics website (see online: http://www.statistics.gov.uk) has a wide range of multiagency data at electoral division and unitary authority for England and Wales that can be downloaded and used to calculate local rates for presentation in tables and maps.

There are some important epidemiological pitfalls that should be avoided in converting these data into disease maps. Firstly to convert Neighbourhood Statistics data, which are presented as number of events into a rate, requires the choice and availability of an appropriate denominator. Secondly if the numbers of events, or population size of an electoral division is small (commonly the case in rural areas of the UK), then the differences between small areas are likely to be due to random variation rather than differences in true underlying risk. Thirdly the appearance and interpretation of a map can vary with choice of data ranges and colour scales used to present the data. An excellent introduction to the subject including discussion of these pitfalls is given in Lawson and Williams (2001).

An example of innovation in the surveillance and assessment of population health using geographical multiagency social, economic, environmental and health data at the small area level is shown in Case Study 3.1.

POLICY AND STRATEGY DEVELOPMENT AND IMPLEMENTATION – COLLABORATIVE WORKING FOR HEALTH

The whole thrust of the new Labour government's policy response to reducing health inequalities lies through multisectoral partnership working between the NHS, corporate local government and other organizations to address the social, economic and environmental determinants of health. A series of measures has been implemented to work towards this aim. In this section we will focus on measures taken in England, but the NHS in Wales and Scotland has published similar policy documents. A useful discussion of the similarities and differences between the White Papers from the three countries is given in an NHS Confederation Briefing Paper (NHS Confederation 1998; see online: http://www.nhsconfed.net).

Firstly the Government took the traditional step of reorganizing the NHS, this time with the aim of enhancing the role of primary care to play a leading role in health improvement and reducing inequalities. Government White Papers were published (DoH 1997) which ended the internal market and established Primary Care Groups in England. These were based on groups of GP practices and where possible coterminous local authority areas of population size around 100 000 to 200 000 people. The boards of Primary Care Groups are multiprofessional, and include GPs, community nurses, pharmacists, optometrists, dentists, local authority representatives and voluntary sector representatives. In addition to responsibilities for local health services, they were given new population health responsibilities to 'improve the health of, and address health inequality in, the local community' (DoH 1999). This was an important step towards integrating the expertise and local knowledge on health and social wellbeing held by primary care practitioners, such as community nurses, into the local planning arrangements to improve health. (See Chapter 7 for further discussion of how community nurses can use baseline data as a starting point for planning health improvement strategies.)

The Government responded to the recommendations of the Independent Inquiry on Inequalities in Health with a White Paper on Public Health entitled *Saving Lives: Our Healthier Nation* (DoH 1999). This document was presented as an action plan to tackle poor health. Its emphasis was clearly to improve the overall health of the population, through partnership working between all sectors with an influence on health, to be monitored nationally through a series of targets to reduce deaths from coronary heart disease and stroke, cancer, accidents and suicide (Box 3.4), with the expectation that local targets will be set locally. However, no explicit national targets were set at the time to reduce health inequality.

Saving Lives: Our Healthier Nation acknowledged the crucial role that nurses have to play in promoting health and preventing illness. Emphasis was given to the role of health visitors, school nurses, midwives and occupational health nurses as

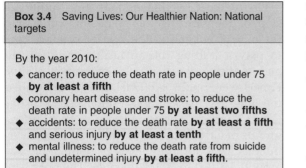

Box 3.4 Saving Lives: Our Healthier Nation: National targets

By the year 2010:

◆ cancer: to reduce the death rate in people under 75 **by at least a fifth**
◆ coronary heart disease and stroke: to reduce the death rate in people under 75 **by at least two fifths**
◆ accidents: to reduce the death rate **by at least a fifth** and serious injury **by at least a tenth**
◆ mental illness: to reduce the death rate from suicide and undetermined injury **by at least a fifth**.

Source: Saving Lives: Our Healthier Nation (1999).

public health practitioners. The Government's view was summarized as 'to develop a family-centred public health role, working with individuals, families and communities to improve health and tackle health inequality'.

Recently the Government has published a consultation document in England on a set of core national health inequalities targets (DoH 2001b). The report reinforces the broader societal and partnership approach required to tackle health inequalities, including the NHS, academic institutions, local government departments, community and voluntary sector organizations, employers, the business community and trade unions. Following the consultation process, national health inequality targets were published in 2002 (see online: http://www.doh.gov.uk/healthinequalities/tacklinghealth.pdf).

From the plethora of government documents, it is possible to pick out five innovations that embody the wider collaborative approach to tackling health inequalities and improving health. These are Public Health Observatories, Health Improvement Programmes, Health Impact Assessment, Health Action Zones and Healthy Living Centres.

PUBLIC HEALTH OBSERVATORIES

The fundamental importance of high-quality public health information required for health and social needs assessment, surveillance and monitoring of disease, monitoring and evaluation, and setting of meaningful targets to reduce health inequality has been recognized by the Government. There are eight Public Health Observatories in England (Source: *Saving Lives: Our Healthier Nation* (1999)), with the following remit:

◆ monitoring health and disease trends and highlighting areas for action
◆ identifying gaps in health information
◆ advising on methods for health and health inequality impact assessments
◆ drawing together information from different sources in new ways to improve health
◆ carrying out projects to highlight particular health issues
◆ evaluating progress by local agencies in improving health and cutting inequality
◆ looking ahead to give early warning of future public health problems.

Further information on the wide-ranging work of the Public Health Observatories can be accessed online: http://www.pho.org.uk

HEALTH IMPROVEMENT PROGRAMME

The White Papers introduced the Health Authority Health Improvement Programme as the strategic planning mechanism to bring the necessary partnerships together to tackle local health inequality and bring about health improvement. Health Improvement Programmes include a comprehensive local health needs assessment to identify health inequalities and set out a range of local priorities for evidence-based action to address them, improve the health of the local population and to improve local healthcare services.

Health Improvement Programmes may address policy areas that have a major impact on social exclusion, such as drugs and alcohol, crime and disorder, community care, asylum seekers and the health of prisoners. Local priorities will also focus on the major groups of diseases, such as coronary heart disease, cancers and respiratory disease and other areas of concern, such as sexual health and injury prevention. Health promotion strategies, such as tobacco control and health protection strategies, such as communicable disease control, noninfectious environmental hazards, healthy transport and housing will be an important output from partnership planning. As with any strategy, a detailed consideration of resource requirements is needed, as well as plans for monitoring and evaluation of the impact of the Health Improvement Programme.

An example of the Gwent Health Authority Health Improvement Programme (Gwent Health Authority 2000) is also available online: http://www.gwent-ha.wales.nhs.uk

HEALTH IMPACT ASSESSMENT

Health impact assessment acknowledges the important effects that a wide range of policies across a wide range of sectors may have on health and may be applied to a policy, a programme or a single project. These might include for example the siting of a new airport runway, road building schemes, new factory developments, or a local planning application.

Health impact assessment has been defined in a number of ways. One definition is:

Any combination of procedures or methods by which a proposed policy or program may be judged as to the effects it may have on the health of a population (Ratner et al 1997).

The overall aim of health impact assessment is to provide a means of ensuring that the potential impact on health is taken into account as part of the decision-making process for policies, programmes and other developments. Health impact assessment may be prospective, in which prediction of the likely health effects is made, concurrent, in which the consequences are assessed as the policy or programme is being implemented, or retrospective, in which the health effects are assessed after policy implementation. Most health impact assessments undertaken to date have been retrospective, but as methodologies become tested, many more prospective studies will be undertaken.

An interesting example of health impact assessment is that of the New Home Energy Efficiency Scheme. The Report (Kemm et al 2001) can be accessed online at: http://www.wales.gov.uk/subihousing/content/energy_efficiency/hiaofhees_e.htm#top

Box 3.5

1. Strategic – to establish the vision and key themes pertaining to its achievement.
2. Governance – to secure the accountability of HAZ activity, and to establish means of monitoring performance and the agreed framework within which the HAZ partners will work.
3. Operational – the activities that will help deliver the vision.
4. Practice – the ability of professionals and others to work with users and communities in new ways.
5. Community – the development of confidence, skills and infrastructure to engage in multisector partnership working.

Source: Barnes et al (2001). Further details are available on the Health Action Zones website at online http://haznet.org.uk

HEALTH ACTION ZONES

Health Action Zones (DoH 1997) were introduced to develop local innovative strategies to tackle health inequalities, deliver measurable improvements in public health and health outcomes and modernize local treatment and care services. They are an innovative approach to public health collaborative action, 'Linking health, regeneration, employment, education, housing and anti-poverty initiatives to the needs of vulnerable groups and deprived communities'. Twenty-six Health Action Zones have been established in England, representing areas of England with some of the highest levels of social deprivation and poor health. They range in population size from 180 000 to 1.4 million people, covering over 13 million people in total. Health Action Zones are co-ordinated by a local partnership board, representing the NHS, local authorities, the voluntary and private sectors and community groups.

A national evaluation of Health Action Zones is in progress. A report of initial findings from a strategic level analysis has been published (Barnes et al 2001) which highlights some of the early difficulties faced in making Health Action Zones work and successes to date. Of interest is the detailed analysis of what collaboration actually means in practice. Five levels are considered necessary (Box 3.5).

HEALTHY LIVING CENTRES

The Healthy Living Centre initiative was set up in January 1999 by the New Opportunities Fund (NOF), the lottery body established under the National Lottery Act. The initiative has a budget of £300 million from lottery funds UK wide. Healthy Living Centres will support national and local health strategies to tackle inequalities in health, including *Saving Lives: Our Healthier Nation* and local Health Improvement Programmes.

Healthy Living Centres aim to promote a social model of health through interventions focused in disadvantaged areas and population groups, for example from Health Action Zones. They will be locally based, and relevant to people of all ages. Their development was seen as an opportunity to develop multisectoral and multiprofessional partnerships across many different organizations to create a valued community resource to provide facilities and services in new ways to people who may not be accessing existing services. This might include, for example, parenting classes or smoking cessation schemes.

Examples of Healthy Living Centre developments across the UK are given in the New Opportunities Fund Quarterly Newsletter 'initiative' and online at: http://www.nof.org.uk and also the Department of Health website online at: http://doh.gov.uk/hlc.htm. A useful evaluation resource for Healthy Living Centres has been published by the Health Education Authority (Meyrick & Sinkler 1999).

Case Study 3.1

The Caerphilly Health & Social Needs Study – information for action

This case study aims to show how a modern collaborative and multidisciplinary public health approach across organizational boundaries can integrate all ten public health functions within local work to achieve positive benefits to the health and social well-being of a local geographically defined population.

The study is based in the county borough of Caerphilly, situated within the former Gwent Health Authority area (Fig. 3.1), one of the 22 unitary authorities in Wales.

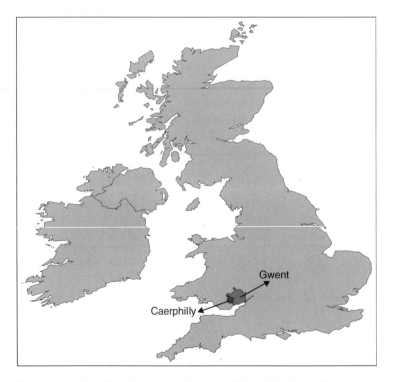

Figure 3.1 Map of the UK to show Gwent and Caerphilly County Borough.

The county borough of Caerphilly was formerly dominated by the mining industry. However the past 20 years has seen a dramatic decline in the traditional heavy industries of coal and, whereas in 1950 there were 29 pits employing 24 000 people, the last of the borough's pits closed in 1990. Throughout this period of pit closure, the borough, and indeed much of SE Wales, suffered major changes in its social and economic structure and high levels of unemployment. Many families are seeing a second generation grow up in unemployment and poverty.

This social and economic decline has resulted in the county borough of Caerphilly containing some of the most deprived electoral wards in Wales and England. Two census wards situated in the Upper Rhymney Valley in the north of the borough are in the highest ranking 5% of wards in England and Wales on both the Breadline Britain and the Work Poverty Indices (Glennerster et al 1999).

In order to take forward the new public health agenda set out in the Welsh Public Health Strategy Green Papers *Better Health Better Wales* (Welsh Office 1998a) and the *Strategic Framework* (Welsh Office 1998b), Gwent Health Authority and Caerphilly County Borough Council made commitments to partnership working. Both authorities had started the process of developing local plans to improve health: Gwent Health Authority was leading on the development of the Health Improvement Programme (HIP) (Gwent Health Authority 2000, and Caerphilly County Borough Council had developed a comprehensive public health strategy for the Corporate Plan 1998–2001 (Caerphilly County Borough Council 1998) which included action on community regeneration strategies to address inequalities within the most deprived Upper Rhymney Valley area of the borough.

Planning local initiatives for local targeting of resources to reduce health inequalities requires analysis of epidemiological data on social, economic and environmental determinants of health and health outcomes at the small area level. In order to gain a greater understanding of the health and social needs of the Caerphilly County Borough, the collaboration between the Directors of Environmental Services and Housing (Local Authority) and Public Health (Health Authority) proposed a four-stage study, the Caerphilly Health & Social Needs Study (Box 3.6).

A Study Steering Group was established, with representatives from the Health Authority, the Local Health

---

Box 3.6 Caerphilly Health & Social Needs Study

Aims

◆ To achieve a greater understanding of the relationship between social, environmental and economic deprivation and health in Caerphilly County Borough, in comparison to the other boroughs in the Gwent Health Authority area, and to inform the development of local community regeneration strategies for health improvement and better targeting of resources.

◆ To establish a robust methodology for sharing and joint analysis of information between Gwent Health Authority and Caerphilly County Borough Council, and to inform the development of the health needs assessment information required by the Local Health Group and Local Health Alliance for developing the Health Improvement Programme.

Objectives

◆ To report the descriptive and comparative epidemiology of social, environmental and economic deprivation at the small area level in Caerphilly County Borough and the Gwent Health Authority area, sharing and integrating data from the following Health and Local Authority data sets:

– Census data – local base statistics; local authority data, e.g. free school meals, unemployment;
– Vital statistics (population, births and deaths); Welsh Public Health Common Data set.

◆ To use Geographical Information Software to present profiles of Gwent and the county borough of Caerphilly, to highlight areas of greatest social, economic and environmental need and health outcomes.

◆ Further analysis of the data sets to identify gaps in knowledge, highlight areas for special study and generate hypotheses on the relationship between social, environmental and economic deprivation and health within Caerphilly County Borough which may be tested by further research.

Group (equivalent to a Primary Care Group in England), and, the Local Authority. The steering group therefore had links into general medical practice, community nursing and the Local Health Alliance, which has a wide membership including the Community Health Council, local voluntary groups and local organizations.

The work of the study was undertaken through a Working Group. This included public health specialists and practitioners, including consultants and senior lecturers in public health medicine, research officers in information, epidemiology and GIS, social scientists, and officers from the Directorates of Environmental Health and Housing, Education, and Social Services within the local authority.

Methods

We chose the 1998 electoral division as the area level for analysis, defined by the April 1998 boundary changes to the original 1991 census wards. The total population of the borough is 170 000, living within 33 electoral divisions.

The working group identified new sources of data from the local authority in the Chief Executive's, Education, Environmental Services & Housing and Social Services directorates. Data from the Chief Executive's directorate included Department of Social Security (DSS) claimant count data on means-tested and nonmeans-tested benefits and unemployment counts requested from the National Online Manpower Information Service (NOMIS) database. The Council Tax and Benefits division of the local authority supplied data on the proportion of houses in each council tax band A to H. The Education Department supplied data on educational achievement at Key Stage 4 (GCSE), together with data on free school meal uptake and children with Special Educational Needs. From a five-stage classification on the identification and assessment of Special Educational Needs (14), we aggregated data for stages 3, 4 and 5 where as a minimum, specialists from outside the school, support teachers and the Special Educational Needs co-ordinator.

Sharing of data between the health and local authorities was facilitated by the Gwent Information Exchange Protocol, which takes into account the requirements of the Data Protection Act legislation.

The education and social services data were shared as an anonymous postcoded data set. These postcodes were linked to the electoral division of residence using *Map Info* GIS software. In order to convert the data into electoral division-based rates, population denominators were extracted from the health authority general practice administrative age–sex register and where required, household denominators were taken from the 1991 census. Denominators for the education data were based on school roll data supplied by the National Assembly for Wales Schools Census (Stats 1) return.

A wide range of health data that are routinely obtained and analysed by the Directorate of Public Health in the health authority were used in the study. Among these were mortality data from the Office for National Statistics (ONS) for many different causes of death, including all-causes, coronary heart disease, cerebrovascular disease, respiratory disease, all malignant neoplasms, lung cancer, breast cancer and all accidents and adverse effects. The Welsh Cancer Intelligence and Surveillance Unit supplied data on the incidence of all malignant neoplasms, lung cancer, female breast cancer, colorectal and prostate cancer.

We classified each of the data sets identified by the study into one of six domains: Income, Unemployment, Housing, Health, Education and Social Services. For local planning purposes, thematic maps of all variables were prepared to highlight variation between electoral divisions within the borough. In the maps, each electoral division is assigned to one of five colour scales, based on dividing the range of the distribution of the variable into equal fifths. This enables easy identification of the lowest ranking electoral divisions for any particular variable.

Examples are shown in Figure 3.2. Four maps (council tax bands A and B, children in families on income support, referrals of children to social services and GCSE educational achievement) are shown to illustrate their value in highlighting areas of greatest need and inequality.

How were the study data used?

A Health & Social Needs Profile Report (Gwent Health Authority, Caerphilly County Borough Council 2000) was written and local ownership of the data and the interpretation of the disease maps were obtained through presentations to meetings of the executive directors of the health and local authorities and of the full council. The use of the Profile in population-based health and social needs assessment and a variety of local strategic planning processes has provided the Local Health Group with the means to fulfil its population-based duties of improving health and reducing health inequality in the local community. The Profile is a policy tool for advocating change, enabling local agencies to move forward on the local partnership agenda to improve health and reduce health inequality.

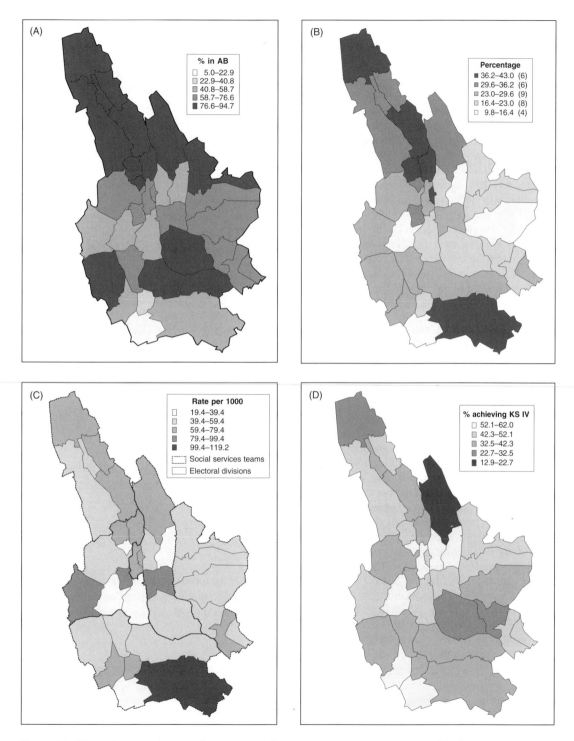

Figure 3.2 Thematic maps of selected variables. (A) Council tax bands A and B (source: CCBC 1999); (B) Percentage of children aged 0–15 living in families claiming income support (source: DSS 1998); (C) Social Services referrals of children aged 0–14, rate per 1000 (source: CCBC 1999); (D) Percentage of pupils achieving at least five GCSEs at grades A–C (source CCBC 1999).

The first use of the Profile was in the Caerphilly LHG Local Action Plan of the Health Improvement Programme (Gwent Health Authority 2000). The local authority also has statutory service planning responsibilities and the Profile enhanced the information used to formulate the Children's Services Plan (Caerphilly County Borough Council Directorate of Social Services 2000a), Social Care Plan (Caerphilly County Borough Council Directorate of Social Services 2000b) and the Housing Strategy and Operational Plan (Caerphilly County Borough Council 2000).

The Profile has also been used by the partnerships in the borough to inform bids to a range of additional funding opportunities including a successful bid to the New Opportunities Fund Healthy Living Centre Initiative and a portfolio of primary care bids to the new Health Inequality fund for the prevention of coronary heart disease. These have been linked to a local community regeneration strategy aimed at addressing the wider socioeconomic factors in one of the most deprived wards in the borough (Caerphilly County Borough Council and Partners 2000). This strategy forms close links between a new primary care centre and the development of proposals for a new community school, community resource centre and transport links.

The Local Government Act 2000 placed a new duty on Caerphilly County Borough Council to co-ordinate the production of an overarching 'Community Strategy' for their area. The duty comes with new powers to promote the social, economic and environmental well-being of local residents. Community planning is well advanced in the borough and has been agreed by a Standing Conference of over 50 partner organizations. To ensure effective community involvement, seven local area forums have been established. The first forums have agreed a local plan of action, informed by the data from the study and consistent with county borough-wide strategic priorities. These plans have been used as a major building block for the Local Partnership's Objective 1 Action Plan (Wales European Task Force 1999). Objective 1 funds are available to the poorest areas within Europe, providing considerable potential to improve health and reduce health inequalities within Caerphilly County Borough.

CONCLUSION

Public health has a long history of action on the wider determinants of health to improve health and reduce health inequality. In the 19th century this focused on improving sanitation and communicable disease control. After a long period of fragmentation of the public health functions and practitioners, public health has been revitalized by government policy initiatives on health inequalities and refocusing of its role and functions in a modern concept of public health – this involves multiprofessional and multiagency working to bring about social change and improvement in population health and reduction of inequality.

This is highlighted in the case study of health and social inequality in Caerphilly County Borough, which integrates public health action across all the defined functions of public health to bring about worthwhile change.

SUMMARY

◆ Public health is about understanding and improving the health of populations or communities.

◆ The most commonly used definition of public health is 'the science and art of preventing disease, prolonging life, and promoting health through the organized efforts of society'.

◆ The Faculty of Public Health Medicine has defined the ten functions of modern public health practice.

◆ Public health is now a modern multiprofessional concept, practised by specialists, generalists and members of society.

◆ The major pressure for the change and innovation leading to the modern practice of public health has been the policy drive to tackle inequalities in health.

DISCUSSION POINTS

1. How can community nurses make a contribution to reducing inequalities in health in their local area? What constraints are there on this public health role?

2. What are the elements of specialist training for community nurses who wish to practice as public health specialists?

3. How can community nurses provide leadership in national and local public health practice?

ACKNOWLEDGEMENTS

I am grateful to my colleagues Professor Stephen Palmer, Dr Edward Coyle, Mr Andrew Jones and Dr John Watkins for interesting discussions on the development of modern public health practice.

REFERENCES

Acheson D 1988 Report of the Committee of Inquiry into the Future Development of the Public Health Function. Public Health in England. HMSO (Cm 289), London

Barnes M, Sullivan H, Matka E 2001 Building capacity for collaboration: the national evaluation of Health Action Zones. Birmingham, University of Birmingham

Beaglehole R, Bonita R 1997 Public health at the crossroads. Cambridge University Press, Cambridge

Caerphilly County Borough Council 1998 Corporate plan of priorities 1998–2001. Caerphilly County Borough Council, Caerphilly

Caerphilly County Borough Council 2000 Housing strategy and operational plan 2000–2003. Caerphilly County Borough Council, Caerphilly

Caerphilly County Borough Council Directorate of Social Services 2000a Review Plan 2000–2001 of the Children's Services Plan 1998–2001. Caerphilly County Borough Council, Caerphilly

Caerphilly County Borough Council Directorate of Social Services 2000b Review Plan of the Social Care Plan 1998–2001. Caerphilly County Borough Council, Caerphilly

Caerphilly County Borough Council and partners 2000 New Tredegar Economic and Community Regeneration Strategy. Support Document for Local Regeneration Fund (LRF) submission. Caerphilly County Borough Council, Caerphilly

Department of Health 1995 Variations in health. What can the Department of Health and the NHS do? HMSO, London

Department of Health 1997 The new NHS: modern, dependable, Cmd 3807. HMSO, London

Department of Health 1998 Independent inquiry into inequalities in health. HMSO, London

Department of Health 1999 Saving lives: Our healthier nation, Cmd 4386. The Stationery Office, London

Department of Health 2001a The report of the Chief Medical Officer's project to strengthen the public health function. Department of Health, London

Department of Health 2001b Tackling health inequalities. The Stationery Office, London

Department of Health and Social Security 1980 Inequalities in health: report of a research working group (The Black Report). HMSO, London

Donaldson LJ, Donaldson RJ 2000 The broad street pump. In: Essential public health, 2nd ed, pp 104–107. Petroc Books, Bodmin

Glennerster H, Lupton R, Noden P, Power A 1999 Poverty, social exclusion and neighbourhood: Studying the area bases of social exclusion. CASE paper 22. Centre for Analysis of Social Exclusion, London School of Economics, London

Gordon D, Shaw M, Dorling D, et al (eds) 1999 Inequalities in health. The evidence presented to the independent inquiry into inequalities in health, chaired by Sir Donald Acheson. The Policy Press, University of Bristol

Gwent Health Authority 2000 Gwent health improvement programme 2000–2005. Gwent Health Authority, Pontypool

Gwent Health Authority, Caerphilly County Borough Council 2000 Caerphilly Health & Social Needs Study: Stage 2. GHA, Caerphilly CBC, Caerphilly

Kemm J, Ballard S, Harmer M 2001 Health impact assessment of the new Home Energy Efficiency Scheme. National Assembly for Wales, Cardiff

Lawson AB, Williams FLR 2001 An introductory guide to disease mapping. Wiley, Chichester

McPherson K, Taylor S, Coyle E 2001 Public health does not need to be led by doctors. British Medical Journal 322: 1593–1596

Meyrick J, Sinkler P 1999 An evaluation resource for healthy living centres. Health Education Authority, London

Ratner PA, Green LW, Frankish CJ et al 1997 Setting the stage for health impact assessment. Journal of Public Health Policy 18: 67–69

Shaw M, Dorling D, Gordon D, Davey Smith G 1999 The widening gap: health inequalities and policy in Britain. Policy Press, Bristol

Stevens A, Raftery J (eds) 1994 Health care needs assessment, the epidemiology based needs assessment reviews. Radcliffe Medical Press, Oxford

The NHS Confederation 1998 Briefing. The White Papers for England, Scotland & Wales. The NHS Confederation, Birmingham

Townsend P, Davidson N 1988 Inequalities in health: The Black Report, 2nd edn. Penguin Books, London

Wales European Task Force 1999 West Wales and the Valleys Objective 1. Single Programming Document for the period 2000–2006. NAfW, Cardiff

Welsh Office 1998a Better health better Wales. Welsh Office, Cardiff

Welsh Office 1998b Strategic framework: Better health better Wales. Welsh Office, Cardiff

Whitehead M 1987 The health divide: Inequalities in health in the 1980s. Health Education Council, London

FURTHER READING

Donaldson LJ, Donaldson RJ 2000 Essential public health, 2nd edn. Petroc Books, Bodmin

This is perhaps the standard introductory text to the principles and practice of public health and offers a comprehensive overview of the subject.

Marmot M, Wilkinson RG 2000 Social determinants of health. OUP, Oxford

A comprehensive summary of the research evidence on the wider determinants of health.

NHS Executive 1999 Public health practice resource pack. NHS Eastern Office, Public Health/Strategic Development Directorates

A useful overview of public health practice at the end of the 1990s.

4

Quality improvement

J. Edwards
E. Muir

KEY ISSUES

- Background and policy context of quality improvement within the UK NHS.

- Defining terms within quality health care.

- The literature and areas of debate.

- Professional regulation.

- Education and CPD.

- Improving quality of community nursing services (where and how to start).

INTRODUCTION

This chapter explores how and why 'quality' has become such a central factor for the future development and improvement of health service provision; it should be read in conjunction with Chapters 1 and 2, where attention is drawn to particular organizational and policy developments that can help to explain some of the contextual issues likely to influence and constrain steps to improve the quality of community nursing services.

It is the current government's commitment to modernizing the NHS (Secretary of State for Health 2000) which incorporates a drive for quality improvement – this with particular reference to enhanced professional regulation, clinical governance and lifelong learning. The term 'clinical governance' was initially introduced in the 1998 White Paper: *The new NHS: modern, dependable*, drawing attention to a national framework for assessing performance and to the related matter of continuous professional development (CPD).

The concept of clinical governance and the high profile given to the term arose in response to widespread public and political concern regarding perceived failures in key areas of healthcare provision – these included cancer screening services as well as individual and unit failures, some of which led to public investigation and occasionally to prosecution. In the light of such investigations, the apparent failure of professional self-regulation became an important and additional government concern. However, both the General Medical Council (GMC) in *Good Medical*

Practice (2001) and The United Kingdom Central Council for Nursing Midwifery and Health Visiting (UKCC) in *The Code of Professional Conduct* (2002) and *The Scope of Professional Practice* (1995) have reaffirmed professional responsibilities and the standards against which doctors and nurses will be judged. This chapter will consider why and how community nurses have a significant role to play in improving both the quality of clinical practice and service provision, and in the implementation of clinical governance policies.

THE POLICY CONTEXT – HISTORICAL PERSPECTIVE

Much has changed since the inception of the NHS, including the expectations of a better-educated public, who are more willing to challenge and who have increasing access to information. However, the exact remit of the NHS continues to remain unclear to most people, that is to say what is/is not possible within allocated budgets is not always clear, either to those providing, or to those receiving, health services. Exploring the development of government health policies can help us understand why some things become the focus of attention and why there are subsequent shifts of interest. The development of a Patients' Charter in the 1980s for instance, represented recognition that patient involvement in decisions about health care was important. However, there was subsequent acknowledgement that in focusing on the *rights* of patients, their *responsibilities* had not been given sufficient emphasis. In more recent policy developments, patient/client involvement continues to play a significant part in quality improvement initiatives. In a Kings Fund Report (1997) for example, successful outcomes of a clinical effectiveness initiative suggest that these were linked to both health professional and patient involvement in the processes.

The politics of health care inevitably involves decision-making to do with taxation and the selection, utilization and management of finite resources. Continuing advances in medical knowledge and technology not only add to the

---

Box 4.1

Corporate governance
Concerned with:

◆ public accountability;
◆ effective management;
◆ sound financial controls.

but
a) not addressing the 'quality' of clinical care and
b) not addressing the different 'quality perspectives' of consumer, provider and clinician.

Clinical governance
Concerned with:

◆ professional autonomy and professionally led change;
◆ reducing wide variation in the quality of services in different parts of the NHS;
◆ introducing clinical audit and audit within primary care.

but
a) not addressing the significance of team functioning and
b) not acknowledging organizational constraints.

---

escalating costs of health care but also to the need to obtain a balance between competing demands such as those of an ageing population with chronic conditions, and those of parents for the technological advances in the care of the newborn. The concept of 'value for money' represents a particular kind of response to problems about how best to allocate scarce resources (see Chapter 26 for a more detailed discussion of this topic) but it is worth noting that *Clinical Governance* has followed *Financial Governance* and *Corporate Governance* in efforts to control costs, target resources, reduce waste and improve the quality of health service provision. Of particular interest to community nurses however, is the potential conflict between policies intended to achieve health service improvement, for example between the concerns of corporate and clinical governance (Box 4.1).

DEFINING QUALITY HEALTH CARE

The term 'quality' is familiar to most people in relation to everyday products and services such as food and clothing, transport and education.

In that sense people have some agreed notion that quality is something desirable and that there is a comparative connotation to phrases such as 'better quality' and 'poor quality'. However, there is an important difference between products and services: making a quality comparison between products can be undertaken before a decision to purchase, using the senses to examine a range of factors such as design, colour and materials, assessing the potential benefits, relative costs and packaging. Assessing the quality of a service however, cannot be undertaken in the same way, since it is only possible to make comparisons after the actual experience of a service. A hairdresser, lawyer or a bus company may develop a reputation about their services but until they are experienced by a customer, it is difficult for an individual to assess the comparative quality, even though cost and options may be clear to a potential user and purchaser. To some extent, assessing the quality of a service is to do with reviewing the opinions of other users but it also involves an assessment of expected personal benefit and convenience, the perceived quality of facilities, general environment and access to qualified people competent to undertake a role or task. In addition, the manner and behaviour of those providing the service is likely to be critical to a positive assessment of quality. However, where the quality of a health service is concerned, there are other significant issues over and above those mentioned above and these are to do with ethical principles (see Chapter 14), a legal framework for practice (see Chapter 13), equity of provision, professional accountability and ensuring user involvement in decision-making.

Some recent attempts to define quality in the NHS have tended to focus on phrases such as 'things that work'; 'things that people want' and 'getting things right first time' (DoH 1998). But such issues, which draw attention to an evidence base to support practice, to communication and clinical competence, would still be expected to take account of the cost and the optimum use of scarce resources in relation to outcomes and to the incidence of error. The purpose of clinical governance processes is to improve outcomes, to avoid adverse situations for patients/clients and

their carers and to achieve greater involvement from them, in the care being provided. Monitoring quality requires both information (to describe the current position, obtaining baseline data) and a system to review that information. The record of care provided by a community nurse could be used, for example, to provide documented evidence of service options being offered to an individual or family and the contributions to the care programme agreed by the individual and/or family to achieve a desirable goal; to the socio-economic circumstances in which clinical decision-making is being undertaken and to the points of progress made towards an agreed goal during a specified time-span. It would be naive however, to imagine that this requires relatively simple changes – it is one thing to try and shift service goals from inputs and processes, to anticipated outcomes that are achievable and measurable. It is quite another to have an information system in place that is capable of describing the current position in relation to agreed service goals, and of making comparisons.

In the early years of the NHS, there had been an underlying assumption that 'quality' was inherent in the ethos and skills derived from education, training and the provision of an infrastructure. However, in the separation of responsibility for key elements of the NHS (renewing and developing buildings; improving facilities and equipment; organizational management; education and training; staff development) the failure to achieve well-integrated provision was essentially predictable. So although an understanding of the relationship between structures, processes and outcomes had been recognized in the 1970s (Donabedian 1981) and the Griffiths Report (1983) had later highlighted a lack of clarity in accountability at a local level, there was a continued focus on through-put/output measures and cost containment. That is to say, although a better understanding of the link between processes and outcomes had been achieved, it did not appear to have resulted in any evidence of quality improvement. Improving the management and efficiency of the NHS during the years of the Thatcher government, did not for example, include a similar level of interest in improving the outcomes of clinical care.

Dawson (2001) suggests that the NHS at that time, '...became much more efficient at providing health care without knowing the extent to which the care given, made any difference to health status'. For community nurses this highlights the importance of being clear about what is expected to happen as a consequence of any intervention and having some idea about how progress towards agreed goals would be recognized and recorded. It also means grasping the essential difference between assessing the benefits of intervention or 'treatment' in response to a diagnosed condition, and assessing the degree to which 'nursing care' contributes to the overall quality of, and satisfaction with, the provision of a service. See below for further discussion of 'care' and 'cure' as important quality elements of a community nursing service.

The DoH (1998) document *A First Class Service: Quality in the new NHS* indicated that clinical governance was to become a system of accountability, as well as a system to:

◆ maintain and improve standards
◆ maintain professional self-regulation
◆ promote and manage CPD.

Here a number of related and explanatory processes have been identified, such as supporting the necessary research on which to base practice, promoting clinical audit cycles, developing skills in the management of change and in risk management, identifying and analysing 'near miss' reports and providing education for lifelong learning supported by programmes for CPD. Such processes help to highlight both individual and management responsibilities for maintaining and improving the quality of service provision and, in addition, to clinical governance being seen as a model for delivering the Government's health improvement programme (HIP) evident in the National Frameworks for Coronary Heart Disease (NHS Executive 2000) and for Mental Health (NHS Executive 2000). Critical questions raised by the UKCC in 'Accountability in Practice' (2001) for example, include:

◆ how is 'good' practice being promoted?
◆ how is 'poor' practice being prevented?

◆ how is unacceptable practice being addressed?
◆ how and what is being learned from things that go wrong?

In addressing other questions about why there has been such a growth of interest in improving the quality of care, the literature points to evidence of geographical variation in health care, to variation between different parts of the NHS, to the incidence of error and to the cost of providing poor quality, or ineffective, care. This has led to attention being much more focused on the development of mechanisms, such as clinical audit, to ensure the most efficient and effective use of scarce resources. A supportive educational initiative from the RCN (1989), for example, linked quality improvement to the setting of standards and clinical audit, pointing out that without agreed standards, it is not possible to compare what 'is being done' with what 'ought to be done'. However, the value of maintaining an effective audit programme was subsequently questioned (Maynard 1991) and it was not until later that an increasing concensus developed, which linked the improved use of research-based evidence together with a more efficient use of available resources, to consistently improving outcomes. Some well-publicized health service failures, such as the detection failures in some cancer screening services mentioned earlier, the unacceptable mortality rates of a specific paediatric surgical unit and the failure to detect the abnormal number of deaths associated with one general practitioner, also helped to push quality improvement to the top of the agenda. In the light of such publicity, particular importance must be given to the changes in the regulatory machinery for healthcare professionals, set out by the DoH (2001) in *Modernising Regulation in the Health Care Professions* and in the proposals appearing in the Health Services Reform Bill (2001) following consultation concerning a new Health Care Professions Regulatory Board and a new Nursing and Midwifery Council.

In the White Paper *The new NHS: Modern, Dependable*, mentioned previously, a statutory duty in respect of the provision of quality services was introduced, drawing attention to the responsibility of chief executives for quality and the promotion of quality improvement initiatives; to the need for developing a national framework for assessing performance; to issues related to CPD in the context of a philosophy of lifelong learning; to clinical audit, risk management and dealing with complaints. By 1999 the NHS Executive had set out a minimum series of actions for health authorities and Trusts to ensure that structures would be in place for quality assurance control. Rolling action plans for Local Health Groups/Primary Care Groups had already appeared in the previous year (Modernising Health and Social Services: national priorities guidance 1999/2000 to 2001/2002).

It is important however, to remember that the primary concern of clinical governance policies is patient safety. The priorities identified for protecting the public from poor performance include:

◆ the identification and dissemination of information about 'best practice'
◆ examining and learning from adverse events, openly and promptly
◆ recognizing and dealing with poor/unacceptable performance at an early stage
◆ adopting a developmental perspective
◆ setting up and managing initiatives to support CPD.

Each of these priorities has clear implications for improving the quality of community nursing services, even if the steps to achieve them are managed differently and prioritized according to local concerns and current developments. Each priority also suggests that there are individual responsibilities as well as management responsibilities.

With reference to patient safety, it is also worth remembering that the economic burden of iatrogenic injury (injuries that are avoidable, including the negative consequences of everyday clinical practices arising from healthcare management) is significant, imposing a considerable burden on hospitals and care in the community. It is against this backcloth that the previously mentioned conflicts can arise between the two driving forces behind clinical governance

policies: the desire to save money on the one hand and the desire to do the very best for patients/clients on the other. For nurses and health visitors in primary care and community settings, Sorrie (2000) highlights the significance of feeling sufficiently confident about the aims of any policy development, ensuring that the goals of any related nursing programme are clear and explicit and that '… they include a mechanism for monitoring efficacy'. With regard to the above four priorities for example, it is as important to understand both the 'why' and the 'how' of a community nursing programme of care, as it is to have an acceptable and supported forum for taking the next steps in achieving important learning from adverse events, in dealing with unacceptable performance and in establishing a framework for CPD.

Watson (2000) reinforces the importance of grasping the underlying philosophy of a policy shift, pointing out that no amount of clinical governance will suffice if there is a weak link in the chain and that it is often the nurse who is insufficiently prepared to understand the principles. Such comments underline the role of continuing education and training, to the significance of professional leadership and to the role of professional portfolios in helping to identify gaps in knowledge, skill or experience, for future service developments. Mandatory education and qualification requirements for specialist community nursing practice are well established but there is now a requirement to maintain a more active CPD record. This is not only for the validation of qualifications, further training and experience but also to enable a community unit or primary care team to:

◆ link staff skills and competencies to current and planned developments
◆ identify future education and training needs, including those to do with the development and introduction of guidelines and protocols
◆ use the CPD record as the basis for agreeing a plan for professional development to meet required clinical standards and for contributing to performance appraisal.

The significance now given to a philosophy of 'lifelong learning' should also reflect the culture shift from 'blame and shame', to one of openness and learning from experiences of adverse events – including the importance of early detection of 'high-risk' situations and their review. This is as much to do with exploring, reflecting on and learning from community nursing care that has 'broken down', (or resulted in undesirable outcomes) as it is to do with providing a supportive work environment with strong professional leadership (see Chapter 27 for further discussion of professional leadership). It is one thing however, to be aware of the need for evidence-based practice. It is quite another to be able to access and review the quality of that evidence, and to plan and manage the changes necessary to improve the standard of community nursing practice.

In more general terms, it is unlikely that the goals of clinical governance can be achieved without modifications to the educational curriculum for those seeking a community nursing qualification. It was the improved understanding of the interplay between organizational systems within the NHS for example, which has helped to illuminate the contribution of systems to the development of risky and adverse events (DoH 2000b), highlighting the benefits of interprofessional learning and the commonality of problems and issues facing most health professionals. Community nurses of the future will only be able to make optimum contributions to the NHS, and to primary care in particular, if they have a better understanding of how healthcare systems work, of the factors which predict impaired performance and of how best to assess the capacity and limitations of the service provided.

An important part of future educational provision should thus be concerned with increasing the capacity of community nurse leaders to understand the NHS as an organization, to be better able to contribute to community nursing policy development and to plan and monitor quality improvements to a service. This includes being able to explain the options and limitations of current resources available to them, particularly as a means to enhance consumer involvement in decisions affecting their care; to assess the risk of a service breakdown and to recognize and respond appropriately to adverse events.

CULTURE AND QUALITY IMPROVEMENT

One of the key issues of clinical governance identified by Scally and Donaldson (1998) was the achievement of a culture change within the NHS – culture being loosely defined as 'the way things are done around here' (Walshe 2000). Others have also recognized that the 'developmental agenda of culture change' has a much greater significance than any top–down system of directives, or any pressures to agree standards for achieving sustained improvement in the quality of care. That is to say, both the professional development of individuals and the overall development of the primary care team (or other unit providing a health-related service) need to be on the agenda for quality improvement. While Walsh and Small (2001) support this developmental focus, they also highlight the potential dangers in perceiving clinical governance as being concerned with adherence to checklists, or with establishing ways to enforce compliance. They remind us of the inherent dangers in blindly following protocols and guidelines without adequate reference to clinical judgement and the importance of being able to maintain a balance between procedures identified as 'best practice' and involving a patient/client in healthcare decisions, who may ultimately reject advice, or a proposed intervention.

The importance of baseline information cannot be overemphasized as the basis for quality improvement: being able to describe the range and type of services provided in relation to the demographic characteristics of the population served; having some basic performance measures such as 'who gets what and how frequently' and the proportion of a specified population group who take up preventive services. Walsh and Small (2001) also recommend having a profile of the clinical and nonclinical practice or unit staff, in terms of skills, qualifications and special expertise. Such an exercise provides valuable opportunities to highlight gaps and achievements, to test the robustness of IT systems, to examine the degree to which available skills and qualifications match the plans for primary care developments, potentially highlighting some priorities for individual and team development.

In a review of adverse events in the NHS, the DoH (2000a) clearly illustrated 'why' and 'how' cultural changes would be critical for appropriately addressing the evidence of existing inadequacies. Examples of these 'inadequacies' included complex, hierarchical and inflexible work environments which contribute to the failure to improve quality, and the separation of professional groups which prevent the proper integration of health care. Dawson (1997), for example, argues that it is the 'different worlds' and their associated hierarchies within the NHS that have helped to prevent effective communication, contributing to poor teamwork and to inefficient planning. For example, failure to involve different professional groups in the planning of changes likely to affect them, has sometimes meant that different elements of a quality service have not been adequately 'joined up', for instance the primary care of older people, of those with significant disabilities and of those becoming parents for the first time. Policy documents suggest a range of actions to contribute to the quality agenda that are as much to do with ensuring the involvement of nurses, midwives and health visitors in policy development and strategic planning, as to do with continuous professional development, innovation in education (to promote clinically based learning), clinical supervision and ensuring access to evidence-based information.

Examples of other cultural factors likely to impede quality improvement are evident from the views of senior health professionals when recently asked to list the 'unwritten rules' operating within the NHS. These included:

◆ 'don't challenge the system'
◆ 'don't admit to mistakes'
◆ 'pass problems up the line'
◆ 'it is wrong to seek answers or to consult others'
◆ 'we need to appoint someone first'
◆ 'we haven't the right training for this'

◆ 'the number of hours worked = value of outcome'
◆ 'change = money + increased stress'
◆ 'consultant time is more important than anyone else's' (Cullen et al 2000).

Evidence of similar kinds of barriers to promoting clinical governance processes in primary care settings have included attitudes to policy developments, the absence of protected time and limited resources. However, given the additional evidence of apathy and anxiety (Wilkin et al 2000) it seems reasonable to assume that there have also been planning and educational failures, as well as a failure to provide support and facilitated guidance in the implementation of clinical guidance policies, including those to do with how best to deal with poor performance.

With reference to the emphasis placed on evidence to support practice, recent systematic reviews undertaken by Foy et al (2001) found that barriers to the adoption of evidence-based care fell into three broad bands:

◆ the characteristics of the guidelines themselves, where for instance the perceived relevance and the practicalities of implementation in particular settings, influenced attitudes;
◆ the characteristics of individuals facing the need to change – their beliefs about and attitudes towards clinical governance processes, as well as their perceptions of current skills or abilities; and
◆ the characteristics of the healthcare environment in which quality improvement initiatives are to be implemented.

The implications of such barriers for those involved in the implementation of clinical governance policies seem to support the need for a developmental approach where there is a continuing and important role for researchers, for those designing and producing evidence-based guidelines, for clinical leadership, for educationalists and for service managers. Of particular interest is the evidence of beneficial effects from involving those who have had positive experiences of changing practice, or those who have special skills in facilitating change or illuminating the benefits of change. Such resources can become real strengths in the hands of those designing and planning implementation strategies for clinical governance (Kitson et al 1998), who themselves require support and protected time, as well as educational resources.

Insight is also needed into the nature of the leadership required for moving the quality improvement agenda forward – away from the traditional 'command and control' philosophy. For example, after putting together a development programme, the NHS Clinical Support Team asked NHS Chief Executives to send 'staff who will be missed, not staff who can be spared' (Cullen et al 2000)! The key characteristics sought included people who were not only capable of designing and delivering quality improvement projects but also had a wide knowledge of the organization, the respect of their colleagues, the trust of senior staff and a commitment to hard work. More opportunities now exist for nurses to participate in Leadership Development and such opportunities are likely to incorporate:

◆ a multidisciplinary approach
◆ exploring the concept and value of emotional intelligence
◆ the significance of involving those likely to be affected by a quality improvement project, at the planning stage
◆ examining how best to assess performance and reviewing baseline measures currently being used to assess achievement
◆ how best to undertake a review of records, or other relevant documents, as a means to explore the degree to which current programmes of care are in line with local policies and priorities
◆ access to computer-based sites for reviewing and analysing available evidence on which clinical practice should be based.

The relationship between clinical governance and improving the quality of care lies in part with the setting and monitoring of standards. Sanderson (2000) suggests that this means ensuring that:

◆ all health professionals have the necessary training and education to acquire the skills and behaviour for working co-operatively with others;

◆ the culture changes mentioned above are supported by timely and accurate information which allows staff to compare their clinical performance with an agreed standard. (It will however be critical to ensure that measures of performance are those that address the important elements of quality care, rather than adopting measures that are relatively easy to count. For example, it would be relatively easy to count the number of housebound patients with leg ulcers who are in receipt of a district nursing service but more time consuming and difficult to count the proportion who have a clear record of an evidence-based and standardized assessment procedure, even though it is the latter which is more closely linked to a successful outcome of clinical nursing care.);
◆ the clinical care provided has an adequate evidence base;
◆ opportunities are provided and used to learn from the experience of an adverse event (e.g. failure to observe a significantly deteriorating condition, or set of circumstances; failure to maintain complete, contemporaneous and legible records; failure to provide up-to-date accurate information when it is sought) in order to reduce the risk of it being repeated and that patients/clients and their main carers understand and are able to participate as much as they wish, in the decision-making related to their care.

THE WAY FORWARD

It is not really possible to implement relevant aspects of clinical governance policies without the development of clinical standards; that means having a clear idea from peer review what comprises 'reasonable practice' and being able to describe 'reasonable practice' with a logical basis (see Chapter 13 for further discussion). In some important ways, 'reasonable practice' is about attitudes and behaviour, communication and working co-operatively with others. But there are also clear links with skills in reviewing research-based evidence, in being able to access computer-based information and being familiar with the role of the National Institute of Clinical Excellence

(NICE), with the work of the Commission for Health Improvement and with the guidance from professional bodies like the NMC and the RCN.

For community nurses to be actively involved in quality improvement requires them to be familiar with the policy context, to understand the concepts of quality and clinical governance and to grasp the implications for their service and its contribution to primary health care. There are of course legal implications surrounding confidentiality and the monitoring of information – again see Chapter 13. There are also differences between families in their response to health problems and to people perceived to be figures of authority. This means that community nurses need to agree how best to characterize a group of people in receipt of a specified programme of care, in order to take account of predictable factors which could influence the outcomes of care. It would be unreasonable for example to have the same goals for all individuals/families with a comparable problem, where a proportion have been defined as 'hard to help' or 'resistant to help'. Unlike hospital-based services – where a person may be diagnosed and treated successfully but remain dissatisfied with the overall experience – community nursing services must be acceptable and valued to attain the co-operation and involvement of patients/clients and their carers. Satisfaction with the experience of a community nursing service is thus likely to be dependent on such quality indicators as:

◆ the setting/environment in which the service is located – convenience, accessibility, comfort, facilities and resources
◆ health professionals – friendly and approachable, available and accessible, well qualified and experienced, reliable, providing answers to questions with timely and useful progress reports
◆ organization and management – readily available information, e.g. about appointments and about other relevant and locally available resources, efficient use of time, reasonable waiting time, records up to date and available.

The above quality markers flag up three important factors influencing the quality of service provision (see Chapter 15 for further discussion about team functioning and team development):

1. *technical factors* such as clinical expertise, clinical supervision and training;
2. *interface factors* such as having a shared vision, the manner in which the service is delivered and perceived, as well as aspects of communication, including interpersonal relationships and teamwork; and
3. *environmental factors* such as ease of access, comfort, adequate information and explanation, efficient organization of the facility.

For the community nurse, analysing the quality of service provision will inevitably go beyond assessing the clinical effectiveness of an intervention to take account of that most elusive of concepts: *caring*. In a review of quantitative instruments designed to measure 'caring', Beck (1999) for instance, reinforces the view that different elements of 'caring' (caring as a human trait; a moral imperative; a therapeutic intervention; an effect and caring as interpersonal communication) may be more significant than others depending on the circumstances. This underlines the importance of contextual information when making comparisons about the effectiveness of community nursing care.

TAKING THE FIRST STEPS TO QUALITY IMPROVEMENT

Three approaches provide examples for taking steps to improve the quality and clinical effectiveness of a community nursing service: i) reviewing a specified community nursing programme of care; ii) focusing on personal development with reference to the professional portfolio; and iii) adopting a project approach.

UNDERTAKING A SYSTEMATIC REVIEW OF ONE PROGRAMME OR ELEMENT OF A COMMUNITY NURSING SERVICE

Suggested questions to be addressed:

◆ Is there a clear description of the population group for whom the programme of community nursing care is provided – one that will allow assessment and comparison of the proportion and characteristics of those who are currently in receipt of clinical care?

◆ What is the basis for prioritizing individuals/families and is there a logical justification?

◆ Is the programme of care based on a systematic review of currently available evidence?

◆ Has the specialist community nursing team been involved in the development of a protocol or guidelines?

◆ Are the goals of the programme defined in measurable and achievable terms and are they focused on outcomes?

◆ Is there a system in place to monitor the efficacy of the programme over an agreed timespan?

◆ Can the current record system provide evidence of progress towards stated goals, or of quality markers such as individual and/or family involvement in decision-making?

FOCUSING ON PERSONAL DEVELOPMENT

This will involve some initial reflection on personal and professional development within the context of your current position and plans for the future. It will also involve making sure that you are familiar with the local priorities for clinical governance in primary care, as well as the employing Trust's priorities for developing your particular community nursing service.

Continuing professional development (CPD) should involve gaining the knowledge and skills that are necessary for achieving and maintaining high standards of practice. This promotes job satisfaction, requires familiarity with how high standards of community nursing care are recognized and gaining sufficient confidence to become involved in the development of protocols, challenging them when it is perceived to be in the best interests of patients/clients. Consider the most appropriate occasion to raise CPD planning with your team leader or line manager.

Using your professional portfolio provides the opportunity to identify achievements but it can also, for example, help to focus on key tasks for improving clinical effectiveness associated with

future plans for primary care development, including the skills necessary for more effective leadership and for obtaining and analysing up-to-date evidence.

ADOPTING A PROJECT APPROACH

Identify a practice-based topic that has been raised recently and appears to cause some concern with reference to the effectiveness of clinical care, or to the organizational arrangements of service delivery. Satisfy yourself that there is sufficient interest in improving the situation.

Then undertake relevant background reading so that you can produce a short introductory paper to be given to colleagues prior to the next suitable meeting, making sure that it explores the basis for concern and the justification for change, together with options for improvement. If there is sufficient interest in making a change, make sure that everyone likely to be affected by any proposal is involved in the planning stages, that the responsibilities for key tasks are divided out fairly and that there is an agreed timescale for reviewing and monitoring progress. Invest enough time in the planning phase. That means not moving forward unless there is agreement about the main purpose and objectives and about who will take responsibility for what.

CONCLUSION

The current government's commitment to modernize the NHS includes a drive to improve the 'quality' of the service, in particular focusing on enhanced professional regulation, clinical governance and lifelong learning (including CPD). There is a focus on the involvement of patients including their responsibilities rather than focusing purely on their rights as 'consumers' which predominated in the 1980s.

The concept of 'value for money' is now aimed at clinical governance rather than corporate governance or financial governance, with the NHS being seen and measured as a service not a product. For clinical governance to work there has been an effort to change the culture of the NHS with a developmental focus to rid itself of the 'blame culture' and other inadequacies which had existed previously.

The clinical effectiveness of community nursing services can only be enhanced by carrying out systematic reviews of each element/programme in the service, focusing on the continuing professional development (CPD) of individual nurses and adopting a project approach to change.

SUMMARY

◆ The concept of value for money is now aimed at clinical governance rather than corporate or financial governance, underlining the significance of quality measures related to the setting and monitoring of standards in clinical practice.

◆ For clinical governance policies to work effectively, efforts are being made to change the culture of the NHS focusing on professional and service development rather than the inadequacies associated with locating and blaming an individual for errors or inadequate care.

◆ The clinical effectiveness of community nursing services can only be enhanced by carrying out systematic reviews of each element and programme of the service, with special reference to the usefulness of information services, the nature of service objectives and the processes to do with maintaining high quality and preventing poor-quality provision.

DISCUSSION POINTS

1. Locate the relevant Trust documents which explain the local approach to clinical governance, consider the implications for your service and identify gaps in understanding that need closing.

2. What quality standards are currently adopted for your community nursing service and to what degree are these relevant to clinical effectiveness and other clinical governance guidelines?

3. How is unacceptable practice being addressed by your community nursing team and by the employing Trust – how do arrangements match with clinical governance concerns for the dissemination of 'good practice' guidelines, openness and learning from adverse events?

REFERENCES

Beck CT 1999 Quantative measurement of caring. Journal of Advanced Nursing 30(1): 24–32
Cullen R, Nicholls S, Halligan A 2000 Reviewing a service – discovering the unwritten rules. Clinical Performance and Quality Health Care 8(4): 233–239
Dawson J (ed) 2001 Clinical effectiveness in nursing practice. Whurr Publishers, London and Philadelphia PA
Dawson S 1997 Inhabiting different worlds: how can research relate to practice? Quality in Health Care 6: 177–178
Department of Health 1998 A first class service: Quality in the NHS. DoH, London
Department of Health 2000a An organisation with a memory. Report of an expert group on learning from adverse events in the NHS chaired by the Chief Medical Officer. DoH, London
Department of Health 2000b The NHS Plan: a plan for investment, a plan for reform. DoH, London
Department of Health 2001 Modernising regulation in the health care professions. DoH, London
Donabedian A 1981 Criteria, norms and standards of quality: what do they mean? American Journal of Public Health 71(4): 409–412
Foy R, Walker A, Penney G 2001 Barriers to clinical guidelines: the need for concerted action. British Journal of Clinical Governance 6(3): 166–174
GMC 2001 Good medical practice. Published and delivered to all those on the Register
Griffiths Report 1983 NHS management enquiry. DHSS, London
Kings Fund 1997 Turning evidence into everyday practice. The Kings Fund, London
Kitson A, Harvey G, McCormack B 1998 Enabling the implementation of evidence based practice: a conceptual framework. Quality in Health Care (7): 149–158
Maynard A 1991 The case for auditing audit. Health Services Journal 101(526): 26
RCN 1989 Standards of care: a framework for quality. Scutari, Harrow
Sanderson H 2000 Information requirements for clinical governance. Clinical Performance and Quality Health Care 8(1): 52–57
Scally G, Donaldson LJ 1998 Clinical governance and the drive for quality improvement in the new NHS in England. British Medical Journal 316: 1917–1918
Secretary of State for Health 1997 The New NHS: modern and dependable. HMSO, London
Sorrie R 2000 Making clinical governance work in primary care: the practicalities. Journal of Clinical Governance 8: 60–62
UKCC 1995 The scope of professional practice. UKCC, London

UKCC 2001 Accountability in practice produced in association with professional nurse. UKCC, London

UKCC 2002 Code of professional conduct, 3rd edition. UKCC, London

Walshe K 2000 Developing clinical governance: leadership, culture and change. Journal of Clinical Governance 8: 16–20

Walsh MJ, Small N 2001 Clinical governance in primary care: early impressions based on Bradford South and West Primary Care Group's experience. British Journal of Clinical Governance 6(2): 109–118

Watson R 2000 Educational effectiveness to support clinical effectiveness in nursing. Clinical Effectiveness in Nursing 4(4): 149–151

Wilkin D, Gillan S, Coleman A 2001 The National Tracker Survey of Primary Care Groups & Trusts 2000/2001: Modernising the NHS? Kings Fund, University of Manchester, London

FURTHER READING

Antrobus S, Kitson A 1999 Nursing leadership: influencing and shaping policy and nursing practice. Journal of Advanced Nursing 29(4): 746–753

Chambers R 1998 Clinical effectiveness made easy – first thoughts on clinical governance. Radcliffe Medical Press, Oxford

Dawson J (ed) 2001 Clinical effectiveness in nursing practice. Whurr Publishers, London

Muir Gray JA 1997 Evidence-based health care. Churchill Livingstone, Edinburgh

Parsley K, Corrigan P 1994 Quality improvement in nursing and health care. Chapman Hall, London

UKCC 2002 Professional self-regulation and clinical governance. Obtainable from the NMC website at www.nmc-uk.org or free from the NMC Distribution Dept

The public health framework

This section develops the contextual themes of policy development, public health and clinical governance and how these affect the role of community nursing. It explores in more detail the knowledge base of epidemiology and the role of screening for disease prevention – an important aspect of primary care. The politics of poverty and social welfare are also raised in this section and can usefully be linked to later discussion surrounding a community development perspective. Community nurses are encouraged to consider their role in reducing health inequalities within a local context, exploring how working with other agencies can help to ensure patients / clients receive integrated health and social care.

The first chapter reviews the role of epidemiology in understanding the origins and processes of disease and draws attention to the different types of data that provide clues concerning causal relationships. The advantages and disadvantages of different kinds of research studies are discussed and subsequently linked to their relevance for community nursing practice, with reference to particular examples of disease. The chapter develops with general and specific considerations for different approaches to prevention, supported by examples, and goes on to examine the role of screening in disease prevention. The contribution of community nursing is underlined with special reference to the wide range of people their services reach.

The second chapter explores poverty in relation to health and healthcare policy and provision, emphasizing the focus of the NHS on reducing health inequalities. A detailed analysis of the factors which link poverty with health inequality is provided, pointing out the limitations of the NHS, using examples of the way the NHS helps to perpetuate inequality by failing to be responsive to the needs of the most vulnerable. The developing politics of poverty is reviewed and linked not only to the importance of adopting a social and economic model of health, but also to the strengthening shift of emphasis to a public health perspective and its link to the future development of primary health care.

The final chapter in this section moves the issues surrounding health inequality forward by examining the concepts of 'health gain' and 'health improvement'. Community nursing services are encouraged to explore how best to contribute to health improvement and how best to address the problems of measuring health gain in the context of a drive to improve efficiency and effectiveness. The community development perspective is introduced and consideration is given to the different skills required for involving local people and working with other agencies. Some useful online references are provided which draw attention to the practicalities of putting theory into practice.

5

Epidemiology and disease prevention

M.L. Burr

KEY ISSUES

◆ Preventing disease should be the concern of all health professionals, particularly nurses who work in the community.

◆ To prevent a disease we need to know its aetiology and natural history, and it is helpful to understand the epidemiological evidence on which this knowledge is based.

◆ It is becoming increasingly possible to prevent diseases by screening healthy people; nurses in the community need to understand the issues involved, since people will expect them to give information and advice on this subject.

INTRODUCTION

Epidemiology is the study of disease in the population rather than in individuals. This chapter will show how epidemiology has contributed to our understanding of the aetiology and natural history of various diseases, and how this knowledge has enabled us to adopt practical measures to prevent the onset or progress of disease. Nurses who work in the community are in a good position to understand the population aspects of health and disease; they are also very favourably placed to help in preventing disease, whether by participating in specific programmes or in the ordinary course of their work. A primary healthcare team with a co-ordinated approach can make a unique contribution to disease prevention.

AETIOLOGY

THE CONTRIBUTION OF EPIDEMIOLOGY

The epidemiological approach has been very useful in investigating the causes of disease. Sometimes the cause of a disease in an individual is not in doubt: if a person is bitten by a rabid dog and then succumbs to rabies, we can reasonably conclude that the bite caused the disease. But many diseases do not have such a clear-cut relation between cause and effect. We may observe that a certain disease is more prevalent in one geographical area than another, and suspect that the explanation lies in some aspect of the inhabitants' environment, lifestyle, or socioeconomic status. But it is unlikely that there is any one factor that is invariably associated with the disease. It may be the case that air pollution, or cigarette smoking, or lack of exercise, or some aspect of the diet, while neither necessary nor sufficient for the disease to occur, increases a person's risk of getting it, other things being equal. The study of epidemiology enables us to identify such 'risk factors' and assess the degree to which they contribute to causation, though it seldom allows us to be sure why a particular person acquired that disease. Different epidemiological methods will be briefly reviewed to illustrate how they can do this.

ECOLOGICAL STUDIES

There are many types of data, collected routinely, that can give useful clues about causal factors. Death rates from various diseases are published for different countries, and for areas within those countries. For many diseases these rates show geographical variations and time trends which suggest that there are factors that make the diseases more common in some places or at some times. It may then be possible to show that the mortality rate is related (positively or negatively) with some factor that is present to different degrees within the various populations. For example, in a study of six American cities the death rates for cardiovascular disease and for lung cancer were strongly related to air concentrations of fine particles, suggesting that air pollution increased mortality (Dockery et al 1993). This kind of study is termed 'ecological'; it examines relationships between groups rather than individuals.

CROSS-SECTIONAL SURVEYS

The cross-sectional survey takes a 'snapshot' of a population at one point in time. It is particularly useful in determining the prevalence of chronic conditions in different groups of people. The results may suggest aetiological links, for example, by showing that chronic obstructive pulmonary disease is more common among smokers than nonsmokers. Similarly, a repeat survey conducted

after several years may reveal a rise in prevalence that suggests possible environmental causes to be explored. During recent decades, repeat surveys of asthma in many parts of the world have shown an increase in its prevalence (Burr 1993). These observations have stimulated research to discover the cause of this increase.

CASE–CONTROL STUDIES

The case–control study asks why some people have acquired a disease (cases), while others from the same population have not (controls). Thus it starts with diseased people and enquires about their past exposure to possible causal or protective factors, and makes the same enquiries about similar people who are free from the disease in question. By comparing the two groups it can be seen whether the disease is associated (positively or negatively) with the factors. The controls may be matched individually with the cases for age and sex, or they may be a broadly similar group. They may be taken from the general population or from groups of patients with conditions that are thought to be unrelated to the disease and factors under investigation. The case–control design has been very useful in investigating numerous aetiological links, e.g. lung cancer and cigarette smoking; phocomelia and thalidomide in pregnancy; Reye's disease and aspirin. One example using computerized data in primary care was a study in two London practices to see whether patients with asthma were more likely than controls to live near a busy road; they were not (Livingstone et al 1996).

COHORT STUDIES

A cohort is a group of people who are defined at one point in time and followed up thereafter. Cohort studies are particularly useful in aetiological research, since the potential causal and protective factors can be ascertained before their effects have appeared. This information is much more accurate than that derived retrospectively in a case–control study and is not biased by knowledge of the outcome. A classic example is the study of smoking in British male doctors set up by Doll and Hill in 1951. During the next 40 years, cigarette smoking was associated with greatly increased mortality rates from numerous diseases; giving up smoking, even in middle age, substantially reduced the excess risk (Doll et al 1994). The main drawback of cohort studies is their size, duration, and cost. Occasionally it is possible to avoid the long delay between baseline and follow up by using a historical cohort. This is a group identified at some point in the past and followed up to the present time; the baseline observations are derived from records, so that this approach is possible only where adequate records exist. Barker (1995) discovered the records of birth weights and other details of babies born during the first half of the 20th century, and has followed up the individuals concerned. In this way, various indices of nutritional state in early life have been found to predict diabetes, heart disease and other conditions in middle age.

RANDOMIZED CONTROLLED TRIALS

The best evidence for causality is provided by the randomized controlled trial (RCT). Unlike the observational studies considered so far, this has an experimental design: suitable subjects are randomly allocated to two or more groups, which receive different interventions or none at all. Differences between the outcomes of the groups can thus be attributed specifically to the interventions. RCTs are most frequently used to evaluate drugs, but the technique can be employed to investigate the effects of other factors such as diet, or the manner in which a service is delivered. Many trials have been conducted that were too small to yield clear results, but if all the RCTs investigating a given topic are identified their results can be combined by the technique of meta-analysis, which may then reveal an overall effect. For example, many trials have investigated the effect of reducing or modifying dietary fat on the incidence and mortality of cardiovascular disease. Most of these trials showed little or no effect, but a meta-analysis revealed a 16% reduction in cardiovascular events, rising to 24% in trials with at least 2 years' follow up (Hooper et al 2001). It was concluded that there is a small but potentially important reduction in cardiovascular risk when dietary fat intake is reduced or modified.

RELEVANCE TO COMMUNITY NURSING

There is growing emphasis on the importance of 'evidence-based medicine'. In consequence, RCTs are increasingly undertaken to provide the evidence on which policies for prevention and treatment should be based. It is quite likely that any health professional will be directly or indirectly involved in a controlled trial at some time in his or her career, so that we all need to have some understanding of the principles involved. Community nurses are likely to know about, or be asked to assist in, any survey taking place in their locality. As part of a primary healthcare team they may even have an opportunity to initiate a study in order to investigate a problem, particularly relating to some local issue. Epidemiological studies can be quite easy to carry out, especially given the wealth of computerized data in primary care.

NATURAL HISTORY – THE CONCEPT

The concept of the natural history of a disease is perhaps not entirely familiar to health professionals, who usually meet the disease only when it causes symptoms, and view its subsequent progress in terms of its response to treatment. But a knowledge of its natural history is central to an understanding of prevention, screening, prognosis, and whether treatment is needed. Most diseases pass through a succession of phases: pathological inception initiates a presymptomatic period leading to clinically manifest disease, which may progress through various stages (sometimes with remissions and relapses) to spontaneous recovery, permanent disability or death. Treatment may modify this course of events to a greater or lesser extent.

THE HOW AND WHY OF NATURAL HISTORY

Epidemiology can provide information about natural history mainly by means of cohort studies. A large group of persons is followed up over time, and the onset and progress of a disease is monitored. For the less common diseases it is necessary to start with newly diagnosed patients. The course of the disease can be related to various factors recorded at baseline and during follow up, to investigate their prognostic significance. It would obviously be unethical to withhold treatment that is known to be effective merely in order to find out what happens in its absence, so the treatment can be considered as one of the potentially prognostic factors. Sometimes a group of patients who refuse treatment will agree to be followed up, and this approach can yield valuable information, although such patients are unlikely to be wholly representative of all those with the disease.

Various questions about the course of diseases and risk factors can be tackled in this way. For example: To what extent do overweight and obesity in childhood predict these conditions in adult life? Is a blood pressure in the upper part of the 'normal' range during adolescence a predictor of clinical hypertension in middle age? What proportion of persons with newly diagnosed noninsulin-dependent diabetes will eventually become insulin dependent or acquire other conditions associated with diabetes, and can we identify those whose risk is greatest? Such questions need to be answered if we are to prevent serious illness before it has become irreversible.

AN EXAMPLE – THE ATOPIC DISEASES

The atopic diseases (atopic eczema, asthma and allergic rhinitis) have an interrelated natural history that illustrates several relevant principles. These conditions are quite common, especially during childhood, and are easy to study by means of questionnaires and simple tests. They are therefore very suitable topics to be investigated by following up newborn infants ('birth

cohorts') or population samples of any age, in whom the onset and course of these conditions can be monitored. Several large cohort studies have been conducted. It is clear that the three conditions are associated with each other within individuals; there is a tendency for babies who have eczema to acquire asthma during childhood and hay fever in adolescence (the 'allergic march'). It can be shown that other evidence of an atopic disposition (such as positive skin prick tests or a high serum IgE concentration) and increased airway responsiveness commonly precede the onset of clinical asthma. The onset of wheeze after the age of 2 years, but not before, predicts allergic asthma during later childhood. This suggests that different factors (infection and allergy, respectively) predominate in the cause of wheezy illness before and after the age of 2 years (Burr 1993).

The investigation of the course and prognosis of asthma requires a cohort of people with the disease to be followed up for as long as possible. The cohort should be selected so as to represent the whole spectrum of the disease. It is obviously much easier to select patients who attend clinics than to identify people with all degrees of asthma by means of a population survey, so most follow up studies have been based on patients referred to hospital doctors. Such studies may show the factors that predict the outcome of more severe asthma, but they are uninformative about the milder and more common forms, and are therefore unhelpful in providing an overall picture of the disease as it occurs in the population. Remission of asthma occurs most often in the second decade of life, and is uncommon after the age of 30 years. The initial severity is an unfavourable predictor, and so is the degree of airway responsiveness. The disease is liable to recur after a symptom-free interval; relapse rates increase with age up to the age of 70 years (Bronnimann & Burrows 1986). The underlying atopic disposition, as shown by skin tests, persists whether symptoms are present or not.

One such cohort study was undertaken by a London general practitioner, who identified asthmatic children in his practice between 1948–52 and followed them up for at least 20 years (Blair 1977). The advent of computerized records opens up excellent opportunities for cohorts to be defined and followed up in primary care.

Studies of the natural history of atopy show that the course of asthma is to some extent determined during early life, before its first manifestations have appeared. It is to this period that attempts to prevent it should therefore be directed. Similar observations could be made about many other conditions.

PREVENTION

GENERAL CONSIDERATIONS

The chief practical incentive for studying the aetiology and natural history of a disease is so that it can be prevented. For many diseases, prevention is plainly better than cure. Cure may be impossible, or only partial, or uncertain, or at the cost of treatment which can be almost as bad as the disease. As more is discovered about causation, it becomes increasingly possible, at least in principle, to prevent conditions (such as atheromatous cardiovascular disease and many cancers) for which there is no entirely satisfactory cure.

Prevention may be better than cure, but in some ways it is less straightforward in its application. People who suffer from a disease may reasonably expect to receive treatment that will improve their symptoms. But people who feel perfectly well do not necessarily want to be told to change their lifestyle or take medication in order to prevent an illness that may never happen anyway. The onus is on the health professional to show why such interventions are advisable and to be sure that they are likely to do more good than harm. Preventive measures often confer benefit only on a minority of those who undertake them, since most of those who are 'at risk' would not in fact acquire the condition being prevented in any case. Thus the benefits of prevention can be demonstrated in groups of people rather than in individuals, and require epidemiological techniques for their evaluation.

Nurses and other health professionals who work in the community are in a good position to understand the need for disease prevention and to make it happen. They see a much wider range of people than their hospital colleagues do. They are likely to have a 'feel' for local health problems, and can probably anticipate difficulties that may arise in attempting to put preventive principles into practice in their area. As part of primary healthcare teams they can help to formulate local policies on how community nursing resources should be used in disease prevention, given the characteristics of their caseload and the practice profile.

PRIMORDIAL PREVENTION

To some extent the causes of disease lie in the patterns of life of the whole population. The term 'primordial prevention' refers to the avoidance of social, cultural and economic conditions that are known to contribute, if indirectly, to an increased risk of disease. For example, a few years ago it was taken for granted in the UK that in any gathering of people there would be some who were smoking cigarettes, and the others would just have to put up with breathing smoke-laden air. Awareness of the hazards of passive as well as active smoking has led to a change in public attitudes and policies, so that trains, aircraft, offices and other public places are now usually smoke free. What was previously regarded as inevitable is now unacceptable. The health effects of this cultural change are probably substantial in terms of respiratory and cardiovascular disease.

Other examples of this type of prevention include the phasing out of propellants that damage the ozone layer (with implications for the incidence of skin cancer); policies on food, housing, road traffic and air pollution; and general measures to tackle poverty and deprivation. The health effects of primordial prevention tend to be indirect and nonspecific, so they are difficult to quantify; the infant mortality rate and the expectation of life at birth are two general indices of the health of a population that seem to reflect overall trends in these underlying factors.

PRIMARY PREVENTION

Primary prevention means reducing the incidence of a disease by addressing the specific factors that increase or decrease the risk of getting it. There are two ways in which primary prevention can be applied, known as the population and the high-risk individual strategies respectively, depending on whether it is directed to the whole community or to those individuals whose risk is greatest.

The population strategy addresses the causal factors within the whole population, so as to reduce the average risk. Although this approach overlaps with primordial prevention, it involves a more direct connection between the preventive measures and the condition being prevented. For example, children are immunized against a range of diseases, some of which (e.g. tetanus) the vast majority would never get anyway. But tetanus is such a serious disease that it is well worthwhile immunizing them all to protect the few. By contrast, virtually all children would catch measles in the absence of immunization, so each child benefits from being immunized; in addition, when the proportion of children immunized reaches a certain level, 'herd immunity' will lead to the eradication of the disease from the community. Thus in both cases the preventive programme should be directed to the population rather than to individuals.

Tetanus immunization illustrates a situation where everyone is at risk but only a few (who cannot be identified in advance) will actually benefit from an intervention; wearing seat belts in motor cars is another example. Even if it is possible to distinguish degrees of risk among individuals – for example, in the case of ischaemic heart disease – the population strategy has considerable advantages. Risk of the disease could be reduced by eating less saturated fat and more fruit and vegetables. The population strategy promotes these changes in the whole community, aiming to change everybody's eating habits, even if only to a small degree. Reducing the population mean intake of saturated fat, and in consequence the mean serum cholesterol concentration, may have little effect on any one individual's risk of disease and yet make an important impact on disease in the population: it has been estimated that each 1% reduction in the average cholesterol level would produce a 3% fall in the incidence of ischaemic heart disease (Rose 1992). The

advantages of this strategy may be summarized as follows:

◆ Eating habits tend to be community-based; it is difficult for individuals to eat a different diet from that of their families and friends.
◆ The effect is more likely to be permanent than a modification of an individual's diet.
◆ It is not always easy to identify the high-risk individuals.
◆ Even if the high-risk individuals are successfully targeted, much of the incidence of the disease occurs among those who are at only average risk, since they are more numerous, and only a population strategy will benefit them.

The North Karelia Project was one of the first attempts to reduce cardiovascular mortality by means of a population-based intervention. It was set up in response to a petition, signed by all North Karelian members of the Finnish Parliament and many other people, calling for national aid to reduce the very high cardiovascular mortality in the area. The intervention comprised a wide range of elements tackling the various factors known to cause cardiovascular disease. The dietary aspect emphasized the need to reduce the consumption of saturated fat and increase that of fruit, vegetables and dietary fibre. It involved the farmers, the food industry, dairies, grocers and canteens; a high-profile public education programme gave advice about food choice and the growing of vegetables. These efforts were rewarded by a decline in average serum cholesterol levels, from 7.1 mmol/l in men and 7.0 mmol/l in women in 1972 to 6.3 and 6.2 mmol/l, respectively, in 1982. In comparison with concurrent changes in a neighbouring county (Kuopio), cholesterol levels showed a significant net decline in North Karelian men and a nonsignificant net decline in the women. Significant net reductions also occurred in smoking prevalence among men, and in mean blood pressures among men and women. From 1974 to 1979, male coronary heart disease (CHD) mortality declined by 22% in North Karelia and by 12% in Kuopio; cardiovascular and all-cause mortality similarly showed a greater annual decline in North Karelia than elsewhere in Finland for both men and women (Puska et al 1985).

There can be little doubt that modest dietary changes within the whole population produce health benefits, but they are not easy to bring about. They are liable to have complex implications for the food industry, farming, the retail trade and politics. Even if they occur, it can be very difficult to demonstrate that the changes and benefits were due to any particular intervention. RCTs are not really suitable for evaluating the population strategy. Doubts may be raised as to whether the reference area was truly comparable, and it is virtually impossible to confine the changes to the study area. Thus mean levels of serum cholesterol and blood pressure declined in Kuopio from about 1977, and since the mid 1980s they have been comparable in the two areas. Similar community-based interventions in the United States have shown few statistically significant net effects: the changes tend to be less than expected in the intervention areas, and more than expected in the control areas (Winkleby et al 1997). The view has been expressed that community interventions are not cost-effective, and health promotion should be refocused towards those at very high risk of disease (Ebrahim & Davey Smith 1998). (See Chapter 27 for further discussion on health promotion.)

In comparison to the population strategy, the high-risk individual strategy certainly has some advantages:

◆ It is easier to implement, since many of the high-risk individuals are already in contact with health professionals.
◆ The intervention can be tailored to the individual.
◆ The subjects are more likely to be motivated to undertake the appropriate changes than those whose risk is lower.
◆ The health professionals are also more motivated.
◆ The effect of a given intervention can be demonstrated by means of an RCT.

One example of this approach is the identification and treatment of people with high blood pressure. For some years, it has been known that control of hypertension confers a reduction in cardiovascular mortality, especially that of stroke

(Collins et al 1990). It has therefore increasingly become the practice for doctors and nurses to measure the blood pressure of any person (particularly someone who is middle-aged or older) who consults them for any reason. This illustrates one method of screening in order to find high-risk people, a subject that is dealt with in more detail below. Another example of the high-risk individual strategy is the prevention of coronary events by prescribing statin drugs for people whose serum cholesterol concentrations are high (Shepherd et al 1995) or whose high-density lipoprotein cholesterol levels are low (Downs et al 1998). The effectiveness of this intervention is not in doubt, but issues arise as to the cost per year of life gained and the appropriate screening policy to find those who should be treated.

The importance of both strategies for primary prevention is acknowledged in the National Service Framework for Coronary Heart Disease (DoH 2000). It calls for policies to reduce the prevalence of coronary risk factors in the population, with reference to smoking, healthy eating, physical activity and obesity. It also requires primary care teams to identify all people at significant risk of cardiovascular disease who have not yet developed symptoms, and offer them appropriate advice and treatment to reduce their risks. Charts and computer programs are available that show whether an individual's risk of a CHD event exceeds 30% over 10 years, on the basis of factors such as age, gender, cholesterol, hypertension and diabetes. For such persons, blood pressure should be maintained below 140/85 mmHg, serum cholesterol should be reduced, and other risk factors should be addressed appropriately.

SECONDARY PREVENTION

Secondary prevention means preventing the progression or recurrence of a disease that has already affected a person. For example, if someone has suffered from a myocardial infarction, secondary prevention aims to prevent another attack. The advantages of the high-risk individual strategy operate to an even greater degree – the subjects and health professionals are likely to be very highly motivated, and the intervention is targeted towards those who are most likely to benefit from it. The principal disadvantage is, of course, that some damage has already occurred and may not be entirely reversible.

Three RCTs have shown that treatment with statins reduces the risk of reinfarction and (in two of them) death among patients with angina or a history of myocardial infarction (Sacks et al 1996, Scandinavian Simvastatin Survival Study Group 1994, The Long-term Intervention with Pravastatin in Ischemic Heart Disease (LIPID) Study Group 1998). The National Service Framework for Coronary Heart Disease therefore recommends statins and dietary advice to lower serum cholesterol in persons with diagnosed CHD or other occlusive arterial disease, together with low-dose aspirin, attention to the modifiable risk factors, and other treatment as appropriate. Statins appear to reduce the incidence of CHD events by the same proportion (about a third) whatever the initial risk may be, so the benefits are greatest in those at highest risk. The National Service Framework therefore gives priority to statin therapy and other preventive measures among persons with existing CHD.

Secondary prevention is usually directed to the detection and treatment of disease in its early stages, so as to prevent its progression to a point where it causes serious illness, permanent handicap or death. This may involve detecting the disease before it has caused any symptoms, for example, finding and treating preinvasive cervical cancer by means of cervical smears. The large-scale detection of early disease (screening) is thus an integral part of much secondary prevention.

TERTIARY PREVENTION

Even when disease is well established and irreversible, it is often possible to prevent complications and reduce the degree of disability that is incurred. This is termed tertiary prevention, and can be very important in determining the quality of life of the patient. One example is the prevention of pressure ulcers in elderly patients undergoing hospital treatment. Most pressure ulcers develop in the first 2 weeks after admission (Bridel 1993), when medical and nursing attention is usually preoccupied with the condition for which the patient was admitted. When the patient is discharged from hospital, a pressure ulcer has profound consequences in terms of mobility, quality of life and health service costs. In most cases it is far easier and more cost-effective to prevent a pressure ulcer than to cure it. Prevention is therefore immensely important, yet the incidence is still disturbingly high. There is inadequate information about the best method of predicting which patients will acquire pressure ulcers and how to prevent them (Cullum et al 1995).

In tertiary prevention it is particularly important to anticipate preventable complications, so that preventive measures can be directed to the patients at greatest risk. It is also very important to avoid defeatism in the patient, nurses and other health professionals; permanent handicap will be minimized if a hopeful attitude is maintained. This is the secret of successful rehabilitation, the context in which tertiary prevention is mainly practised.

SCREENING

GENERAL CONSIDERATIONS

Screening has recently been defined as 'a public health service in which members of a defined population, who do not necessarily perceive that they are at risk of, or are already affected by, a disease or its complications, are asked a question or offered a test to identify those individuals who are more likely to be helped than harmed by further tests or treatment to reduce the risk of disease or its complications' (UK National Screening Committee 2000). It is important in primary prevention to identify high-risk individuals, and in secondary prevention to detect a disease before the person has become aware of it or has taken any action about it. The above definition draws attention to the fact that screening is designed to reduce risk rather than to eliminate it completely; it also recognizes the possibility that the screening procedure may actually cause harm.

There are certain criteria that should be met before a screening programme is introduced. The disease should be serious and fairly common; there is a trade-off between these two criteria, in that it may be worth screening for a condition that is rare but very serious if undetected (e.g. phenylketonuria), and for one that is relatively mild but very common (e.g. minor visual defects in children). The natural history must be understood, and there needs to be a reasonably long period during which the disease can be detected before it usually presents spontaneously. The test should ideally have a high sensitivity (the ability to detect the abnormality when it is present) and a high specificity (the ability to identify the absence of the abnormality when it is not present). These features are inversely related; the cut-off point at which the test result is considered to be abnormal may have to be adjusted so as to produce an acceptable balance between falsely reassuring people who are at risk (which defeats the object of the exercise) and unnecessarily worrying people who are not at risk (which brings it into disrepute). The test also needs to be simple, cheap, safe and acceptable. Appropriate and timely treatment must be available, and adequate facilities are needed. Most important of all (but often overlooked), there must be some benefit to the person in having the abnormality detected at an earlier stage than would have otherwise been the case. This benefit may take the form of a better outcome (e.g. a greater chance of survival) or less unpleasant treatment (e.g. avoiding radical surgery).

TYPES OF SCREENING PROGRAMMES

There are two ways in which screening can be conducted: opportunistically and proactively. Opportunistic screening is illustrated by the measurement of blood pressure in any adult who consults a doctor or nurse for any reason. Since most people consult a health professional at some time every year, most of the population could be covered, with major health benefits in terms of reduced risk of stroke and heart disease. This approach has the obvious limitation of being suitable only when the test requires little technology.

Where more sophisticated methods are required, the screening procedure has to be organized in a proactive manner. Members of a target population are invited to attend for testing in a systematic programme that will cover the whole of that population over a defined period of time. One example is the National Breast Screening Programme, which sets out to offer breast screening to all women aged 50–64 years over a 3-year period. This type of screening requires an efficient system of delivery, including up-to-date information about the names and addresses of persons eligible for screening.

EVALUATION OF SCREENING PROCEDURES

There are several aspects of a screening procedure that require evaluation. The qualities of the test itself, as carried out in 'field' conditions, need to be carefully appraised. Its sensitivity and specificity should be ascertained amongst the kind of people to whom it will be offered. Its acceptability must be assessed; there is no point in setting up a screening procedure that will not be used, and what is acceptable in one culture or age group may not be in another. As far as possible, the procedure should be made a 'positive experience' so that people will return for repeat screening when the time comes.

It is particularly important to evaluate the screening procedure as a whole, asking such questions as: 'To what extent will people be better off if they are screened than if they are not?' 'How many people will actually be worse off (physically or psychologically) by being screened?' 'How much does it cost to save a single life or prevent some adverse event by screening?' The only satisfactory way of evaluating screening procedures is by means of RCTs, which will show the difference in outcomes (good and bad) brought about by screening. Such RCTs can take one of two forms. One method is to screen an appropriate population, and randomly divide those who are positive to the test into two groups, one of which is treated while the other is not. The outcome is then recorded in both groups, and the difference (if any) can be attributed to the screening procedure. This approach is ethically justifiable only if there is genuine uncertainty as to whether the treatment is beneficial for people who are positive to the test. If the screening test measures a continuous variable such as blood pressure, a 'positive test' is defined somewhat arbitrarily as a blood pressure above a certain level. A higher level of blood pressure also needs to be defined, above which it would not be ethically acceptable for treatment to be withheld. Between these two limits is the area of clinical uncertainty that can be investigated by an RCT. Another example of this type of evaluation is provided by the two primary prevention trials of statins already referred to, which recruited their subjects by means of screening programmes (Downs et al 1998, Shepherd et al 1995).

In some situations it is unethical to withhold treatment for anyone with a positive test – for example, if the test detects a qualitative abnormality indicative of early cancer. The appropriate method of conducting a trial is to randomize people to be screened or not to be screened. The outcome is then compared in the screened and unscreened groups. RCTs of breast cancer screening have taken this form.

The first approach is more sensitive, since the risk of the subjects who are randomized is much higher than in the second approach. It can therefore be conducted with a smaller number of people. There is, however, the issue of what should be done about people with borderline results. Would it be right to ignore a blood pressure that falls just below the cut-off for a 'positive' result, or should the person concerned be told about it and invited to return at a later date so that it can be treated if it crosses the line? In that case, the trial may not accurately reveal the effect of the screening procedure, since the control group is subject to some degree of intervention that would not have occurred in an unscreened population.

Whichever type of trial is used, it is important that it should be conducted at a stage well before the screening programme becomes widely available. Once a screening test is in general use it may be considered unethical to deprive anyone of its supposed benefits. Screening for cervical cancer was introduced without an RCT anywhere in the world, and it would now be impossible to evaluate cervical screening in this way.

In addition to the evaluation that should precede the widespread introduction of screening, it is also important to maintain some ongoing evaluation, since conditions may change since the original trials were conducted. Quality control of the tests and treatment must be built into the system. There should be some mechanism for detecting adverse effects (including anxiety) caused by the programme. It may become possible to distinguish between subgroups that are particularly likely to benefit from screening and subgroups that are particularly liable to be harmed by it. It is also desirable to see whether those most likely to benefit are in fact making use of the service; cervical screening has tended to be least used by those sections of the population who are at greatest risk of cervical cancer. The reasons for this imbalance need to be investigated and addressed.

CURRENT ISSUES

At any given time there will be some diseases for which a screening programme is feasible but has not yet been introduced. The UK National Screening Committee (2000) has recently made recommendations about screening for certain conditions. In some cases, the evidence does not seem to justify the introduction of a screening programme at present. For example, prostate cancer (a common and serious disease) can be detected at an early stage by the prostate-specific antigen (PSA) test, and treatment offers a better chance of cure when it is given early rather than late. But the PSA test is rather inaccurate and can needlessly lead to anxiety and unpleasant investigations; moreover, the disease often progresses so slowly in elderly men that it causes them no harm, whereas the treatment is traumatic and liable to have unpleasant side-effects (impotence and incontinence). This is an example of a screening process that, while technically effective, may do more harm than good.

Screening for abdominal aortic aneurysm is feasible and of potential benefit. An RCT funded by the Medical Research Council provides some evidence on which a decision can be taken as to whether a screening programme should be set up. The situation regarding ovarian cancer is uncertain where a 12-centre trial is in its early stages. Screening for diabetic retinopathy appears to offer real benefit, and proposals are currently being considered to set up an appropriate programme.

THE ROLE OF COMMUNITY NURSES

Community nurses can contribute to the success of screening programmes in several ways:

◆ undertaking opportunistic screening, e.g. measuring and recording blood pressure in patients they see for other reasons;

◆ screening high-risk groups, e.g. maintaining registers of patients at high risk of CHD and ensuring that their serum cholesterol has been measured;

◆ being able to answer questions that are raised by patients and members of the public, who expect a nurse to advise them about whether a screening procedure will be worthwhile and what will be involved.

CONCLUSION

All health professionals should be concerned to prevent disease and disability. Community nurses are particularly well placed for this purpose, since they deal with a wide range of people, including those whose risk of serious conditions can fairly easily be reduced. Opportunities arise to play a part in preventing disease, particularly by means of health education. It is important to be well informed about the current state of knowledge, since people may turn to a nurse for advice and explanation.

SUMMARY

◆ Nurses who work in the community are well placed to understand the population aspects of health and disease.

◆ Epidemiology has provided us with much of our understanding of the aetiology and natural history of disease.

◆ Epidemiological methods are easy to apply, particularly now that so much information in primary care is computerized.

◆ Preventing disease is part of the responsibility of all health professionals, especially those in primary healthcare teams. It operates at the population level and among high-risk individuals, and at all stages of disease.

◆ Screening is becoming increasingly important in disease prevention. It raises complex issues, and community-based nurses will be expected to provide information and advice to members of the public about these matters.

DISCUSSION POINTS

1. How would you reply to a young smoker who said 'My grandfather smoked like a chimney and lived to be 92'?

2. What advice would you give to a man aged 60 who is wondering whether to have a screening test for prostate cancer?

3. You are a practice nurse who runs an asthma clinic. Many of your patients believe that their symptoms are aggravated by the fumes emitted from a local factory. How could you investigate this problem?

4. How might you encourage people in a deprived urban area to eat more fruit?

REFERENCES

Barker DJP 1995 Fetal origins of coronary heart disease. British Medical Journal 311: 171–174

Blair H 1977 Natural history of childhood asthma: 20-year follow-up. Archives of Disease in Childhood 52: 613–619

Bridel J 1993 The epidemiology of pressure sores. Nursing Standard 7(42): 25–30

Bronnimann S, Burrows B 1986 A prospective study of the natural history of asthma: remission and relapse rates. Chest 90: 480–484

Burr ML 1993 Epidemiology of asthma. In: Burr ML (ed) Monographs in Allergy, vol 31: Epidemiology of Clinical Allergy. Karger, Basel, pp 80–102

Collins R, Peto R, MacMahon S, et al 1990 Blood pressure, stroke, and coronary heart disease. Part 2, short-term reductions in blood pressure: overview of randomised controlled trials in their epidemiological context. Lancet 335: 827–835

Cullum MN, Deek J, Fletcher A, et al 1995 The prevention and treatment of pressure sores: how effective are pressure-relieving interventions and risk assessment for the prevention and treatment of pressure sores? Effective Health Care 2(1): October 1995

Department of Health 2000 National Service Framework for Coronary Heart Disease. Modern Standards and Service Models. Department of Health, London

Dockery DW, Pope CA, Xu X, et al 1993 An association between air pollution and mortality in six U.S. cities. New England Journal of Medicine 329: 1753–1759

Doll R, Peto R, Wheatley K, Gray R, Sutherland I 1994 Mortality in relation to smoking: 40 years' observations on male British doctors. British Medical Journal 309: 901–911

Downs JR, Clearfield M, Weis S, et al 1998 Primary prevention of acute coronary events with lovastatin in men and women with average cholesterol levels. Journal of the American Medical Association 279: 1615–1622

Ebrahim S, Davey Smith G 1998 Health promotion for coronary heart disease: past, present and future. European Heart Journal 19: 1751–1757

Hooper L, Summerbell CD, Higgins JPT, et al 2001 Dietary fat intake and prevention of cardiovascular disease: systematic review. British Medical Journal 322: 757–763

Livingstone AE, Shaddick G, Grundy C, Elliott P 1996 Do people living near inner city main roads have more asthma needing treatment? Case-control study. British Medical Journal 312: 676–677

The Long-term Intervention with Pravastatin in Ischemic Heart disease (LIPID) Study Group 1998 New England Journal of Medicine 339: 1349–1357

Puska P, Nissenen A, Tuomilehto J, et al 1985 The community-based strategy to prevent coronary heart disease: conclusions from the ten years of the North Karelia Project. Annual Reviews of Public Health 6: 147–193

Rose G 1992 Strategies of prevention: the individual and the population. In: Marmot M, Elliott P (eds) Coronary Heart Disease Epidemiology: from Aetiology to Public Health. Oxford University Press, Oxford, pp 311–324

Sacks FM, Pfeffer MA, Moye LA, et al 1996 The effect of pravastatin on coronary events after myocardial infarction in patients with average cholesterol levels. New England Journal of Medicine 335: 1001–1009

Scandinavian Simvastatin Survival Study Group 1994 Randomised trial of cholesterol lowering in 4444 patients with coronary heart disease: the Scandinavian Simvastatin Survival Study (4S). Lancet 344: 1383–1389

Shepherd J, Cobbe SM, Ford I, et al 1995 Prevention of coronary heart disease with pravastatin in men with hypercholesterolemia. New England Journal of Medicine 333: 1301–1307

UK National Screening Committee 2000 Second Report of the UK National Screening Committee. Department of Health, Social Services & Public Safety, Northern Ireland; The National Assembly for Wales; The Scottish Executive. Department of Health, London

Winkleby MA, Feldman HA, Murray DM 1997 Joint analysis of three U.S. community intervention trials for reduction of cardiovascular disease risk. Journal of Clinical Epidemiology 50: 645–658

FURTHER READING

Beaglehole R, Bonita R, Kjellström T 1993 Basic epidemiology. World Health Organization, Geneva

This book gives a good general outline of epidemiology. It is well-written and easy to understand, with plenty of examples.

Department of Health 1993 Targeting practice: the contribution of nurses, midwives and health visitors. The health of the nation. Department of Health, London

This booklet covers a wide range of examples of ways in which community nurses can influence disease prevention.

Last JM 2001 A dictionary of epidemiology, 4th edition. International Epidemiological Association, Oxford

This is a reference book for epidemiological terminology.

National Screening Committee 1998 First report of the National Screening Committee. Health Departments of the United Kingdom

This report contains the first edition of The NSC Handbook of Population Screening Programmes; it gives a good outline of the principles of screening, including ethical and social issues. The Second Report (see References) updates these principles and deals with several specific screening procedures in more detail.

Perkins ER, Simnet I, Wright L 1999 Evidence-based health promotion. John Wiley and Sons, Chichester

This book deals with a wide range of topics in health promotion, many of which are relevant to community nurses. It covers theoretical and practical aspects.

6

Structural issues relating to poverty and health

H. Jefferson

INTRODUCTION

This chapter considers how the welfare system, and the NHS in particular, deals with the effects of poverty on the health of the public. This is done through the examination of key documents and reports, which have influenced policy decisions and service delivery. It seeks to identify the role Government has had in shaping policy direction; the structures that are proposed and those that have been developed, in order to deliver the policy agenda.

HOW POVERTY IS VIEWED IN HEALTHCARE POLICY

Traditionally, in terms of healthcare provision, poverty has equated to the need to reduce inequalities in health and to control disease. Public health policy has been driven by Marxist ideology (O'Brien & Penna 1998, Porter 1998); however, the ideologies of mainstream 'acute' welfare policy have changed over the past 20 years, while Marxism has been rejected. Public health policy has become marginalized and out of step with the current ideological thinking.

Factors such as socioeconomic and demographic trends, work patterns, disease patterns, epidemiological trends (CMO 1998, Fink et al 2001, WHO 1998), health risks (Giddens 1999), and the effects of globalization (Held 2000, Yeates 2001) have again brought to the fore the need to take public health seriously and to start developing

---

Box 6.1 The components of health inequalities

◆ Socioeconomic factors
◆ Gender
◆ Place of residence
◆ Ethnicity
◆ Access to the welfare system and services
◆ Education
◆ Employment
◆ Housing
◆ Social cohesion (exclusion)
◆ Disability.

This is manifested through, for example:

◆ unskilled labour (work force)
◆ racism
◆ exclusion
◆ fragmented families
◆ law and order and safety issues
◆ mental health needs
◆ child poverty.

---

clear, comprehensive and consistent strategies in health care to reduce health inequalities. With this is the need to demonstrate real achievement regarding the Health for All 2000 Alma-Ata Agreement (WHO 1978) through improvement in population health. We cannot continue to afford treating illness while ignoring illness prevention. Already the UK NHS has fallen from 18th place in the world to 24th (Boseley 2001). In addition to this, inequalities in health have not reduced in the past 40 years (CMO 1998) and the gap between rich and poor continues to increase (Shaw et al 2001).

Inequalities in health go far beyond the remit of the NHS and indeed tackling health inequalities requires comprehensive policy formation across government agencies if it is to have any chance of success. The recognition that policies that reduce poverty require government-level cross-departmental collaboration in development and implementation is relatively new, even if at the local level interagency collaboration in public health has been operating, ad hoc, for some time.

While the health service is required to tackle the components of health inequalities (Box 6.1) in terms of providing services to families and children and those with mental health problems and disabilities, it must also ensure that service provision is not disadvantageous in its delivery.

However, the NHS is itself responsible for perpetuating inequalities by employing some of the poorest-paid people in the country, adopting, if covertly, racist policies, and often putting people at risk (Acheson 1998). This means that for the NHS, reducing inequalities goes far beyond the need to review its clinical service configuration and delivery but must also include its internal employment and organizational policies.

STRUCTURAL ISSUES

The term 'structure' refers not only to the obvious physical construction and organization of services but also to the underlying patterns of thought, health need, behaviour and social organization that accompanies how the service is delivered. In the context of this chapter these structural issues are to be investigated through public health and NHS policy, policy direction, government and agency responsibilities as well as wider influences that effect service delivery. New configurations and delivery will in turn affect the role, function and development of community nursing.

HISTORICAL BACKGROUND

Concern about the public's health and the reduction of poverty is not a new phenomenon. It has been an issue for the church and state for many centuries either for moral reasons or for economic ones. Periodically crises have arisen such as war, disease, plague, high levels of death and morbidity, which have focused the minds of policy makers on the health needs of the population. The Public Health Act (1848) was passed as a direct result of campaigning to improve sanitation and since then a public health function has been part of the responsibility of those providing health and local authority services (Acheson 1988, Allsop 1995, Baggott 2000, Calman 1998, CMO 1998, Hamlin & Sheard 1998).

By the 1970s concerns were again beginning to grow about the still-increasing gulf between wealth and health even after 25 years of a national health service. This prompted the call for an inquiry, led by the Secretary of State for Social Services (Labour) into the nation's health.

THE NEW RIGHT AND PUBLIC HEALTH

THE BLACK REPORT

Black and his colleagues were asked to consider differences in health status among the social classes and identify the factors which might contribute to these differences. They were asked to analyse this material in order to identify possible causal relationships and to assess the implications for policy, including identifying what further research should be initiated. The review was started in 1977 and completed in 1980 and the findings showed that:

… the poorer health experience of lower occupational groups applied at all stages of life … The class gradient seemed to be greater than in some comparable countries … and was becoming more marked. During the twenty years up to the 1970s covered in the Black Report, the mortality rates for both men and women aged 35 years and over in occupational classes I and II had steadily diminished while those in IV and V changed very little or had deteriorated (Townsend et al 1992, p. 2).

In addition, those belonging to the manual classes did not use the health services as much as the other classes, yet they had more need of the healthcare system.

In terms of identifying the influencing factors, the Working Group concluded that the following socioeconomic factors were key:

◆ income
◆ work
◆ environment
◆ education
◆ housing
◆ transport.

All were found to affect health and all favoured the better off. These, however, largely remained outside national health policy.

The Working Group made 37 recommendations which concentrated on three broad policy areas: a) giving children a better start in life; b) encouraging good health through preventative and educational action; and c) reducing the risks of early death for those with disabilities. This was to be achieved through:

◆ improving the welfare infrastructure
◆ developing primary and community service delivery
◆ tackling the wider health inequalities through benefits, better working conditions and new schemes
◆ developing an integrated policy and delivery strategy
◆ re-allocating resources based on need
◆ improving GP services in areas of high ill-health
◆ ensuring Health and Social Services moved closer together in terms of integrated planning, joint funding and resource allocation and focusing on the development of community care.

Government responsibility was identified as improving public health through addressing the structural and environmental factors outside the control of individuals such as tobacco advertising and the need to reduce child poverty. This would require government commitment and coordination in relation to policy formation.

The report was submitted to the new (Conservative) government in 1980, but it proved unpopular, as it did not sit well with the New Right views on social responsibility. It was dismissed on financial and effectiveness grounds.

THE HEALTH DIVIDE

By the mid 1980s there was a need to update the picture. New dimensions of health, other than just social class and mortality, were being identified and measured. These new measures included 'quality of life' measurement and other indicators of wealth such as housing tenure, car ownership, employment status, gender and ethnic origin.

The *Health Divide* report found a lack of action on the *Black Report* recommendations by the

Government, however there was considerable activity locally and professionally, in terms of research into inequalities supported by health, local government, voluntary agencies, etc. 'Nevertheless, without a national commitment all this has, understandably, had piecemeal results.' (Townsend et al 1992, p. 17). The report also noted that, 'successive governments seem disinclined to accept investment in health as a necessary assumption of planning...' (ibid). In fact governments seem to see 'welfare expenditure ... as something different from economic growth and efficiency' (op. cit., p. 18), in other words they saw no detrimental (negative) relationship between ill-health and inequalities in health and the state of the economy. Therefore there was no perception of a causal link (in a negative direction) yet they could argue that economic growth must be a prerequisite for spending more on health and welfare. The Government refused to see the hidden costs to the economy of an unhealthy workforce.

The *Health Divide* did not confine its analysis to the UK only but looked at how we rated against other European healthcare systems. In taking a European perspective, Whitehead looked at complex issues such as economic crises and pollution as well as other welfare systems. Her findings were supported by reports from WHO which also showed widening inequalities in Europe in the 1980s. She highlighted the fact that in Britain we compounded our situation by our contradictory approach to policy development. On the one hand we were developing policies to promote public health but also developing other policies without thought for the impact that these might have on the health of the public.

Whitehead's work reinforced the message of Black and colleagues and strengthened the evidence that 'health inequalities between social groups are genuine and cannot be explained away as artefact...' (op. cit., p. 397). Also the 'evidence that socioeconomic circumstances have a major impact on health is now extremely strong...' (ibid).

In terms of policy Whitehead recommended that better indicators of social inequality were needed and improved measures of health to aid planning and evaluation of policies, along with increased recording and auditing of socioeconomic factors and improved resource allocation, access and quality of care to reduce *inequality in health* caused by *inequality in health care* (op. cit., p. 398). In terms of fair and equitable health services, the findings showed, for example, that there was still poor provision of services in deprived areas, where unskilled people used the GP more. This was compounded by inherent inequalities in the existing NHS reforms and resource allocation/reward systems as well as poor quality standards (see Chapter 4 for further discussion of quality and quality improvement).

The *Health Divide* attracted a wider audience than was expected but then it coincided with growing public concern over inequalities in health as shown in the Archbishop of Canterbury's Commission on Faith in the City, which came to similar conclusions. Although the report was criticised by the Government as being biased and Marxist, the findings were borne out by bodies such as the British Medical Association (BMA), the Faculty of Public Health Medicine (FPHM), the World Health Organization (WHO) and, perhaps most damning of all, by internal DoH reports.

THE REPORT OF THE COMMITTEE OF INQUIRY INTO THE FUTURE OF THE PUBLIC HEALTH FUNCTION (ACHESON REPORT – 1988)

Unlike the *Health Divide*, this was a government commissioned inquiry (Acheson 1988) established by the Secretary of State for Social Services in January 1986. The rationale for the inquiry was to consider the future development of public health medicine and to review the control of communicable diseases. Changes to these services would take place in line with the implementation of general management (Griffiths Report 1983). The inquiry was restricted in its focus, reviewing the work of the current clinical and related services, to establish how the public health function could be strengthened (Allsop 1995, Baggott 2000). The panel did not look directly at issues of poverty and health. Having defined public health as, 'the science and art of preventing disease, prolonging life and promoting health through organised efforts of society' (Acheson 1988, p. 1), the members concentrated on examining ways of improving the surveillance measures of population health through evaluation of existing health services and the encouragement of policy development which promoted and maintained health.

The inquiry noted that one of the problems undermining the roles of the public health doctors in the NHS was the confusion over the public health function of local authorities (LA's) and health authorities (HA's). Both had responsibilities for public health since 1948 but unlike the LA, the medical role had changed with each NHS restructuring and had been eroded over time. The LA role and responsibilities had been more constant, however there was significant overlap between the two bodies. In addition to this, they noted that the NHS had not concentrated on providing services which looked at lifestyle issues such as smoking, drinking and diet.

The Inquiry made 39 recommendations that sought to clarify the role, function, educational requirements, skills and title of doctors working in public health medicine; the organizational structures that would support the medical function and how these would inter-relate with LAs and also how communicable disease notification, monitoring and advice would be improved.

THE FIRST ATTEMPT AT A PUBLIC HEALTH STRATEGY

In 1992 the Government and Department of Health published their own internally promoted Public Health Strategy, stimulated by continued pressure to recognize the links between socioeconomic factors and ill-health and the need to incorporate public health into mainstream welfare ideology.

THE HEALTH OF THE NATION

The Health of the Nation: A Strategy for Health In England (HOTN) (DoH 1992) was a White Paper driven by the following ideas:

◆ a commitment, in the widest sense, to the pursuit of health

◆ NHS reform, adopting a strategic approach to health promotion and prevention
◆ responsibility for delivering the targets must lie primarily with individuals and families, not the Government.

It was also a late response to the Alma Alta declaration (WHO 1978) and the *Targets for Health for All* (WHO 1985) requirements, set out in the 1970s. However, unlike the WHO, *HOTN* failed to make allowance for inequalities in health and the effect of socioeconomic factors on health.

The strategy was almost immediately undermined by the fact that the behaviours required to reduce the incidence of illness were not addressed. For example, the incidence of CHD, strokes and lung cancer can be reduced by stopping smoking, however while local 'Smoke Stop' initiatives were set up, the Government refused to take policy action on banning smoking advertising. In fact, this reluctance to ban smoking advertising has remained with successive governments (DoH 2001d). In addition to this, the message on diet was not getting through and the consumption of alcohol was rising (CMO 1998, 2001b). Screening services for cancers, particularly breast cancer and cervical cancer were found to be patchy across the country. Some Trusts and HAs did not see the provision of screening programmes as a priority, seeing them as expensive for little gain. However there have been improvements in the current cancer strategy, which stemmed from the *HOTN*.

In the case of mental illness, a series of high-profile cases did not help public confidence regarding the impact of policy development (Utting 1994). Over sexual health, the control of gonorrhoea was in fact less of a problem than the incidence of chlamydia in young sexually active girls, yet this did not appear in the strategy. The strategy also failed to make inroads into teenage pregnancy rates and in the case of drugs, proved largely ineffective, because cultural issues such as attitudes to drug taking and use of recreational drugs were not addressed. Accident figures also did not reduce significantly (CMO 1998).

In 1998 an assessment of *The Health of the Nation* was undertaken (DoH 1998a). It was welcomed as the first central strategy for health improvement in England. However, it was deemed flawed both conceptually and operationally because it lacked cross-government, cross-agency and local support. Health authorities did not use it as a framework for their purchasing of services and it had little impact on Trust performance, particularly in the Acute Trusts. Local authorities saw it as dominated by medical conditions, which excluded them. It served only to emphasize the different agendas and cultures in the NHS and LAs and did nothing to bring them closer together. Finally there was a lack of guidance on how to interpret and operate the strategy locally and few incentives to do so. It was recommended that a new strategy be adopted which operated within a social, economic and environmental context and had a foundation built on collaboration.

THE ROLE OF PRIMARY CARE IN IMPROVING PUBLIC HEALTH

The development of primary care services has been addressed in a series of documents (DoH 1987, 1996a–d, Griffiths 1988), firstly in order to develop them in line with the internal market principles of the New Right and then as the means of operating the *HOTN* strategy through development of GP-run health promotion services. More recently, primary care has been developed as the main vehicle for the delivery of the New Labour healthcare agenda, strengthening the health promotion function initiated through *HOTN* while removing the internal market system (DoH 1997a,b, NHSE 1998a,b). Primary care now forms the backbone of NHS and public health delivery (DoH 1999e, 2000, 2001b, NHSE 1999a,b). This is to be further strengthened by the merging of health and social care (DoH 1997a, 1999b, 2001b, House of Commons 2000), through the proposed development of Care Trusts by 2003 (DoH 2001b). This will bring together not only health and social care policy but also joint service design and delivery particularly around the issue of Urban Regeneration Projects that can utilize the skills of social and voluntary organizations along with the NHS, to improve social conditions and reduce

poverty-related illnesses. These requirements are built into the function of Primary Care Trusts (PCTs) and Care Trusts and will be developed, monitored and measured through bodies and systems such as the Health Development Agency (HDA), the Modernizing Agency, CHI, the Performance Assessment Framework (PAF) and the National Service Frameworks (NSFs). PCTs and Care Trusts will therefore be the major structure for the delivery of the public health agenda and the merging of health and social care responsibilities will increasingly force the NHS to recognize and respond to the wider determinants of health. Indeed, if followed to its logical conclusion, these policy changes could shift the whole concept of what constitutes health care in the future.

THE NEW LABOUR GOVERNMENT

New Labour welfare policy is characterized by 'integrated care' (DoH 1997b, p. 1), collaboration, comprehensiveness, consistency, modernization and community-focused care, where services will be restructured to make primary care the gateway to healthcare delivery. It is to operate through a 'third way', positive welfare model (Giddens 1998) which is neither traditional left or right, but combines private and public sector service provision, while advocating social responsibility. Part of this responsibility is to tackle ill-health and inequality through ensuring that the NHS works 'locally with those who provide social care, housing, education, and employment' (DoH 1997b, p. 1) and to this end, the Government has taken on the role of developing a new NHS infrastructure to support and deliver this agenda.

New Labour welfare policy is also becoming increasingly characterized by confusion, inconsistency in policy decision-making and a lack of clarity over what the new NHS will look like at the end of the ten-year reform strategy (DoH 2000). In terms of poverty reduction, there is much rhetoric and, so far, no evidence of improvement. In fact the gap between the rich and poor continues to increase (Shaw et al 2001). Reform timescales and structures keep changing (DoH 2000, 2001b) and there is no clear sense of how, practically, health and social care structures integrate with other related areas such as education, housing, employment, etc. or how this transition is to be supported. Bits of detail have emerged as subsequent government documents have been published, but nowhere is this drawn together to provide a clear picture. The recently published Wanless Report (Wanless 2002) is an attempt to address this, however it is too early to know how acceptable this will prove with politicians and public. Outlined below are key documents and reports that seem to be shaping the public health agenda and outlining the main structures for delivery.

CMO ON THE STATE OF THE PUBLIC HEALTH 1997 (1998)

This is an annual report (CMO 1998) published by the Chief Medical Officer (CMO), however in that year it coincided with the retirement of the CMO and the 150th anniversary of the 1848 Public Health Act. Calman used this report to reflect on the success of public health policy over the last 150 years and to look to the future. He acknowledged that there had been improvements in areas of infant and postneonatal mortality, an improvement in life expectancy, improved cervical screening, an increase in immunization uptake and a continued fall in deaths from coronary heart disease (CHD), however there were also adverse trends such as the rise in obesity in adults and the rise in smokers between 11–15 years of age. Calman noted that despite the 'improvements in many key indicators of the health of the population, it remains of much concern that substantial inequalities in health persist: indeed, for some measures the gap between socio-economic groups has widened' (CMO 1998, p. 12). In fact:

Social class inequalities in death rates – as judged by the gradient in mortality between highest (I) and lowest (V) social classes – do not appear to have decreased over the past 40 years … (op. cit., p. 102)

This was a damning indictment of the successive failures of governments to get to grips with the real issues surrounding inequalities and prompted the incoming Government to act.

ACHESON REPORT (1998)

With the arrival of New Labour and the failure of the *HOTN* strategy to improve public health, Sir Donald Acheson was asked to undertake an independent review of inequalities in health in England in July 1997. The Report (Acheson 1998) made 39 recommendations covering socio-economic determinants of health, inequalities in health and inequalities in health related to gender and ethnicity. In terms of policy decisions to reduce inequalities in health, Acheson recommended that: (i) all policies likely to have an impact on health should be evaluated in terms of their impact on health inequalities (health impact assessments); (ii) high priority should be given to the health of families and children; and (iii) further steps should be taken to reduce inequalities and improve the living standards of the poor. Acheson also argued that future policies should be 'upstream' – i.e. wide ranging in their benefits (cross boundaries) and 'down stream' – narrower and more focused. He identified 12 areas for future policy development namely:

- poverty, income tax and benefits
- education
- employment
- housing and environment
- mobility
- transport and pollution
- nutrition and the Common Agricultural Policy
- mothers, children and families
- younger people and adults of working age
- ethnicity
- gender
- equity within the NHS.

The report was considered comprehensive and far reaching by public health specialists. It also identified the status of UK public health compared with other EU countries and raised the uncomfortable issue that the NHS contributes to inequalities and poverty. Despite the report being commissioned by the Government few of the Acheson recommendations appear directly in the NHS policy *Saving Lives: Our Healthier Nation* (DoH 1999a), which gave a confused and disappointing message in terms of the government view on the need for comprehensive and holistic welfare policy. The *Acheson Report* was overshadowed by the publication of *Saving Lives,* although most public health professionals felt that it offered the better strategy for improving population health. Although Acheson's findings were responded to and used to develop government policy, it was to be New Labour's second term before action became evident. Meanwhile *Saving Lives* was launched and amounted to a modification of *Health of the Nation* with the same built-in flaws.

SAVING LIVES: OUR HEALTHIER NATION (1999)

This White Paper (DoH 1999a) was published late due to a series of embarrassments, the most high profile being Bernie Ecclestone's contribution to Labour electoral funds and the refusal of the Government to ban tobacco advertising. Yet improving the NHS and public health had been a keystone in the New Labour Manifesto including the appointment of a Minister for Public Health. To reduce embarrassment, the White Paper was launched by the Prime Minister with cross-departmental signatory support. It was seen as the NHS part of an action plan for tackling inequalities in health, concentrating on four areas: cancer, coronary heart disease (CHD), mental illness and accidents while also, supposedly, recognizing that social, economic and environmental factors were important in affecting health. As with *The Health of the Nation, Saving Lives* was medically focused and target based. In order to operate the policy there would need to be structural improvements in the design and delivery of services through improved service partnerships, local developments, changing of professional roles, setting and improving standards of care and measuring overall service performance (DoH 1999b) (see Box 6.2). It would be realized by individuals improving their own health, being supported by their local communities working in conjunction with local organizations.

Improved health was to be community focused with the NHS being re-oriented 'to ensure for

---

Box 6.2 Structural Issues Identified – Saving Lives 1999

Achieved through:

◆ £21 million being identified for development
◆ tackling smoking
◆ integrating government and local government
◆ stressing that health improvements will be a key role for the NHS
◆ pressing for higher health standards (not just for the privileged).

Delivery:

◆ Healthy Citizens programmes
◆ NHS Direct
◆ Health Skills (help selves and others)
◆ Expert Patients (programme to help you manage your condition)
◆ joint partnerships with LA and NHS such as Health Action Zones (HAZ), Healthy Living Centres (DoH 1999f), etc.

Approach:

◆ HAs would focus on improving health
◆ PCG/Ts would have new responsibilities for public health
◆ The NHS and LA/local government would work together to improve community health.

---

the first time ever, health improvement will be integrated into local delivery of health care' (DoH 1999a, p. 3). This at least was a start to linking public health issues to the mainstream 'acute focused' policy documents (DoH 2000, 2001b), by acknowledging that some of the existing and developing structures already proposed would also serve to deliver the public health agenda. However, new and specific structures were also identified such as the setting up of the Health Development Agency and the Public Health Development Fund, as well as looking to improve public health information, promote research and to review changes needed in education and training to improve professional skills though the findings of a health audit.

Saving Lives was not without its critics. Duggan (1999) for example, noted a number of paradoxes: firstly, that *Saving Lives* establishes targets that focus exclusively on health trends and risks, rather than the social and cultural concerns that set the context within which healthy public policy is developed; secondly, the three-way 'health' partnership proposed between Government, communities and individuals fails to be convincing in terms of the partnership being one of equals; thirdly, that inequalities are seen as the major contextual challenge for healthy public policy, yet *Saving Lives* sets no overall targets for the reduction of poverty; and fourthly, that there is a failure to harness commitment because there is no analysis of the contribution to be made to the overall strategy by national and local agencies, in attempting to improve health. In addition, there was no coherent framework for planning and operating the partnerships seen to be so important for success.

REDUCING INEQUALITIES: AN ACTION REPORT (JUNE 1999)

This report (DoH 1999c) is the government response to Acheson's Inquiry. In this the Government acknowledged that the Acheson Inquiry helped to inform the White Paper, *Saving Lives*, but that the tackling of the 'root causes of ill-health are so varied, we cannot deal with them by focusing on "health" alone. We must tackle in the round all the things that make people ill. Therefore, in this report we set out the action to be taken across Government- and through partnerships between various local and regional organisations in England – to reduce health inequalities.' (op. cit., p. 3) and to 'tackle the *causes* of poverty and social exclusion not just alleviate the *symptoms*' (op. cit., p. 5). This will be achieved by focusing on creating a fairer society through building healthy communities (see Box 6.3).

Delivery and evaluation will be through the National Service Frameworks (NSFs) and the NHS Performance Assessment Framework. In addition to this there will be a review of NHS resource allocation to look at how avoidable health inequalities can be reduced. The NHS will review its employment procedures with the aim of ensuring it has a representative workforce and reduces incidents of racial harassment. Directors of Public Health will include, in their Annual Reports, an assessment of health needs and inequalities to support local agencies in taking action. Clinical quality will be monitored through NICE and clinical governance (see Chapter 4).

Box 6.3 Structural Issues Identified – Reducing Inequalities 1999

- ◆ Building Healthy Communities through New Deals for Communities, A Single Regeneration budget, use of HImPs, PCTs, HAZs, Healthy Living Centres, the New Opportunities Fund and the Social Exclusion Unit.
- ◆ Policies in turn will be subjected to health impact assessment (DoH 1999d).
- ◆ Education and Early years through Sure Start Programmes, improved educational standards, Healthy Schools Programme, Health Skills, Citizenship as part of National Curriculum and Personal, Social and Health Education, improved sport and physical activity.
- ◆ Employment – New Deals for Employment, healthy workplace initiative, Occupational Health strategy for England, family friendly policies.
- ◆ Housing – space and amenity standards, smoke alarms, new Housing Inspectorate, tackling fuel poverty and promoting home energy efficiency.
- ◆ Homeless people – cutting homeless sleepers by 2/3 by 2002 – Homeless Action Programme.
- ◆ Reducing crime.
- ◆ Transport and Mobility – reducing road accidents by 2010 through a comprehensive national road safety strategy, 5-year local transport plans, walking and cycling initiatives, concessionary fares, vehicle emissions, vehicle excise duty, speed policy.
- ◆ Public Health Issues such as nutrition, fluoridation, reducing tobacco and alcohol consumption, mental health issues with a focus on women, young men, ethnic minorities; teenage pregnancy – wanting to half rates of conception among under 18s in England by 2010 and setting a downward trend for under 16s.
- ◆ Appointing a Minister for PH, and setting up a Public Health Development Fund and Health Improvement Beacons.

This appears to be the first really serious attempt by the Government to identify a proposed infrastructure for improving public health, drawing on central NHS policy; yet much of this detail is not included in *Saving Lives*, therefore adding to the confusion of the Government's message on population health, and further undermining the official NHS strategy by showing how it was not integrated with other government policy. It also suggests that *Saving Lives* was policy developed 'on the hoof' by a new and inexperienced government and it is only now, some years into the government tenure that a considered approach to policy development was beginning to emerge.

GOVERNMENT RESPONSE TO THE SELECT COMMITTEE (PUBLIC HEALTH) (JULY 2001)

This document (DoH 2001c) sought to highlight and challenge the embedded confusion that was rapidly becoming the main characterization of the government approach to public health, in particular its organization and coordination of a public health strategy.

Ironically, the very energy and zeal which the Government brought to bear in the battle against inequalities has, to some extent, undermined their policy goals. Health Action Zones developed too slowly to spread all the money allocated to them in their first year. Each of the initiatives we have reviewed seems to have its own merits. The difficulties have arisen more from their quantity and lack of integration. We believe that the problems in implementing some of the public health initiatives to date are not necessarily short-term glitches that will be solved over a period of time. Instead, we believe these difficulties reflect more profound systemic and structural problems which relate to the lack of co-ordination between different Government Departments, statutory agencies, elected authorities and the voluntary sector... (op. cit., p. 9).

The Select Committee concluded that:

[The] ... interrelationship between several major strands of government policy needs to be made much clearer. For example, there are the neighbourhood renewal strategy, Sure Start, the various zone-based initiatives, as well as planning mechanisms such as HImPs, community plans, and regional development strategies. Each has its own goals and targets and measures of success. People need to be able to understand the relationships among them ... We endorse this view and recommend that the Government clarifies how the various strands of policy are connected to provide a more coherent policy framework. Otherwise there is a risk of serious failure in partnership working. Paradoxically, the danger of so many partnerships in existence is that a new order of fragmentation will occur (op. cit., p. 28).

The Select Committee recommended that the public health function remain with the Department of Health but with the proviso that if they did not take it more seriously then it might be transferred outside their control (op. cit., p. 42). This was a veiled threat to the Government and the Department of Health to get its house in order and an expectation that new guidance in the second term of government would properly address this if credibility were not to be further damaged.

CMO STRENGTHENING THE PUBLIC HEALTH FUNCTION (MARCH 2001)

This project (CMO 2001a) was started by the CMO, Kenneth Calman in 1997 and should have been published in 1998 along with *Saving Lives: Our Healthier Nation*, however the Government delayed publication. It was only with the pressure of public health groups and the House of Commons Select Committee Report (DoH 2001c) that it was published. However it was published with modifications in the details. It focused on 'public health in its broadest sense ...' (CMO 2001a, p. i) and on the need to develop a public health infrastructure 'to help change the social, economic, and environmental factors which lead to poor health. It helps address social exclusion, inequalities in health and provides support to local authorities and re-oriented NHS in ensuring that local partners focus on improving health as well as services quality ...' (ibid).

The first chapter outlines how this report is both a final report and links directly to the Government's 'health strategy and modernisation programme for health and local authority services' (op. cit., p. 1) as laid out in the *NHS Plan*. However there are caveats put upon the report by stating that proposals that would need structural and legislative changes were excluded from this report due to the timescales needed for legislative changes, the disruption that structural changes would cause and the fact that organizations would need to work in a 'joined up' fashion (ibid). While it is not entirely clear what point is being made here, it is implying that any changes are going to take time (beyond this term of office) and that whatever is developed will have to work within the existing structural constraints of the mainstream NHS and local authority organizations. Just why the above are excluded does not make sense, as dealing with legislation and structural change will be central to an effective public health strategy and implementation plan. Hence the nature of government intent remains unclear.

Many of the structures and organizational requirements already identified in the previous document (DoH 1999c) are restated (see Boxes 6.2 and 6.3), however additional and modified structures and detail are included (see Box 6.4) and it is recommended that this report be read in detail.

Box 6.4 Structural Issues Identified – Strengthening the Public Health Function (2001)

- A new Opportunities Fund (lifelong learning)
- Improved health surveillance
- Regional Public Health Observatories
- The Health Development Agency (supporting local public health forums)
- A new information strategy
- Disease registers
- Neighbourhood statistics service website
- A task force to focus on health inequality targets
- A national research and evidence-based strategy for public health (DoH 2001a)
- NHS Learning Network
- 'Beacons' to be identified in the NHS and local government
- National forum of non-government and public health organizations – access to expertise
- Regional Directors of Public Health (DoH 2001b)
- Co-terminous boundaries between health and local government
- Resourcing PH skills in the NHS and LA
- Voluntary sector involvement in identifying needs, supporting community participation and promoting 'self health care'
- Impact assessments to be carried out on fuel, poverty and the New Deal
- Local Strategic Partnerships (DoH 2001b)
- A need for a framework for public involvement
- Community development approaches in education and training
- Development of community plans – involving local people and run by local councils
- A National Strategy for Neighbourhood Renewal
- A Healthy Community Collaborative (Modernising Agency).

Delayed publication and the lack of hard, practical detail on how these changes were going to be achieved was unhelpful. The report was big on 'comfort phrases' but without much substance with which to affect levels of commitment. It stated a desire to strengthen and make tangible public involvement but there was no sense of how this would be supported or what infrastructure would be developed to ensure proper public involvement was possible. It was also not clear what power, authority or influence the non-governmental public health organizations national forum would have on policy direction and service structures, or what would happen if the Government priorities and the public priorities differed markedly. How this would be resolved was unclear, and given the experience of the past, it is quite likely that there will be differences in perspectives. It does not bode well for a practical public health strategy if there

is continued disagreement between policy and operation. In addition to this, it is difficult to conceptualize what this will look like in 5 or 10 years time as no 'picture' is offered, suggesting that perhaps the Government is not clear itself about what it wants the welfare system to look like in the future. What is clear is that to develop and maintain these structures will be costly and time consuming.

TACKLING INEQUALITIES (AUGUST 2001)

This consultation document (DoH 2001d) attempted once again to clarify the government and NHS approach to public health. It was a disappointing document in that it offered nothing new or different and neither did it deal with issues raised by the Select Committee, or other critics. It noted that the Government would look at banning smoking advertising but, once again, no timescale for action was offered. This continued to undermine the efficacy of the *Smoking Kills* White Paper (DoH 1998b) and to cause confusion over government commitment to make radical inroads into improving the nation's health.

The response to this consultation document was published in June 2002 (DoH 2002). The Government is required to be much clearer about its public health strategies on, for example, anti-poverty and neighbourhood renewal and its responsibilities to creating cross-government infrastructures to support service development and delivery. On 20 November 2002, Alan Milburn announced the end of tobacco advertising and offered financial incentives to PCTs to reduce smoking in the population. He also announced the establishment of a new Health Inequalities Unit and that the Prime Minister would be taking a personal lead on the 'cross cutting review on health inequalities' in this year's Spending Review. The impact of these measures on improving the population's health will be observed with interest and government commitment judged on the outcome.

CONCLUSION

There is no doubt that progress has been made to clarify public health priorities and to start creating a cross-government, cross-agency infrastructure to deal with these issues. However the reality is that progress has remained slow and issues raised by Black and Whitehead some 20 years ago still remain unresolved today. While local agencies work, piecemeal, to improve the welfare of their local communities, the Government continues to lag behind in its commitment to really tackle the underlying causes of poverty and ill-health. Given the recent internal tensions between government ministers over the future funding and resourcing of the NHS, coupled with increased dissatisfaction with the NHS performance, there is a real danger that progress on tackling poverty will stop, as attention once again returns to the problems of the 'acute' NHS sector. In addition to this, the involvement of the UK in the war against terrorism, post September 11 2001, means that attention has turned to foreign policy rather than internal domestic policy, letting the Government 'off the hook' by both deflecting criticism of internal policy decisions and reducing the momentum for progress on poverty reduction. Who knows what the implications of external world events will be, either through terrorism or threats from new diseases (CMO 2002) but, ironically, if it is bad enough, this could be what finally forces us to address the determinants of the nation's health.

SUMMARY

◆ Public health policy has been marginalized over the past 20 years with a rejection of Marxist policies, with a focus on the 'acute' welfare policy.

◆ Inequalities in health have not reduced in the last 40 years, indeed the gap between the rich and the poor is growing.

◆ The New Right in the form of successive Conservative governments and New Labour have failed to address issues raised by numerous governmental and nongovernmental reports, in particular failing to respond to the link between health and poverty. Although the current New Labour government have made more of an effort, at least to say the right things, delays and a lack of cohesive planning have resulted in disorganization and an unclear path ahead.

DISCUSSION POINTS

1. Given the structures that are being developed in the NHS, how do you think they can be utilized in practical terms to reduce poverty and health inequalities? What is the role of community nursing in this?

2. What influence do you see 'globalization' having on welfare policy in the UK and how might this affect the ability of the UK to improve health and reduce health inequalities?

3. What are the *real* incentives for the Government and the NHS to reduce poverty and health inequalities?

REFERENCES

Acheson D 1988 Public health in England – The report of the Committee of Inquiry into the future development of the Public Health Function (The Acheson Report). HMSO, London

Acheson D 1998 The independent inquiry into inequalities in health report. The Stationary Office, London

Allsop J 1995 Health policy and the NHS: Towards 2000, 2nd edition. Longman, London

Baggott R 2000 Public health – Policy and politics. Macmillan Press Ltd, Basingstoke

Boseley S 2001 NHS healthcare lags in world efficiency list. The Guardian, 10 August 2001, p. 8

Calman K 1998 The 1848 Public Health Act and its relevance to improving public health in England now. British Medical Journal 317: 596–598

Chief Medical Officer 1998 On the state of the public health 1997. Department of Health, London

Chief Medical Officer 2001a The report of the Chief Medical Officer's project to strengthen the public health function. Department of Health, London

Chief Medical Officer 2001b Annual report of the Chief Medical Officer 2001. Department of Health, 2001

Chief Medical Officer 2002 Getting ahead of the curve. Department of Health, London

Department of Health 1987 Promoting better health – The Government's programme for improving primary care. HMSO, London

Department of Health 1992 The health of the nation – A strategy for health in England. HMSO, London

Department of Health 1996a Primary care – The future. The Stationary Office, London

Department of Health 1996b Primary care: The future – Choice and opportunity. The Stationary Office, London

Department of Health 1996c The National Health Service: A service with ambitions. The Stationary Office, London

Department of Health 1996d Primary care: Delivering the future. The Stationary Office, London

Department of Health 1997a The NHS (Primary Care) Act. The Stationary Office, London

Department of Health 1997b The new NHS: Modern, dependable. The Stationary Office, London

Department of Health 1998a The health of the nation – a policy assessed. Two reports commissioned for the

Department of Health from the Universities of Leeds and Glamorgan and the London School of Hygiene and Tropical Medicine. The Stationary Office, London

Department of Health 1998b Smoking kills. The Stationary Office, London

Department of Health 1999a Saving lives: Our healthier nation. The Stationary Office, London

Department of Health 1999b The Health Act 1999. The Stationary Office, London

Department of Health 1999c Reducing health inequalities: An action report. DoH, London

Department of Health 1999d Health impact assessment – Report of a methodological seminar. Department of Health, London

Department of Health 1999e Primary care groups: Taking the next steps. HSC 1999/246: LAC (99) 40. Department of Health, London

Department of Health 1999f Healthy living centres. Department of Health, London

Department of Health 2000 The NHS plan: A plan for investment, a plan for reform. The Stationary Office, London

Department of Health 2001a A research and development strategy for public health. Department of Health, London

Department of Health 2001b Shifting the balance of power within the NHS: Securing delivery. Department of Health, London

Department of Health 2001c Government response to the House of Commons Select Committee on Health's second report on public health. Department of Health, London

Department of Health 2001d Tackling health inequalities: Consultation on a plan for delivery. Department of Health, London

Department of Health 2002 Tackling inequalities: The results of the consultation exercise. Department of Health, London

Duggan M 1999 Saving lives! Will it? UKPHA Report no 2, Autumn 1999

Fink J, Lewis G, Clarke J (eds) 2001 Rethinking European welfare. Sage Publications in association with The Open University, London

Giddens A 1998 The third way: The renewal of social democracy. Polity Press, Cambridge

Giddens A 1999 Runaway world – How globalisation is shaping our lives. Profile Books, London

Griffiths R 1983 NHS management inquiry Griffiths Report. DHSS, London

Griffiths R 1988 Community care: Agenda for action. HMSO, London

Hamlin C, Sheard S 1998 Revolutions in public health: 1848 and 1998? British Medical Journal 317: 587–591

Held D (ed) 2000 A globalizing world? Culture, economics, politics. Routledge/The Open University, London

House of Commons 2000 Health and Social Care Bill. London: The Stationary Office. Presented to the House of Commons on 20 December 2000

Milburn A 2002 Tackling health inequalities, improving public health. Alan Milburn's Speech to the Faculty of Public Health Medicine, Royal College of Obstetricians and Gynaecologists, 20 November 2002, London

NHSE 1998a The New NHS: Modern, dependable – Establishing primary care groups. HSC 1998/065, 9 April 1998

NHSE 1998b The new NHS: Modern, dependable – Primary care groups: Delivering the agenda. HSC 1998/228: LAC (98) 32. 8 December 1998

NHSE 1999a Working together: Human resources guidance and requirements for Primary Care Trusts. NHSE, Wetherby

NHSE 1999b Primary Care Trusts: Establishment, the probationary period and their functions. NHSE, Wetherby

O'Brien M, Penna S 1998 Theorising welfare. Sage Publications, London

Porter S 1998 Social theory and nursing practice. Macmillan, Basingstoke

Shaw M, Dorling D, Davey Smith G 2001 Did things get better for labour voters? Premature death rates and voting in the 1997 election. Townsend Centre for International Poverty Research, University of Bristol, Bristol. www.social-medicine.com/townrep2.html

Townsend P, Davidson N, Whitehead M (eds) 1992 Inequalities in health – The Black Report, 2nd edn. Penguin, London

Utting W 1994 Creating community care – Report of the Mental Health Foundation Inquiry into Community Care for People with Severe Mental Illness. The Mental Health Foundation, London

Wanless D 2002 Securing our future health: Taking a long-term view (final report). The Public Enquiry Unit, HM Treasury, London

World Health Organisation 1978 Primary health care: Report of the International Conference on Primary Care. WHO, Alma-Alta, USSR, Geneva

World Health Organisation 1985 Targets for health for all. Copenhagen, WHO Regional Office for Europe

World Health Organisation 1998 Health 21 – An introduction to the health for all policy framework for the WHO European Region. Copenhagen, WHO Regional Office for Europe

Yeates N 2001 Globalization and social policy. Sage Publications, London

FURTHER READING

Baggott R 2000 Public health – Policy and politics. Macmillan Press Ltd, Basingstoke

This book provides a useful background into the subject of public health policy, giving a historical and contextual view as well as considering the public health issues of today.

Chief Medical Officer 2001 The report of the Chief Medical Officer's project to strengthen the public health function. DoH, London

This is an informative current Government supported key document on Public Health that attempts to identify how the current structures being developed by the NHS will support the reduction of poverty and health inequalities.

Yeates N 2001 Globalization and social policy. Sage Publications, London

This is a readable book, which provides a useful introduction into the world and language of 'globalization' and examines the effect that this will have for nation states' welfare policy.

Sontag S 1991 Illness as a metaphor and AIDS and its metaphors. Penguin, London

Both these essays examine the use of metaphors in health and the mythologies surrounding disease such as TB, cancer and AIDS. These metaphors have coloured how we describe, talk about and how we rationalize disease, including associating disease with personal blame. These myths and metaphors still influence our decisions about welfare priorities.

7

Frameworks for health improvement

E. Gould

INTRODUCTION

How does the concept of achieving health improvement and delivering health gain affect the way health professionals practice? Moving from an individual to a collective focus, how can we use communities as a frame of reference? This chapter aims to clarify the prerequisites for achieving health improvement particularly in a community setting.

Firstly, it is important to know where you are starting from and in order to do that it is necessary to agree on a definition of health and to establish the current health status of the population served. In addition to this, information is needed about the availability of local resources to meet health problems and how the community itself perceives its own health needs.

Secondly, agreement is needed about what improvements in health your community nursing service, or your primary care nursing team is trying to achieve, given the key local determinants of health. From a thorough understanding of the starting point, goals or targets for improving health should emerge, which are appropriate, measurable and achievable (see Chapter 16 for an interesting examination of professional leadership and the management of change).

Thirdly, options need to be discussed concerning how to get from the starting point to the destination with reference to the most effective use of scarce community nursing resources. The 'route' taken will depend upon the availability of strategies known to be effective together with their cost, their social and clinical acceptability, and their practical feasibility. Along the route there will be challenges to overcome such as the lack of evaluation of many healthcare interventions; the difficulties of defining relevant outcomes; the need for multiagency collaboration and for monitoring progress and highlighting good practice. Each of these elements is a complex area of study in its own right. As a practitioner the key to achieving health gain is to remain constantly critical of what you do, why and how you do it, and questioning whether there are more effective ways of maximizing health benefit.

Working with individuals is one thing, working with collectivities in a community framework is quite another. The skills are not necessarily interchangeable (Gould 1998) and community nurses should be mindful that the approaches they may use with individuals can actually be counterproductive when working alongside communities. Here the emphasis must be on subsidiarity, a concept outlined in this chapter.

WHAT DO WE MEAN BY HEALTH IMPROVEMENT?

THE CONCEPT OF HEALTH GAIN

Fashions in the vocabulary of health services come and go. Each major reform and reorganization has brought with it new vocabulary. In the UK, the NHS reforms of 1998 (DoH 1998) brought the phrase 'health improvement' to the fore. Each health authority was required to produce, in partnership with service providers and with local authorities, a Health Improvement Programme (HIP). This would be an overarching service plan to address the health needs of the population and achieve health gain. Health improvement, health gain: a different vocabulary but to all intents and purposes, the same concept.

The expression 'health gain' appears to have originated in a strategy for improving the health of the people of Wales (Welsh Office 1989). It was cited in that strategy as being the key criterion for judging the effectiveness of a health service and

found increasing popularity in other health service documents (DoH 1991). It ˌ ˌ ˌ ˌ ˌu currency in the UK at a time of extensive organizational change (DoH 1989). This included the introduction of an internal market whereby, as the guiding principle, those who manage services (the providers) competed to contract services with those who commission them (the purchasers). Whilst these changes have themselves been overtaken by new reforms, other drivers such as efficiency, cost-control, accountability have remained.

In 1948 with the introduction of the NHS, Aneurin Bevan said that his role as a politician was:

… To give you all the facilities, apparatus and help I can and then leave you as professional men and women to use your own skill and judgment without hindrance … (Bevan 1975)

This early faith in subjective clinical judgement has given way to an ever-pressing need for providers of health services to justify how they make use of resources in terms of both effectiveness and efficiency. That is to say doing the right things (clinically effective things) in the right way (cost-effectively using resources). The term 'health gain' has largely become synonymous with effectiveness. Is an intervention effective in advancing and maximizing the health potential of an individual? Is it effective in raising the overall health of a population? Health gain is fundamentally about productivity in relation to health care, resulting in a better outcome than would have been achieved without the intervention (See Chapter 26 for a more detailed discussion of 'value for money'). This may be in terms of reducing the risk of mortality, i.e. the recipient of the service lives longer, and/or reducing the severity or duration of morbidity, i.e. the quality of life of the recipient is improved.

The slogan which exhorts health services to 'Add years to life and life to years' may seem straightforward enough but actually conceals many complex issues. Health gain is a vague term in which many other concepts overlap. As Hunter (1993) points out:

Health gain is something of a catchall notion insofar as it embraces a number of issues and initiatives that are derived, sometimes loosely, from the National

Health Service (NHS) reform agenda. Developments in needs assessments, in health outcomes, in listening to local people, in health services research and development programmes, and in articulating a health strategy, all in one way or another flow from and impact upon health gain.

MEASURING HEALTH STATUS

Measuring improvements in health status itself implies an underlying agreement about the nature of health (Bowling 1997). However, as Seedhouse (1986) has pointed out, health is not a word with a single uncontroversial meaning. Negative definitions of health relate to the absence of disease or illness, and health problems as medical problems. Traditional indicators of negative health status include measures of mortality, disease incidence and sickness data. This may still be the most appropriate way in which to measure the health status of severely compromised populations where many of the basic prerequisites for health, such as peace, shelter, food, education, income, are absent. But in less extreme situations, measurement of health status requires an underlying concept of health which is positive, as in the original World Health Organization definition – 'A state of complete physical, mental and social wellbeing, and not merely the absence of disease or infirmity'. Whilst this may be challenged as an unachievable ideal, it set health into a broad context, moving away from a wholly medical paradigm. The need to see health in a social, economic, cultural and environmental context can be considered central to the concept of health gain. Seedhouse (1986) has suggested that amidst all the various theories and conflicting approaches to defining health, a significant common factor can be found:

All theories of health and all approaches designed to increase health are intended to advise against or prevent the creation of, or to remove, obstacles to the achievement of human potential.

By this token, achieving health gain is about *addition,* the adding of years to life and life to years but it can also be seen as a *subtraction,* breaking down the barriers to improved health status.

INTRODUCING THE BROADER PERSPECTIVE: DETERMINANTS OF HEALTH AND THE NEW PUBLIC HEALTH

Seeing health in a social, cultural, economic and environmental context, influenced by multiple determinants, is central to the concept of health gain. The determinants of health are many and varied and there is still much to understand about the ways in which these determinants interact. The influences of age, sex and heredity combine with factors relating to individual lifestyles which become embedded in individual social circumstances, living and working conditions. These in turn sit within the broader context of the socioeconomic, cultural and environmental conditions of society as a whole.

Given these varied determinants and their interrelationship, it should be apparent that initiatives to improve health cannot be considered as the exclusive territory of health professionals. The concept of a multiagency approach to health protection and improvement was termed the *New Public Health* (Ashton & Seymour 1988). A decade later this approach had become part of establishment thinking. Partnership working, interagency collaboration, health alliances are a political as well as a strategic and operational necessity. Consider, for example, the inputs that may contribute to road traffic accidents and the benefits to health gain which could result from changes in habits or policies, with consequent reduction in accidents:

♦ *Individual*: Stress; alcohol and drug abuse; the use of mobile telephones; driving experience.
♦ *Socioeconomic*: Resources for safety measure implementation; traffic engineering; vehicle requirements; transport policies.
♦ *Cultural*: Attitudes toward: alcohol use/driving; legal system/penalties; seat belt legislation.
♦ *Ecosystem*: Terrain; climate; population densities.

This multifactorial approach inevitably challenges the centrality of health care in determining health status. McKeown and Lowe (1966) suggested that changes in the health status of the British population during the second half of the 19th century and early part of the 20th century were largely due to rising incomes and material advances: better food, housing, education as opposed to the effects of medical discoveries. Although their views have been challenged, there remains this recognition (Hunter 1993) that health status is not the result of health care alone but that other policy fields and services may be more important and instrumental in achieving certain aspects of health gain (see Chapter 6 for more detailed discussion of the health impact of social and contextual factors).

PLANNING FOR HEALTH IMPROVEMENT

How can we plan for health improvement given its multifactorial nature?

KNOWING THE STARTING POINT

Health needs assessment

The need to undertake epidemiological assessments in order to inform both short-term and strategic health planning is not something new. Prior to the reorganization of the NHS in 1974, Local Authority Medical Officers of Health had a statutory obligation to produce annual Public Health reports describing the health profile of the local population, analysing contributory factors and making recommendations for disease prevention and health promotion. These were largely discontinued after 1974 although following the Black Report (Townsend et al 1988) there was a revival of interest in local health problems which linked social and economic conditions with health status. The Annual Report of the Director of Public Health Medicine on the state of public health in a particular region or district was reinstated in 1988. The completion of a community health profile has been a requirement of post-basic community nursing courses, while every medical general

practice is required to submit an annual report of the practice population together with performance data, albeit using a disease-orientated approach. It would however be a waste of resources for every community nurse to complete a local profile when the critical issue is agreement about what is needed and why, and finding out what is already available.

There are a number of guidelines available on how to compile a health profile (Twinn et al 1990) but there is no universal prescription of exactly what information needs to be included; that will depend on the precise aim of the profile. Pickin and St Leger (1993) provide a useful guide to the sources of demographic and health data one could include in a comprehensive assessment of health status. Others such as Burton (1993) use a definition of community profiling that is a more general description of the social, environmental and economic aspects of a given area. Broadly speaking, the measurement of health status identifies health problems in a community and requires information on:

◆ Demography
  – age/gender distribution
  – ethnic groupings
  – household/family type.
◆ Disease patterns
  – mortality measures – death rates: crude and age specific
  – summary mortality statistics – standardized mortality ratios; life expectation
  – morbidity – short-term self-limiting illness to long-term chronic disease.
◆ Determinants of health (modifiers)
  – socioeconomic factors – e.g. unemployment, housing, transport
  – environmental factors – e.g. atmospheric pollution
  – ethnic factors – e.g. the racial effects on disease prevalence of sickle cell anaemia in those of Afro-Caribbean origin
  – cultural factors – e.g. religious beliefs within a community.

There are ways in which a profiled population may have specific characteristics of interest to specialist health services. For example, women who have undergone breast surgery, or individuals who have continence needs. The principles are the same in that 'hard' data are needed for planning – quantified information about the structure and characteristics of the group, as well as 'soft' data that may be concerned with group perceptions of their needs and priorities.

Measurement of health status can be part of the wider process of health needs assessment, a process given prominence following the introduction of the NHS reforms (DoH 1989). Pickin and St Leger (1993) describe this process as one of exploring the relationship between health problems in a community and the resources available to address those problems in order to achieve a desired outcome. There are a number of needs assessment methodologies representing both medical and socioeconomic models (Frankel 1991, Stevens & Raferty 1991). The life-cycle framework starts with a population and looks at the needs of that population as it passes through life stages (Pickin & St Leger 1993); a locality approach divides a population into geographical areas. Another approach is to use a framework of predetermined health gain targets (Hamilton-Kirkwood & Parry-Langdon 1993).

The underlying reason for any health needs assessment is the need to plan how best to match available resources to existing problems in the most effective way, agreeing priorities and setting some short- to medium-term objectives – and this, after all, is something practitioners do every day!

KNOWING WHERE YOU WANT TO BE

Targeting

Determining the starting point of our 'journey' to achieve health improvement requires the incorporation of health needs assessment into a current profile of health status – but this is not without its complexities. Agreeing on appropriate goals, which are measurable, acceptable and achievable both to the community and to those who provide services, is the next step. Increasingly the process for this has been the setting and monitoring of targets. In 1985 for example, the World Health Organization produced its strategy based on the overall aim of *Health for All* by the year 2000

(WHO 1985), a goal which it had adopted at the 34th World Health Assembly in 1979. This strategy took the form of 38 specific targets with an emphasis on health promotion and disease prevention. Since then targets have been used as a focus in many strategic documents (DoH 1991, Welsh Health Planning Forum 1991a, 1991b).

Harvey (1992) assesses the arguments for and against target setting which may be summarized as follows:

◆ Arguments for targets
  – Targets are quantified indicators of achievement or failure.
  – Targets inspire action and a sense of purpose.
  – Targets stimulate debate and highlight the nature of major health problems in a population.
  – Targets encourage rational purchasing of health services.
◆ Arguments against targets
  – Targets overemphasize the destination at the expense of how to get there.
  – Targets encourage guesswork.
  – Targets overemphasize health issues which are readily measurable at the expense of equally significant issues which are measurable only with difficulty.
  – Targets can be overoptimistic and lead to distortion.
  – Targets based on secular trends ('We'll get there even if we do nothing!') lead to complacency.

There are everyday circumstances where individual practitioners develop their own targets, but without some agreed service goals the value of the community nursing contribution can be lost. Agreeing and setting goals which are appropriate to local health status and needs, which are acceptable to the community and make reference to locally agreed priorities, can make it easier to agree a mechanism for monitoring progress. But to take things a step further, communities themselves need to be involved in the target setting: who better than the recipients of an intervention to judge its effectiveness against targets they themselves have set? In reality, targets are often imposed from without, by a central agency responsible for strategy or for funding. A major part of this debate must be the extent to which communities have health 'done' to them, passive recipients and consumers and not active coproducers of their own health.

CHOOSING A ROUTE

Generally speaking there are two healthcare strategies for achieving health gain: preventive strategies and therapeutic strategies. Preventive strategies aim to improve health through action on lifestyles and environments and include the implementation of screening services and immunization programmes. Therapeutic and rehabilitative strategies aim to provide services to meet existing health deficits. The type of strategy that is employed will depend on the health gain you are trying to achieve, but all strategies will present challenges relating to:

◆ the need to move from input to outcome measures
◆ attribution and the need for multiagency collaboration recognizing that improvements in health do not depend on health services alone
◆ benchmarking – the need to obtain baseline data and to monitor practice and processes.

Moving from input to outcome measures

The focus on health gain has moved the emphasis on the evaluation of health services from service inputs (the use of resources) and throughput (activities or processes of care) (Beck et al 1992) to outcome measures. Was the outcome worthwhile: did the intervention achieve what it was intended to achieve: overall did the intervention do more good than harm? However, the linking of health gain with performance management has, to a certain extent, denied the importance and quality of the processes involved. In health care (and particularly in nursing care) we cannot separate process and outcome into distinct compartments: the process is embedded in the outcome.

The evaluation of interventions in terms of their outcome is difficult to perform for several reasons

and the complexity of outcome measurement is well documented (Beck et al 1992, Holland 1983). Long et al (1992, 1993), for example, describe the serious practical difficulties in measuring the outcomes of some types of service:

◆ Those with 'low level effects' – consultations without clinical interventions. This is a feature of many community nursing contacts where the use of interpersonal skills to support clients is often difficult to evaluate.
◆ Those where the start and end of a treatment or intervention are unclear, for example in rehabilitation programmes.
◆ Those where several interventions are being conducted simultaneously.
◆ Those where many variables are intersecting over the longer term. This is often the case in health promotion activity where it may be virtually impossible to demonstrate a causal link between a health-promoting intervention and a specific outcome.

Clark and Henderson (1983, p. 274) have described the difficulty in attributing an outcome to a particular intervention in the field of preventive health where a positive intervention aims for a negative outcome by saying that:

It is logically impossible to prove causation for an event which did not happen; the best one can do is to replace proof by an estimate of probability.

Immunization of a child against polio should for example prevent it from contracting the disease but there are intervening variables such as organism virulence and aspects of individual and community susceptibility that are also likely to influence the probability of infection.

Establishing evidence of causal associations between an intervention and an outcome is important if we are to decide which interventions are likely to achieve health improvement and which are not. However, there is an acknowledged lack of research-based evidence to support many healthcare interventions which have become part of accepted health services provision (Cochrane 1972). For evaluation to have scientific rigour it requires the use of research methods which have the following approximate hierarchy for reducing bias:

◆ clinical impressions
◆ cases/case-series without formal controls
◆ studies with historical controls
◆ case–control studies
◆ nonrandomized concurrent controls
◆ randomized controls.

This positivist approach dominates in the natural sciences including epidemiology. But where does it leave us in terms of evaluating the outcomes from community interventions with a predomination of human interactions? Adamson et al (2001, p. 26) in their review of best practice in community regeneration write:

Judgements of the effectiveness of community based strategies are notoriously difficult (Breitenbach 1997), especially when framed within the quantative approaches required by the majority of funding agencies.

They go on to make the following points:

◆ Monitoring and evaluation techniques must be participative and directly involve the community in measuring and determining the level of change.

◆ Monitoring and evaluation must aim to balance the quantitative indicators conventionally required for public accountability with qualitative indicators which are meaningful to the community and demonstrate change in the daily experience of life in deprived communities.

◆ Monitoring and evaluation should set out a number of clear and accessible 'benchmarks' which measure the quality of life in a community and which should provide a standard to which all communities aspire to (ibid, p. 27).

Interagency collaboration

The integrating, synthesizing focus of health gain may constitute its chief appeal for those anxious to mobilize healthy alliances which deliberately seek to blur professional and organisational boundaries (Hunter 1993, p. 103).

A focus on health gain and health improvement has changed the tone of policy documents and reframed organizational approaches to service

delivery. Legislation has given the financial flexibility to introduce pooled budgets and funding which can only be accessed through a partnership approach (e.g. Sure Start). However, collaboration at a policy level is outside the influence of most individual practitioners: their everyday work involves multiagency working at a practical teamwork level. But here too the collaborative approach is not without its difficulties. Issues such as the following can mean that the meeting of client/community needs is subordinated to the assertion of professionalism:

◆ interprofessional rivalry
◆ authority/power differentials
◆ conflicting agendas
◆ differing priorities
◆ role ambiguity
◆ differing resource inputs.

McMurray (1993) for instance asks:

What mechanisms exist in the community to promote collaboration between health care providers, the education, the environment, industry and housing sectors? Are community-wide concerns represented by the different sectors on committees and task forces? What are the gaps in efforts across the sectors?

The need to share information, agree on divisions of labour, be clear about core competencies and ensure policies have a common aim, are the basic requirements of multiagency collaboration on an everyday level. In this way health gain targets may be seen as an appropriate way of identifying goals and providing the starting point to agreeing the activities and processes likely to achieve desirable outcomes.

Networks or hierarchies?

How do we deliver health improvement when the players involved are so distributed across organizations and geographical locations? Once the concept of health gain is accepted, it is quite clear that the old ways of managing through hierarchies and recognized chains of command do not have the flexibility to deliver complex care arrangements. Partnership working means that new approaches are needed.

Where colocation of partners is possible, the approach should be one of integrated teams (Elwyn & Smail 1998, Ovretveit 1993). At a strategic level in situations of both complex demand and supply, fully networked organizations have proven advantages over hierarchies (Jones et al 1997). Developments in communications and information technology will have a marked effect on the coordination of care in distributed environments: this means that practitioners in health and social care may well find themselves working in virtual organizations (Hedberg et al 1997).

WHY CHOOSE A COMMUNITY FRAMEWORK?

CURRENT THINKING ON HEALTH INEQUALITIES

As mentioned above, a key feature of health policy development in recent years has been the need to deliver health improvement/health gain. In parallel with this has been concern over the growing health divide and the need for health improvements which reduce the differentials in health status between social classes. These differentials in health status indicate that some groups enjoy substantially better health and longer life expectancies than others (Benezeval et al 1995) and that in almost all developed societies, people lower down the social scale can have death rates two to four times higher than those nearer the top (Wilkinson 1996). In the UK the Government has made the reduction of inequalities in health a duty of public agencies at all levels and in all sectors (Whitehead et al 2000). The implications warrant brief discussion if we are to consider the community perspective in relation to health improvement.

The 'Black Report' (DHSS 1980) proposed a typology which has become a starting point for many subsequent considerations of health inequalities. Four categories of explanation were put forward: artefact, social selection, behavioural/cultural, and materialist. Post-Black, researchers have explored the issues of, for instance, social capital (Kawechi et al 1997, Kunitz 2001) and identity (Karlsen & Nazroo 2000) as determinants of health.

Behavioural and cultural explanations behind health inequalities have attracted much interest. There is no dispute that health-damaging behaviours contribute to poor health outcomes: during the 1980s for example, the focus on the individual behavioural explanation of health inequalities resulted in a UK policy emphasis on personal health education. This approach gave little recognition to the fact that individual behaviours are conditioned by and embedded in the sociocultural context. Hence the lack of success in achieving behaviour change in disadvantaged groups in relation to health behaviours. To put it bluntly, as those in the higher socioeconomic groups take up health promoting-behaviours, those in the lower socioeconomic groups do not, resulting in a further increase in the health divide. In addition to influencing health-related behaviours, material and social circumstances impact directly on health status. At a fundamental level poverty restricts the capacity to purchase sound housing or good food. These material determinants of health are widely acknowledged.

However, there is increasing recognition, as Bartley et al (2000) point out, that income alone will not explain social differences in leisure preferences. These leisure and lifestyle preferences involve behaviours that impact on health through exercise, nutrition, substance misuse and so on. Wilkinson (1996) suggests that part of the association between people's material circumstances and their health appears as a relationship between relative income, or social position and health. Above a certain level of average income, it is not the amount of income but the way it is distributed which matters. Marmot's classic exploration of health inequalities amongst British civil servants (Marmot et al 1991, Marmot & Davey Smith 1997) suggested the significance of psychosocial working conditions and showed that position in the office hierarchy correlated strongly with mortality risk.

It becomes clear, if health status reflects a combination of complex interactions between factors at the individual and collective level, why a community approach to health improvement has become so much favoured. But first we need to think about what is meant by the term 'community'.

TOWARDS A DEFINITION OF COMMUNITY

It has been pointed out that whilst a weakness of discourses on community is the largely uncritical way in which the term is used, at the same time it is the very imprecision of community which gives it 'both its power and its appeal' (Labonte 1998). Geographical communities based on a locality or neighbourhood; a demographic group, e.g. older people; communities of identity – a leisure pursuit for example; institutional communities of the school or the workplace.

As mentioned above, the focus on the individual behavioural explanation of health inequalities resulted in a UK policy emphasis on personal health education during the 1980s. The disease prevention approach, smoking cessation, exercise and 'healthy eating' continued to predominate with its emphasis on individual responsibility. This is not to say that this work has been confined to the one-to-one encounter and health promoters have used social marketing, health fairs, school-based programmes, group work as ways of communicating health behaviour messages. In that sense, a community becomes the vehicle or the medium through which health promoters deliver specific interventions. This work has its place but this approach can perpetuate a victim-blaming culture with further alienation and disempowerment of already demoralized communities. The community development approach – and there is no single theory of community development – is fundamentally about improving the capacity of collectives to address their social, economic and political needs; many of which, as already outlined, have an impact on health status. A helpful model of community development practice is to be found again in the work of Labonte (1998) who identifies key characteristics of each strategic 'sphere' of practice from personal care, through the support of group development to community organizing, coalition building and advocacy to political action. Practitioners may work in all these spheres at the same time or concentrate their efforts in one: what matters is that they bring the appropriate skills to each sphere of work. Community nurses accustomed to one-to-one interactions will find that capacity building is likely to require a different set of professional tools.

INVOLVING COMMUNITIES

Communities and the individuals within them are not just the passive recipients of health care; the need to involve the users of health services in decisions about those services has been recognized as a fundamental principle of primary health care (See Chapter 4 for further discussion of this quality issue). The Health for All by the year 2000 philosophy (WHO 1981) put the community at the centre of health systems, defining need, setting priorities, planning and evaluating services.

During the late 1960s and early 1970s, community participation was promoted in the developing world (Conyers 1982) as a way of expanding accessibility to health services without necessarily increasing the costs. It arose from the failure of existing health services to provide adequate care at realistic cost and the increasing realization that improved health status was often linked to environmental, social and cultural issues. These could be better dealt with by communities themselves rather than by a narrowly defined health sector. Participation by individuals and communities was suggested as a process of consciousness-raising and empowerment, in the belief that power gravitates to those who solve problems (Freire 1972).

Community participation is the logical conclusion to involving people in health service planning; in the context of the UK NHS this involvement is less extensive. It has been argued (Ong et al 1991) that despite the fact that responsiveness to local views is a theme in the 'modernization' of the NHS, clients/patients/communities are more likely to be seen simply as consumers of health services. Their views are sought in terms of their satisfaction with the care provided rather than as contributors to service development. Efforts to assess local perspectives through traditional patient-satisfaction surveys have also been questioned (Dixon 1993) and increasingly a variety of qualitative sociological research methods are now being used to involve local people in service planning decisions (Popay & Williams 1993). Systematic research strategies such as Rapid

Appraisal (Ong et al 1991) bring together individual research techniques in attempts to understand how people perceive their health needs. Such perceptions are based on underlying value systems which may be at variance with the values systems of those who provide the services. Local communities have been shown, for instance, to have different priorities from those of providers (Ruffing-Rahal 1987) in so far as their perceived health needs are concerned.

Whilst there are sound democratic and moral reasons for involving communities in the decision-making process, the process itself is not straightforward. Hunter (1993) asks whose values should count – those of clinicians, politicians, managers or the public? An agreed value system and a correlation, or at least a compromise between the perspectives of the community and the providers, is essential if a health gain strategy is to be acceptable and workable.

ON SUBSIDIARITY AND EMPOWERMENT

The changed political climate and the emphasis on partnership have increasingly seen policies premised on the empowerment of individuals as productive members of their own communities. These policies are informed by the growing body of research concerning social position, social capital, self-determination and their effects on health status. '*Sure Start*' aims, for example, through interventions directed at preschool children and their parents, to increase the self-determination of individuals from disadvantaged homes.

'*Health Action Zones*' (Powell & Moon 2001) and '*People in Communities*' (c.f. Adamson et al 2001) use the language of empowerment in relation to developing the health of communities and thus the individuals who comprise them. However, we need to exercise caution in putting forward community empowerment as the answer to the problems of growing health inequalities and social exclusion.

The idealized community … serves more as a justification for a decline in state welfare programs than any authentic community empowerment (Labonte 1998)

Parachuting in 'empowerment' in the guise of well-intentioned professionals tends to lead to unsustainable processes and outcomes. Policies which 'do health' to people will fuel passive consumption. Policies which disguise social control as empowerment will also cast the individual as a health consumer powerless to actively play a part in the production of their own health. Grace (1991, p. 341) usefully reminds us that:

(the) ideology of empowerment … effectively masks its collusion with the contemporary form of political economy, consumer capitalism.

What is needed is to move towards policies based on the concept of subsidiarity. This involves not 'handing out' or the delegating of power but 'ruling and unifying only with the consent and agreement of equal partners' (Norton & Smith 1997). Subsidiarity allows excluded communities to access the competencies and capabilities of the professional classes but on mutually negotiated terms.

THEORY INTO PRACTICE

COMSCAN

The COMSCAN project (www.wales.gov.uk/keypublications) worked with Primary Health Care Teams using rapid appraisal techniques to bring a community perspective to a number of specific health issues. From teenage pregnancy to chronic obstructive pulmonary disease, the teams 'investigated' the full range of stakeholder views and came up with proposals to modify/develop their own practices in line with their 'findings'. Access the web address above for full details of 20 projects.

ARTS FACTORY

Radical initiatives such as Arts Factory (http://www.artsfactory.co.uk) use the concept of subsidiarity to engage in health improvement. Founded on principles derived from the craft, ecology and community development movements, this enterprise returns productive capacity to local people: '(they are) tired of being labelled as some sort of problem and want to be part of the solution.' (Arts Factory 2000).

CONCLUSION

A substantial proportion of this chapter has been devoted to identifying some of the implications of using health gain as the underlying value base for health service provision. In addition the chapter has touched on the issues associated with a community approach to health improvement. If nurses are to focus on this aspect of their work and engage effectively with communities, whether they are communities of interest or of locality, they will need to develop their understanding of the theories and models of community development practice. This is a complete area of study in itself. Many of the skills nurses can bring to community development are transferable from their more traditional nursing practice: needs assessment, a focus on quality of life, empathy, advocacy and a whole range of interpersonal and communication skills. But they will also have new skills to learn, not least that communities themselves are 'part of the solution' not just part of the problem.

SUMMARY

◆ Health gain is fundamentally about improving health status.

◆ Recognizing the full range of health determinants is fundamental to the concept of health gain and underpins health improvement.

◆ Multiagency collaboration is often essential to achieving health gain, particularly within a community framework.

◆ You have to know where you are before you can decide where you're going: an assessment of current health status, together with available resources, is a prerequisite to the identification of acceptable, appropriate, health gain targets.

◆ Community values and perspectives are essential in planning and implementing a strategy for health improvement.

◆ Subsidiarity rather than empowerment is a key concept in improving health in communities.

◆ Community nurses will need to familiarize themselves with models and theories of community development if they are to engage fully in a community approach to health improvement.

DISCUSSION POINTS

1. What criteria would you use to decide between two alternative strategies to achieve health improvement? Use an example from your own experience.

2. Consider one of the important components of your own professional role. What health gain may be achieved in carrying out that aspect of your work? What outcome measures would be appropriate?

3. Can health promotion tackle risk conditions, whose existence lies in deeply structured and political policies outside the direct control of local community groups? (Labonte 1998)

4. How can communities become 'part of the solution' and not just 'part of the problem' in relation to health improvement?

REFERENCES

Adamson D, Dearden H, Castle B 2001 Community regeneration: review of best practice. National Assembly for Wales, Cardiff

Arts Factory 2000 People power. Mindbomb Issue No.10

Ashton J, Seymour H 1988 The new public health. Open University Press, Milton Keynes

Bartley M, Sacker A, Firth D, Fitzpatrick R 2000 Dimensions of inequality and the health of women. In: Graham H (ed) Understanding health inequalities. Open University Press, Buckingham, UK

Beck E, Lonsdale S, Newman S (eds) 1992 In the best of health? The status and future of health care in the UK. Chapman & Hall, London

Benezeval M, Judge K, Whitehead M 1995 Tackling inequalities in health. Kings Fund, London

Bevan A 1975 In: Watkins B (ed) Documents on health and social services; 1834 to the present day. Methuen, London

Bowling A 1997 Measuring health – A review of quality of life measurement scales, 2nd edn. Open University Press, Milton Keynes

Breitenbach E 1997 Participation in an anti-poverty project. Community Development Journal 32(2): 159–168. Cited in: Adamson D, Dearden H, Castle B 2001 Community regeneration: review of best practice. National Assembly for Wales, Cardiff

Burton P 1993 Community profiling: A guide to identifying local needs. School for Advanced Urban Studies, University of Bristol, Bristol

Clark J, Henderson J (eds) 1983 Community health. Churchill Livingstone, London

Cochrane AL 1972 Effectiveness and efficiency: Random reflections on health services. Nuffield Provincial Hospital Trust, London

Conyers D 1982 An introduction to social planning in the Third World. John Wiley, New York

Department of Health 1989 Working for patients. HMSO, London

Department of Health 1991 The health of the nation. HMSO, London

Department of Health 1998 Putting patients first. HMSO, London

Dixon P 1993 Some issues in measuring patient satisfaction. The bulletin of the Community Consultation and User Feedback Unit. CCUF Link, December. WHCSA, Cardiff

Elwyn G, Smail J (eds) 1998 Integrated teams in primary care. Radcliffe Medical Press, Abingdon

Frankel S 1991 Health needs, health care requirements and the myth of infinite demand. Lancet 237: 1588–1596

Freire P 1972 Pedagogy of the oppressed. Penguin, Harmondsworth

Gould E 1998 All for one, and one for all: Health visiting and public health. Nursing Times 94(1): 32–33

Grace VM 1991 The marketing of empowerment and the construction of the health consumer: A critique of health promotion. International Journal of Health Services 21(2): 329–343

Hamilton-Kirkwood L, Parry-Langdon N 1993 The needs agenda: Health needs assessment. The Bulletin of the Community Consultation and User Feedback Unit, CCUF Link, August. WHCSA, Cardiff

Harvey I 1992 Targets, targets everywhere, the health of South Glamorgan: The annual report of the Director of Public Health Medicine. South Glamorgan Health Authority, Cardiff

Hedberg B, Dahlgren G, Hansson J, Olve N-G 1997 Virtual organisations and beyond. Wiley, New York

Holland W (ed) 1983 Evaluation of health care. Oxford University Press, Oxford

Hunter D 1993 The mysteries of health gain. Health Care 92/93. King's Fund Institute, London

Jones C, Hesterly WS, Borgatti SP 1997 A general theory of network governance: Exchange conditions and social mechanisms. Academy of Management Review 22(4): 911–945

Karlsen S, Nazroo JY 2000 Identity and structure: rethinking ethnic inequalities in health. In: Graham H (ed) Understanding health inequalities. Open University Press, Buckingham, UK

Kawechi I, Kennedy BP, Lochner K, Protherow-Stith D 1997 Social capital, income inequality and mortality. American Journal of Public Health 26(1): 6–15

Kunitz SJ 2001 Accounts of social capital: the mixed health effects of personal communities and voluntary groups. In: Leon DA, Walt G (eds) Poverty, inequality and

health: an international perspective. Oxford University Press, Oxford

Labonte R 1998 Communities for better health. Paper for the Communities for Better Health Master Class, Community Health Development in Wales. Health Promotion Wales, Cardiff

Long AS, Bate L, Sheldon TA 1992 The establishment of a UK clearing house for assessing health service outcomes. Quality of Health Care 1: 131–133

Long AS, Dixon P, Hall R 1993 The outcomes agenda, the contribution of a UK clearing house on health outcomes. Quality in Health Care 2: 249–252

Marmot M, Davey Smith G, Stansfield S, et al 1991 Health inequalities among British civil servants: The Whitehall II Study. Lancet 33: 1387–1393

Marmot M, Davey Smith G 1997 Socio-economic differentials in health: The contribution of the Whitehall studies. Journal of Health Psychology 2: 283–296

McKeown T, Lowe CR 1966 An introduction to social medicine. Blackwell Scientific Publications, Oxford

McMurray A 1993 Community health nursing: Primary health care in practice. Churchill Livingstone, Melbourne

Norton R, Smith C 1997 Understanding the virtual organisation. Barron's Educational Theories, New York

Ong BN, Humphris G, Annett H, Rifkin S 1991 Rapid appraisal in an urban setting: an example from the developed world. Social Science in Medicine 32: 909–915

Ovretveit J 1993 Coordinating community care. Open University Press, Buckingham

Pickin C, St Leger S 1993 Assessing health need using the life cycle framework. Open University Press, Buckingham

Popay J, Williams G 1993 Sociological approaches to collecting information on health needs. In: Pickin C, St Leger S (eds) 1993 Assessing health need using the life cycle framework, Chapter 4. Open University Press, Buckingham

Powell M, Moon G 2001 Health Action Zones: the 'third way' of a new area-based policy. Health and Social Care in the Community 9(1): 43–50

Ruffing-Raffal MA 1987 Resident/provider contrast in community health priorities. Public Health Nursing 4(4): 242–246

Seedhouse D 1986 Health: The foundations for achievement. Wiley, Chichester

Stevens A, Raferty J 1991 Assessing health care needs. A DHA project discussion paper. NHS Management Executive, Department of Health, London

Toronto Department of Public Health (1994) Making communities, Toronto Department of Public Health. Cited in: Labonte R 1998 Communities for better health. Paper for the Communities for Better Health Master Class, Community Health Development in Wales. Health Promotion Wales, Cardiff

Townsend P, Davidson N, Whitehead M 1988 Inequalities in health: the Black Report and the Health Divide. Penguin, Harmondsworth

Twinn S, Dauncey J, Carnell J 1990 The process of health profiling. Health Visitors Association, London

Welsh Health Planning Forum 1991a Protocol for investment in health gain: Cardiovascular diseases. Welsh Office NHS Directorate, Cardiff

Welsh Health Planning Forum 1991b Protocol for investment in health gain: Maternal and early child health. Welsh Office NHS Directorate, Cardiff

Welsh Office NHS Directorate 1989 Strategic intent and direction for the NHS in Wales. Welsh Office, Cardiff

Whitehead M, Diderichsen F, Burstrom B 2000 Researching the impact of public policy on inequalities in health. In: Graham H (ed) Understanding health inequalities. Open University Press, Buckingham

Wilkinson RG 1996 Unhealthy societies; the afflictions of inequality. Routledge, London

World Health Organization 1946 Preamble to the constitution. WHO, Geneva

World Health Organization 1981 Global strategy for health for all by the year 2000. WHO, Geneva

World Health Organization 1985 Targets for health for all – Targets in support of the European Regional Strategy for Health for All. WHO, Copenhagen

FURTHER READING

Bowling A 1997 Measuring health – A review of quality of life measurement scales, 2nd edition. Oxford University Press, Milton Keynes

Minkler M (ed) 1997 Community organizing and health. Rutgers University Press, New Brunswick, NJ

Wilkinson R 1996 Unhealthy societies: The afflictions of inequality. Routledge, New York

The family as a framework for practice

The third section continues to develop important themes for community nursing by focusing on the family and the particular perspective of family nursing. Both sociological and psychological perspectives are adopted to explore the diversity of experiences in family life, aspects of continuity and change and perhaps more importantly the impact of external influences mentioned in previous chapters. Given the emphasis placed on quality assessment and the identification of risk factors as the basis for decision-making and intervention, the family is usefully examined both as a potential source of ill health as well as a resource for enhancing health and quality of life. Particular importance is given to the potential for violence within intimate family relationships and to child protection issues, as well as those to do with older people. Current theory and research is explored in considerable detail as the basis for the community nursing role in child protection.

The concept of 'family' is explored in depth in the first chapter, adopting a sociological perspective to consider changing patterns of family living and the diversity of experiences across time. Special reference is made to the demographic aspects of marriage and cohabitation, to the changing and unchanging roles of women and to current expectations for personal fulfilment. The impact of divorce and the rise in one-parent family households are two issues of particular significance for community nurses given established links with poverty, child and women's health. By questioning the picture of contemporary old age and the predictable problems that arise within families, a third and critical aspect of primary care is also raised.

The psychological perspective adopted in the second chapter alerts the community nurse to the costs and benefits to the individual of family life, to the styles of interaction and life events which can predict positive mental health, or a risk of breakdown in family relationships. The concept of a dysfunctional family is mentioned because of the special challenge for healthcare professionals, an important issue when assessing the value or benefit of community nursing intervention. The following chapter addresses the difficult problem of violence within the family, exploring explanations for abuse to women, children and older people and highlighting the size and extent of the problem and its links with overall physical and emotional ill health. It is a chapter which highlights the importance of team-working in primary care and the importance of agreed processes for assessment, intervention and evaluation. Chapter 10 focuses particularly on the theory and research which underpins community nursing intervention for the prevention of the physical abuse of children.

It looks specifically at sociological, structural and environmental factors which seek to offer explanatory models; but of greater interest for a community nursing assessment is the discussion of interacting variables within the family which predict increased risk. In conclusion different models of prevention are clearly presented emphasizing the importance of the social context in which abuse occurs.

Chapter 12 develops the concept of family nursing, contrasting the difference in focus between the individual and the family for assessment and intervention. It moves away from the traditional problem oriented nursing perspective to one which focuses on identifying the strengths within the family and on family empowerment. Theories supporting a family nursing approach are discussed and the implications of genetic research are raised in terms of implications for future development in the context of primary care and community nursing.

8

The family: a sociological perspective

G. Allan
G. Crow

KEY ISSUES

◆ Continuities and changes in households and families.

◆ Diversity in people's experiences of families.

◆ Influence of external factors on dominant patterns of family life.

INTRODUCTION

While we all talk about 'the family' as though it were obvious and unproblematic, in a very real sense 'the family' as such does not exist. Rather what we have are many different forms of family, each of which gets modified and changed, over time, generally slowly, but sometimes more radically. This point is not as banal as it might seem. Indeed arguably the key to understanding the nature of family life lies in recognizing the interplay between continuity and change which characterizes all aspects of family relationships. It is this notion of the family as dynamic rather than static, variable rather than uniform, which will provide the framework for much of what follows in this chapter.

We can recognize that change occurs within families at a variety of levels. Clearly individual relationships within families change over time. Think here about your relationships with your parents. Whether or not they are still together, the ways they have treated you, their expectations about your behaviour, and the forms of control they have exercised over you, have all altered as you have grown older. In adulthood, your relationship with them is likely to continue but not in anything like the same form as when you were a child. So too relationships between husbands and wives, between brothers and sisters, or any other family members also alter as people age and take on different responsibilities. Most of the time this change is considered routine and normal, though there are occasions, such as divorce or the onset of severe infirmity, when it is more traumatic and requires more rapid adjustment.

But just as relationships between family members alter over time, so too the patterns of family living within a society are liable to change as wider social and economic conditions alter. Traditionally within sociology, a great deal of attention has been paid to the impact that industrialization had on family relationships. For example, there has been much debate around whether industrialization led to the decline of extended family relationships or, in contrast, actually generated the conditions necessary for greater solidarity between extended family members. Such debates are echoed in much popular discourse, though this tends to emphasize the pathological character of contemporary family life and the decline of family values. Thus, we often hear claims that family life has become more insular and less community oriented, or that elderly people do not receive sufficient support from their families. Recently too there has been much emphasis placed on shifts occurring within marriage, though here there are more conflicting views as to how this should be interpreted. Some argue that in comparison to the past – though exactly how far back in the past is often left unspecified – marriage is now a much more equal relationship, a far more genuine partnership than it used to be. Others point to the rising levels of divorce as an indicator that many no longer regard marriage with the sanctity it deserves.

So what has been happening to family life and family relationships? How different are our experiences from those of our grandparents? How much change has there been and how much continuity? In order to examine these issues, this chapter will focus on key aspects of the social organization of family and domestic life pertinent to community nursing. These include marriage, divorce, lone-parent households, and the family circumstances of elderly people. We will begin by examining the contemporary patterning and social organization of marriage.

MARRIAGE AND COHABITATION

Throughout the first two thirds of the 20th century marriage became a more common experience. By the late 1960s approximately 95% of men and women were or had been married by the time they were in their mid-40s. Marriage age also decreased over this period, with the average age of first marriage for men being 23 and for women 21 in the late 1960s. Since the early 1970s though, demographic aspects of marriage and partnership formation have altered markedly. To begin with, age at first marriage has shown a steady increase since the mid 1970s. By 2000 the average age had risen to 29.6 for men and 27.5 for women. In part this reflects the massively increased levels of cohabitation now occurring. In this regard, marriage is becoming less normative as a mode of household and family formation. Until the 1970s, very few couples cohabited prior to marriage, with most of those who did being separated or divorced. By the turn of the 21st century, well over half of all marrying couples had cohabited. Importantly too, many couples now live together without marriage being an explicit project. Indeed, around a quarter of all unmarried women aged 18–49 were cohabiting in the late 1990s (General Household Survey 1998). Thus, while religious and ethnic variations persist (Berrington 1994), behaviour that was censured a generation ago is now accepted by most as an uncontentious and morally appropriate way of developing romantic/sexual relationships.

Along with these changes in the demography of marriage and partnership formation, there is also a widely held belief that the basis of these relationships has been altering. Contemporary ideology, or what Cancian (1987) some years ago termed 'blueprints' of marriage, emphasize the idea of marriage as much more of a partnership between equals than it was in the past. It is now seen as an emotionally closer relationship, based on developing conceptions of personal compatibility, commitment and love. It consequently carries with it a heightened range of expectations, including a greater belief that personal expression and mutual satisfaction provide the central rationale for the relationship. It is this which people forming partnerships and getting married seek. More than their grandparents or even their parents, they want their marriages to encompass a mutual sharing, a union between equals, premised on contemporary images of romantic love as a means to personal fulfilment. In this light, changing terminology is also important. The increased use of the term 'partnership' reflects these changing aspirations, as well as solving the 'dilemma' of what status to give cohabitation.

However despite these ideologies, the basic organization of marriage and 'coupledom' has remained relatively constant. While cohabitation appears sometimes to entail a more symmetrical and equal relationship, once married, couples usually fall into a more standard pattern. Moreover, the division of labour and domestic responsibilities within a marriage, and consequently the division of opportunities and constraints affecting each spouse, become most marked when (and if) the couple have children. In general, men continue to be seen as having the primary commitment to the job market and the main responsibility for securing household finances, while women are assigned principal responsibility for domestic labour, childcare and household management. The patterns here of course are not identical to those occurring in the past. There have undoubtedly been important changes, particularly with respect to wives' employment. For example, in 1961 less than 40% of wives aged 16–59 were in employment. By 2000 75% of married and cohabiting women were employed, with 40% in full-time employment (Social Trends 2001). Equally mothers return to employment much sooner after childbirth than they did even 20 years ago. Yet while most couples now depend on two incomes for their household's standard of living, men's earnings are still seen as 'primary' in a way in which women's are not. In turn, wives are still taken to be the person with primary responsibility for the smooth functioning of household and family matters. (For a fuller discussion of these issues, see Allan & Crow 2001.)

As children age, as wives return to employment and as the couple develop different commitments outside the home, we might expect that some aspects of their division of work are renegotiated. Yet, while there are modifications over time, rarely does such renegotiation appear to lead to radical change (Crompton & Harris 1999). Husbands and older children may help somewhat more in household tasks, but the primary responsibilities for domestic management and familial care usually continue as before. Even following major changes in household circumstances, for example with male unemployment, the renegotiation of responsibilities appears to be limited. In general, the household division of labour continues to be patterned in the ways established early in the marriage.

The continuation of a high division of labour within marriage is linked very strongly to the inequalities which flourish within the job market. Notwithstanding British and European Equal Opportunities legislation, occupations still tend to be highly gendered. For example, the majority of women employees work in a few female-dominated occupations, e.g. as secretaries, nurses, teachers, sales staff and cleaners. Importantly too, the jobs women are in typically pay significantly less than male occupations. For the last two decades, and with very little variation between years, full-time women employees have received approximately 70% of the wages male employees receive, with this relationship being broadly consistent across different skill levels. Part-time employees, the vast majority of whom are married women, usually receive even lower proportional pay (Crompton 1997).

Overall, it is not really surprising that a conventional division of labour continues to be 'negotiated' by most couples. As well as husbands earning more than wives, women are socialized into being more accomplished at domestic activities than men and tend to have child care and other relationship responsibility built more into the construction of their personal and social identities. Of course, in principle a division of labour need not be associated with an unequal distribution of resources within a marriage or other partnership, nor with the dominance of one spouse over the other. Yet research has regularly shown that within most marriages, though not all, this is the outcome. Despite the prevalence of ideologies of coupledom, men have greater control of financial resources, more freedom for leisure and more control over key decisions than their wives do (Allan & Crow 2001). So notwithstanding modifications in employment patterns, in marital ideology, in domestic standards, in childcare practices and the like, the point remains that individual couples construct their marriages within an economic and social context which remains structurally unequal and usually provides men with more options and a greater access to resources than women.

DIVORCE

Divorce is one aspect of family life where there has been a clear change in the last 30 years. Whereas in the late 1960s there were only 45 000 divorces each year, over the last decade there have been, on average, over 150 000. This is a rise in the annual rate from four per 1000 marriages to over 13 per 1000. Each year approximately 150 000 children under the age of 16 experience their parents' divorce, almost a doubling since 1971. Alongside this there has been an expansion in the number of lone-parent families, not all of which arise through divorce of course, and a large increase in the number of step-families. This has resulted in much more diversity in family patterns compared to even a short while ago. It also means that many individuals now experience different forms of family life at first hand, moving say from a two-parent family to a lone-parent one, and then later forming a step-family.

It is difficult to be precise about the reasons for the rise in divorce. Divorce, like marriage, is a legal procedure, so at one level the heightened rate of divorce merely reflects changes in the law, with the 1969 Divorce Reform Act having been especially important. However, the law itself reflects changed marital ideologies; moreover the fact that divorce is made more available does not

of itself explain why people have increasingly chosen it as an option. Three factors seem particularly important. First, as we have already noted, there have been changes in marital 'blueprints'. Increasingly people are expecting continued personal satisfaction from marriage and not just a convenient domestic, sexual and economic arrangement. Indeed, the 1969 Divorce Reform Act – which is still the basis of current divorce law – itself symbolized this. Instead of viewing marriage as essentially a legal contract between two people which could only be terminated if broken by a specific action of one of the spouses, for example adultery or desertion, under the 1969 Act, marriage was understood more as a personal arrangement which could be terminated if it had 'irretrievably broken down', irrespective of what led up to this, or the behaviour of either spouse.

Secondly, increasing divorce rates are feasible only if both spouses normally have access to sufficient material resources to sustain themselves. Of particular importance here are the changes there have been over the last 50 years allowing separated women to maintain a sufficient standard of living independently of their (ex)husbands. The creation of increased employment opportunities for married women has been important in this, as has the availability of social security payments and the protection given in divorce settlements to the housing needs of those caring for children. Thirdly, divorce is now far less stigmatized than it once was. It is seen as undesirable, but no more than an event which has a personal rather than a social significance. Divorce is no longer treated as a moral issue to the same extent as it once was, nor as indicative of questionable character. As divorce becomes accepted as an unfortunate but not unusual occurrence, so it comes also to be seen as a solution to marital difficulties that in a previous era would have been tolerated. It is this 'normalization' of divorce in both legal and social terms which lies at the heart of the currently high levels of divorce.

In understanding the impact which divorce has on those involved, it is crucial that it is viewed as a process occurring over time, rather than as a specific legal event. The factors that lead up to the breakdown of the marriage, and the understandings each spouse has of these, will have an impact on the way in which the divorce and its aftermath are handled. This is particularly important when there are children, for as is now better recognized, divorce represents the ending of a marriage but not the ending of parenting. Legislation governing the Child Support Agency (CSA) has brought the economic implications of this to the fore, but it also applies to the personal relationship each child maintains with the nonresidential parent. American research has indicated the importance for children of maintaining an active relationship with both parents (Richards 1999). Moreover it is in the child's interests that the two parents develop a consistent and co-operative relationship with one another with respect to parenting. This is rarely easy, given the history of hostility and conflict characterizing much pre- and postdivorce behaviour (Smart & Neale 1999). When parents continue to be in conflict over, say, financial arrangements or childcare responsibilities, or indeed when recrimination, jealousy and other strong emotions are still being experienced, it is difficult to develop a mutually consistent and supportive stance in relation to children. Given the tensions and problems which can be generated, it is perhaps not surprising that a third of nonresidential fathers appear to see their children less than once a month (Bradshaw et al 1999).

LONE-PARENT HOUSEHOLDS

Over the last 30 years, the numbers of lone-parent households has increased quite dramatically, both as a result of high levels of divorce and because more children are being born outside marriage. As the numbers have grown, the range and diversity of experiences of those living in such households has also increased. Undoubtedly the majority of lone-parent households have much in common, especially with respect to their poverty and material deprivation. Yet variations in the living conditions, family histories and economic opportunities of different lone-parent households should not be ignored. Just as the routes into, and indeed out of, lone-parenthood

have become more complex, so too the social, economic and domestic circumstances of those involved have become more diverse (Crow & Hardey 1999).

In the mid 1990s it was estimated that there were over 1.6 million lone-parent households in Britain, containing approximately 2.6 million children – roughly 1 in 5 of all dependent children (Haskey 1998). Of these, a little over 100 000 were headed by men. While this is not an insignificant number in itself, the predominance of female-headed lone-parent households warrants emphasizing as it plays a major part in shaping the experience of lone-parenthood. Of the 1.5 million female-headed lone-parent households there are, over 50% stem from divorce or marital separation, with fewer than 100,000 being the result of widowhood. Over a third are headed by single (i.e. never married) women (Haskey 1998). This represents a quite remarkable demographic change since the mid-1970s. Then, fewer than 10% of children were born 'out of wedlock'. By 1998, the figure was nearly 40%, with nearly 90% of teenage mothers being unmarried (Birth Statistics 1978, 1999). However, it is worth noting that approximately half of all mothers recorded as being unmarried on their child's birth certificate are cohabiting with the father when the birth is registered.

The great majority of lone-parent households live in poverty. For example, Marsh et al (1997) found that 80% of lone-parent families in their sample were receiving a means-tested social security benefit, with two-thirds on Income Support, and thus living on the minimum officially considered viable. However the route into lone-parenthood has some bearing on this. In general, lone fathers and widowed mothers tend to be somewhat better off than other lone parents (though not as well off as two-parent households). These groups usually have older children than other lone parents, and as a result fewer problems with the co-ordination and costs of child care. They are also more likely to have employment or pensions which make them less dependent on state benefits, and to be in owner-occupation. In contrast, divorced, separated and single mothers – collectively over 85% of all lone parents – frequently experience high levels of poverty for long periods.

The reasons for this are various. Women's disadvantaged position in employment is one factor. The relatively low pay of many female jobs, especially for women without significant qualifications, means that many lone mothers have little prospect of enhancing their financial position. In addition, the need for flexibility over child care often makes it difficult to co-ordinate employment and parenting responsibilities. When children are at school, part-time employment may become feasible though the financial benefits of this, as distinct from its social and personal advantages, are generally quite limited. In recent years, state policies have been attempting to reduce the numbers of lone mothers in poverty through more generous employment allowances, enhanced provision of childcare facilities, and through ensuring that nonresidential fathers pay higher levels of maintenance for their children. However, despite these initiatives, the great majority of lone-mother households continue to experience poverty (Kiernan et al 1998, Rowlingson & McKay 1998).

As well as being poor, lone mothers tend to be disadvantaged in other ways. For example, they have worse than average housing conditions, with a disproportionate number being in rented accommodation, or sharing their home with other adults. Only about a third of lone-parent families are in owner-occupation compared to three-quarters of all other households with dependent children living in them. So too, a quarter of lone-parent households live in flats compared to one in 20 of other households with children in them (GHS 1998). Equally there is evidence that lone parents, but especially lone mothers, suffer more health problems than other families (Shouls et al 1999). This is not altogether surprising, given the relationship between material well-being and good health. Families in poverty and in poor housing, as so many lone-parent families are, generally experience worse health than those who have adequate resources (see Chapter 6).

Overall, there is no doubt that a majority of lone-parent families are disadvantaged, especially those which are female-headed. Yet while poverty and material deprivation is the norm,

various aspects of lone-parenthood come to be valued by many. Simply in financial terms, some lone mothers are, in Hilary Graham's telling phrase, 'better off poorer' (1987, p. 59), because they now control all the household resources, whereas previously they only received a proportion of the overall larger 'household' income, with their husbands or partners retaining the rest. Equally, while many lone parents experience social isolation and a sense of having to cope with a wide range of demands alone, others value the freedom and autonomy over their use of time, domestic organization and social activities which lone-parenthood offers. For some too, the curtailment of disharmony and marital violence more than compensates for poverty. The point here is not that these more positive aspects of lone-parenthood necessarily counter its negative features, but rather that lone-parenthood is often an ambiguous and diverse experience.

STEP-FAMILIES

Cohabitation and marriage represent major routes out of lone-parenthood, though some take them more readily than others. Generally, single mothers form new unions quicker than those who have been married previously, with age, educational attainment and family size affecting the chances of remarriage for those who have divorced (Rowlingson & McKay 1998). But just as the levels of divorce, births outside marriage and lone-parenthood have increased over the last 20 years, so has the number of step-families formed. According to official estimates, some 6% of families with dependent children were step-families in the late 1990s, with many other children having a nonresidential step-parent (Social Trends 2001). Overall there has been surprisingly little research into step-families in Britain and also little official concern for them. The assumption has tended to be that step-families are essentially similar to other two-parent families.

However the diversity and complexity of step-families make this an oversimplified view. Aside from factors like the age of the children and how long they have known their step-parent, the social roles of step-father and step-mother are ill-defined. There are few guidelines about just how much of a parent a step-parent should be. For example, the extent of the step-parent's involvement, their rights to impose discipline, and the commitment expected between step-parent and child, are all much more open to negotiation than in natural families, so that the potential for disagreement and conflict is that much greater. Equally the 'boundaries' around step-families tend to be more permeable than in natural families, especially where contact is maintained with the nonresidential parent and his or her kin. So too, the different members of a step-family have different family and kinship networks to each other, often resulting in different kinship loyalties. In essence, the symbolic 'unity' of a step-family cannot be assumed in the way it is in natural families. Given these structural dilemmas, it is hardly surprising that step-families appear particularly prone to friction, notwithstanding their members' frequent efforts to present themselves as, in essence, no different from 'ordinary' families.

OLD AGE

There is a strong belief that kinship ties outside the household have become less significant than they once were. In particular, the solidarities that exist across the generations are now seen to be weaker than in the past, with the result that many elderly people are left isolated, leading lonely and largely unfulfilling lives. This picture of contemporary old age is highly questionable.

There are now for example more than four million people over the age of 75 compared to half a million in 1901, an increase which is 16 times that of the general population. Moreover nearly half of all women over 65 live alone. Along with these demographic shifts, there have been important changes in elderly people's social and economic circumstances. In particular, it is becoming increasingly inappropriate to treat the elderly population as homogeneous. The divisions between them are as important as the similarities. For example,

the rise of private pension plans and of owner-occupation since the mid 20th century have exacerbated differences in income and wealth amongst those aged 65 and over. These factors, together with variations in life expectancy, have also led to very important gender differences in the experience of old age (Arber & Ginn 1995, Phillipson 1998).

On the surface, the fact that so many elderly women especially live alone appears to give credence to the claim that elderly people no longer receive the support they deserve and need. Undoubtedly some of these people are very isolated and receive inadequate social support; some will never have married, or have no surviving children to whom they might turn. Yet there are other factors at work here too, which give a rather different picture. In particular, culturally a high priority is often given to maintaining household independence, though there are important ethnic variations in this (Phillipson et al 2001). That is, while there is strong value placed on relationships between genealogically close adult kin being generally supportive, there is also much weight given to the idea that in adulthood, personal and household autonomy takes priority. Kin, including parents and children, should not interfere too much in each other's lives. Here there can be a fine line between supporting and interfering, between assuming some responsibility and maintaining independence (Finch & Mason 1993). Indeed, rather than neglecting their elderly parent(s), it would seem many adult children play a major role in helping them to sustain independent lives as infirmity encroaches.

Of course the nature of the relationship which elderly people have with their children varies a good deal. In part, this will be shaped by the past development of their bond, but it will also be influenced by a range of other personal factors, such as geographical location, employment, other familial and domestic responsibilities, material resources, and health. It is important to recognize here that older age of itself does not have any necessary impact on family relationships. The great majority of older people are relatively fit and active, well able to manage their own lives, and have no reason for fuller involvement with their children than in preceding life stages. As in earlier times, the relationships are likely to be characterized by a degree of reciprocity with both sides providing support of different forms for one another, but without either being in a position of dependence.

It is not old age per se which alters the nature of these exchanges, but rather changes – sometimes gradual, sometimes radical – in older people's circumstances. However, such changes as reduced income, widowhood, and poor health have a differential impact on the older population. Expressed simply, those with most resources, in particular those who have higher levels of private pension and significant investments, are in a better position to sustain their lifestyle and independence through purchasing services privately. Those with fewer resources, a position in which many older women find themselves, especially after their husband's death, are likely to become more quickly dependent on kin for support. In nearly all cases though there is a desire to maintain some semblance of balance and reciprocity in these ties. This can often require careful and quite subtle 'negotiation' if the older individual's sense of self-worth is not to be undermined.

When extensive care is required, it tends to be provided by family members, though usually the responsibility falls most heavily on one particular person. This is typically the spouse where there is one, or another adult living in the same house. Otherwise it is usually daughters or daughters-in-law who are most active in providing informal care. While this has now been much discussed in the research literature on caring (see, for example, Ungerson & Kember 1997), it is still easy for health professionals and others to underestimate the actual level of work which such caring entails and its impact on the lifestyles and well-being of those who do it.

CONCLUSION

There has been little explicit focus in this chapter on issues directly concerned with health behaviour or practice. Other chapters discuss these matters more directly. Its aim has been to provide a broad framework through analysing key aspects of contemporary family experience. However the arguments made in this chapter certainly have relevance for healthcare provision and the work of community nurses. Three particular issues are worth highlighting in conclusion. First, there is growing diversity in household and family patterns, both demographically and materially, with recent increases in cohabitation, divorce and remarriage. In delivering health care, advice and support, the particular circumstances of individual families need to be recognized. Second, the family itself is not a single entity or social unity. It comprises sets of relationships which change over time but which also typically entail a marked division of labour, resources and power. Recognizing these divisions and the impact they have on the experiences of different household members can be important in providing appropriate health services. Finally, it is important that all health workers recognize the extent to which health care continues to be delivered informally, principally by family members and predominantly by females responsible for the household's domestic organization. Despite the changes which are imagined to have occurred, most nonspecialized nursing and health care is carried out by wives, mothers and daughters. At times the burden of such care can be extremely heavy, a fact which should not be downplayed even when those involved give the impression of 'coping'.

SUMMARY

◆ The structure of families is constantly changing; these changes may be sudden or gradual, and although families can be grouped, the differences between different families in the same grouping can be extreme.

◆ Numbers of couples not marrying but cohabiting have increased dramatically over the past 30 years. However the roles men and women have, no matter the legal relationship, still adhere to old 'norms' with men having more options and access to resources.

◆ The divorce rate has escalated over recent decades due to its 'normalization'; however to understand the implications of divorce on family members it must be seen as a long-term event rather than a single occurrence for the family.

◆ Lone parenting, usually with women at the head of the family, has increased over the past two generations and has its own implications with these families more likely to be living in poverty.

◆ Step-families need to be seen, not as being identical to natural families, but as families which can have their own tensions due to divided loyalties, etc.

◆ The old must be seen as people with very different experiences, differing levels of family support and financial security, and therefore different needs.

DISCUSSION POINTS

1. Why might it be useful for community nurses to profile family diversity in the neighbourhood served by the practice team?

2. How would you record family differences in a way which would account for variation in community nursing intervention?

3. Why would it be important to assess in detail care, the impact of caring for a frail older member of the family?

REFERENCES

Allan G, Crow G 2001 Families, households and society. Palgrave, Basingstoke

Arber S, Ginn J 1995 Connecting gender and ageing. Open University Press, Buckingham

Berrington A 1994 Marriage and family formation among the white and ethnic-minority populations in Britain. Ethnic and Racial Studies 17: 517–546

Birth Statistics 1978 Birth Statistics 1976, OPCS, Series FM1, No. 3. HMSO, London

Birth Statistics 1999 Birth Statistics 1998, ONS, Series FM1, No. 27. HMSO, London

Bradshaw J, Stimson C, Skinner C, Williams J 1999 Absent fathers? Routledge, London

Cancian F 1987 Love in America: Gender and self-development. Cambridge University Press, Cambridge

Crompton R 1997 Women and work in modern Britain. Oxford University Press, Oxford

Crompton R, Harris F 1999 Attitudes, women's employment and the changing domestic division of labour: a cross-national analysis. In: Crompton R (ed) Restructuring gender relations and employment. Oxford University Press, Oxford

Crow G, Hardey M 1999 Diversity and ambiguity among lone-parent households in modern Britain. In: Allan G (ed) The sociology of the family: A reader. Blackwell, Oxford

Finch J, Mason J 1993 Renegotiating family responsibilities. Routledge, London

GHS 1998 Living in Britain: Results from the General Household Survey, National Statistics. Stationery Office, London

Graham H 1987 Being poor: perceptions and coping strategies of lone mothers. In: Brannen J, Wilson G (eds) Give and take in families: Studies in resource distribution. Allen & Unwin, London

Haskey J 1998 One-parent families and their dependent children in Great Britain. Population Trends 91: 5–14

Kiernan K, Land H, Lewis J 1998 Lone motherhood in twentieth century Britain. Oxford University Press, Oxford

Marsh A, Ford R, Finlayson L 1997 Lone parents, work and benefits. Social Security Research Report No. 61. Stationery Office, London

Phillipson C 1998 Reconstructing old age. Sage, London

Phillipson C, Bernard M, Phillips J, Ogg J 2001 The family and community life of older people. Routledge, London

Richards M 1999 The interests of children at divorce. In: Allan G (ed) The sociology of the family: A reader. Blackwell, Oxford

Rowlingson K, McKay S 1998 The growth of lone parenthood. Policy Studies Institute, London

Shouls S, Whitehead M, Burström B, Diderichsen F 1999 The health and socio-economic circumstances of lone mothers over the last two decades. Population Trends 95: 41–46

Smart C, Neale B 1999 Family fragments? Polity, Cambridge

Social Trends 2001 No. 31, National Statistics. Stationery Office, London

Ungerson C, Kember M 1997 Women and social policy: A reader. Macmillan, Basingstoke

FURTHER READING

Allan G 1999 The sociology of the family: A reader. Blackwell, Oxford

The essays in this collection cover a wide range of topics relevant to this chapter. It includes sections on Changing Families; Marriage Intimacy and Power; Domestic Organisation; Divorce and Lone-Parenthood; and Family, Kinship and Care.

Allan G, Crow G 2001 Families, households and society. Palgrave, Basingstoke

This book provides an introduction to the sociology of the family, reviewing recent research and highlighting the changes there have been in domestic life. Written principally for sociology students, it develops some of the arguments made in this chapter.

Finch J, Mason J 1993 Renegotiating family responsibilities. Routledge, London

This book provides a thorough discussion of the role of kinship in contemporary Britain. Based on a survey of kinship attitudes and behaviour, the authors highlight the negotiations which occur in assigning kinship responsibilities.

Kiernan K, Land H, Lewis J 1998 Lone motherhood in twentieth century Britain. Oxford University Press, Oxford

This book provides an excellent review of the changing circumstances of lone mothers. It examines the growth of lone motherhood and how public understandings of lone motherhood have altered over time. It also reviews the different ways that the state has responded to the financial and other needs of lone-parent families.

McRae S 1999 Changing Britain: Families and households in the 1990s. Oxford University Press, Oxford

This is a very useful collection of specially commissioned papers, all based on recent research into different aspects of family life. It is particularly useful for understanding patterns of change and continuity in family relationships over the last generation.

Phillipson C, Bernard M, Phillips J, Ogg J 2001 The family and community life of older people. Routledge, London

This fascinating study of the family and community relationships of older people in contemporary Britain contains much of interest to community nurses. It is particularly interesting because it compares the current and past circumstances of elderly people in three different urban locations.

Smart C, Neale B 1999 Family fragments? Polity, Cambridge

This book reports on research into post-divorce family arrangements. In doing so, it engages with recent theorizing about changing family relationships and highlights key aspects of family organization. By focusing on the consequences of marital breakdown, it reveals much about the patterning of contemporary marriage and domestic organization.

9

The family: a psychological perspective

N. Frude

INTRODUCTION

Medicine, as an applied biological science, has traditionally regarded the individual person (or, even, the individual body) as the principal unit of examination, diagnosis and treatment. In most cases attention usually narrows to one or more 'sub-systems' (the respiratory system, the cardiovascular system, etc.). Some physicians, and a majority of nurses, may have maintained a 'whole person' perspective, but traditionally relatively little attention has been paid to wider systems such as the family and the community. In the past few decades, however, there has been a growing acknowledgement of the important influences of wider systems, and 'family medicine', 'family nursing', 'family therapy', 'community medicine', and 'community nursing' have all become well-established disciplines.

In this chapter some of the ways of thinking about families from a psychological perspective will be examined. We need to acknowledge at the outset that there are many other ways of looking at family issues, including those offered by the political, ethical, legal, and sociological perspectives (see Chapter 8 for example). The various perspectives should not be regarded as competing or contradictory, but they do offer distinct analyses by virtue of the different issues they identify and the diverse ways in which they examine these issues. Thus whereas the sociologist is generally concerned with the family as an institution in society, and often emphasizes the relationship between the family and wider systems (the health service, for example, or the benefits system), psychologists are typically more concerned with the interactions and relationships within particular families and how these change as a result of the impact of events such as illness, death, or the birth of a child.

The aim of this chapter is to provide a basic framework for thinking, psychologically, about families, rather than to summarize knowledge about the effects of particular events on families. An extensive review of the impact of illness, handicap, divorce, bereavement, etc. on family life has been provided elsewhere (Frude 1991). In the first part of this chapter the family as the background or context for the individual will be examined to show that family relationships are important determinants of a person's physical health and psychological well-being. The second half of the chapter will focus on the family group or unit. We will examine the nature of 'healthy' and 'dysfunctional' families and consider how different types of families might respond when one of their number becomes ill.

THE FAMILY AS THE CONTEXT FOR THE INDIVIDUAL

THE VALUE OF FAMILY RELATIONSHIPS

Being part of a family brings a number of costs and benefits to an individual. If a person decides that the costs of family membership outweigh the benefits (so that family membership has a negative value), then he or she may decide to withdraw from the family. According to one influential psychological theory ('social exchange theory'), the decisions that people make about their lives, including their family life, reflect their own cost–benefit analyses (Nye 1982, Ruben 1998). This kind of analysis has been used, for example, to explain why people choose to have (or not to have) children, why they may choose to separate, and why older children sometimes choose to return to live with their parents (Rigazio-DiGilio & Cramer 2000, Veevers & Mitchell 1998). A good

deal of research has been aimed at discovering what people want (i.e. the benefits they hope for) from relationships, and what they wish to avoid (i.e. the costs). Some adults who have had an unsatisfactory marital relationship in the past make the judgement that no such relationship in the future would be 'worth it'. The majority of people in this position, however, do look forward to a better relationship in the future and exert considerable effort to find 'the right person'. When interviewed, such people are able to say what they are looking for in a relationship – they are able to provide a list of hoped-for benefits.

It is clear that many marriages and long-term cohabiting relationships eventually end (according to some estimates, around 50% of all those who are currently getting married will eventually divorce). There is also a good deal of conflict and violence within families. Few families, indeed, could be described as completely harmonious. In view of these facts, it might be tempting to conclude that the family is a disaster area and that people would be better off without family ties. However, such a conclusion would be unjustified. We have to consider the benefits as well as the costs, and the love and support as well as the conflict and violence. On average, people value their relationships positively and there is strong evidence that, on the whole, close relationships benefit individuals.

When people are asked what makes them happy, what provides them with satisfaction, and what gives meaning to their lives, they emphasize their close relationships much more than any other aspect of their life, including their occupation, hobbies, health or money (Freedman 1978). This is not to deny that many people blame a key relationship for their unhappiness, or that intimate relationships often provoke the most intense anger, anxiety and sadness, but, on the whole, people do assess the impact of their closest relationships in positive rather than in negative terms. Furthermore, in support of such subjective assessments, there is objective evidence suggesting that, overall, the effects of close relationships are more often favourable than unfavourable.

RELATIONSHIPS AND LIFE EVENTS

It is now well established that psychological and physical health is profoundly affected by life events such as divorce, the birth of a child, bereavement, or moving house. Several lists (or 'inventories') of commonly experienced life events have been compiled, with each item being assigned a weighting to reflect the likely impact of an event of that nature. These inventories can be used to assess how much 'life change' an individual has experienced in the past 6 months, or the past year. Individuals' total life change scores have been found to predict many health outcomes, including susceptibility to infection, the risk of being involved in a serious accident and the risk of cardiovascular disease (Richter & Guthke 1993). Generally speaking, those who have experienced several recent major changes are more vulnerable to physical and psychological illness than those who have not experienced such changes.

A high proportion of the events listed in inventories compiled to assess major life changes (e.g. Holmes & Rahe 1967, Richter & Guthke 1993) are directly related to family life. Such events include the illness of a family member, a bereavement, a child leaving home, marital separation, and sexual problems. Lists of positive events also show a preponderance of family-related items (Argyle & Henderson 1985), and the same is true of minor positive and negative events (sometimes referred to as 'uplifts' and 'hassles' respectively). Compared with those who live in isolation, people who live in a family setting have lives which are relatively full of incident. They experience more 'entrances' (such as the birth of a child) and more 'exits' (the death of a family member, marital separation, or a young adult leaving home). They experience more 'uplifts' (such as birthdays, anniversaries, and school successes), but they also experience more 'hassles' (such as minor illnesses of family members, or family rows) (Harper et al 2000, Maybery & Graham 2001). Many of those who live in isolation are lonely and feel that their life lacks interest, excitement, or involvement. Whereas many early studies stressed the potential danger of exposure to 'excess life change', it is now appreciated that a modest degree of incident and transition may actually promote health.

INTIMACY, WELL-BEING AND HEALTH

Studies that have asked people to report how happy they are, how lonely they feel, and how stressed they feel, have revealed a number of interesting findings. For example, Wood et al (1989) conducted a 'meta-analysis' whereby they re-analysed the findings from 93 previously published studies that had addressed the issue of happiness and positive well-being. They showed that, overall, women reported greater happiness and life satisfaction than men (despite the fact that women are twice as likely to be clinically depressed as men). They also showed that marriage was associated with higher levels of well-being both for women and for men, thus contradicting an earlier suggestion that marriage was associated with greater happiness for men but lower happiness for women (Bernard 1973). Similarly, studies comparing the reported happiness, loneliness, and stress experienced by married people, single people, the widowed, and the divorced, also indicate that those who are currently married have fewer problems and have a greater sense of positive well-being than those in any of the other groups (Frude 1991).

Objective indicators point in the same direction. Overall, married people have better physical health than those who have never married or are divorced or widowed. They are less likely, for example, to suffer from asthma, diabetes, ulcers, tuberculosis, cancer of the mouth and throat, hypertension, strokes and coronaries (Cohen & Syme 1985, Goldman et al 1995). The association between health and being married is even apparent in mortality data. Married people are at significantly less risk of dying at a young age, compared to those who are single, widowed or divorced (Ben-Schlomo et al 1993, Lillard & Waite 1995, Tucker et al 1999).

A broadly similar pattern emerges when the statistics for mental health are considered. When groups of people matched for age, sex and social class are compared in terms of their psychiatric history, morbidity rates are lowest for the married population (Bebbington et al 2000, Bloom et al 1979). General community surveys also reveal that married people experience the fewest psychological symptoms, with an intermediate rate among widowed and never-married adults, and the highest rates among those who are divorced or separated.

Before we conclude that 'marriage is good for you', however, it does need to be stressed that the statistics merely show an average advantage for those who are married. It must be remembered that for many people the marital relationship is oppressive or violent, and that conflict and aggression can jeopardize both physical and psychological health. There can be little doubt that many people would be much healthier if they were to opt out of an unhealthy relationship. Although divorce is often a major stressor, many divorced people adjust to a new lifestyle and end up healthier and better adjusted than many of those who opt to remain in a conflictual or violent marital relationship (Frude 1991).

WHY DO GOOD RELATIONSHIPS PROMOTE HEALTH?

How can we explain the association between a stable, intimate relationship and relatively good health? One explanation is that people who are in a secure relationship are likely to have a greater sense of well-being than those who lack a partner, and that as a result they may be less vulnerable to stress. Another suggestion is that a partner may be useful during critical periods, for example when the individual faces a major life change. One way in which a partner may help is by listening to the person's worries and providing informal therapy. In their study of the social origins of depression among women, Brown and Harris (1978) found that the presence of an intimate and confidant was associated with a relatively low impact of stressful events.

People often 'consult' their partners when they are under emotional strain, and many report that they derive great comfort from their partner's counsel and that it helps them to survive a

crisis. Health and counselling professionals are often a 'last resort' for those who seek help for psychological problems. Relatives, friends, work colleagues, neighbours, volunteer helpers (for example, the Samaritans) and other professionals (for example, ministers of religion) are frequently used as counsellors, advisors and 'sounding boards'. However, when people are asked whom they 'really depend on' when personal problems arise, they are more likely to cite their partner than anyone else (Griffith 1985). Informal psychotherapy is a feature of the majority of marriages and it has been found that those who are satisfied with their partner's 'therapeutic' efforts are likely to be satisfied with the marriage as a whole (Nye & McLaughlin 1982).

The presence of a partner may also contribute to health because of its regulatory effect. Partners, relatives and close friends often encourage a person to comply with certain 'rules' and help them to refrain from dangerous activities (Tucker & Mueller 2000). Thus a partner will often keep a watchful eye on an individual's smoking and drinking, encouraging them to eat well, to exercise regularly, to attend for medical checkups and to comply with medical advice. People who are socially isolated do not receive the mixture of encouragement and censure that helps others to check any excessive or dangerous behaviour. Although it may not be experienced as pleasant or useful being on the receiving end of frequent 'nagging' about the need to lead a healthy and ordered life, it is undoubtedly beneficial for many people. Those who do not have a partner to support them in this way are more likely to lead disordered lives and to expose themselves to danger. Thus many of those who are newly divorced eat and sleep irregularly, smoke, and drink to excess.

THE FAMILY UNIT

So far, family relationships (especially marital relationships) have been considered in terms of their costs and benefits to the individual. Thus we have maintained an individual perspective, considering the family as a 'context' or 'backdrop' that can help to explain variations in health and well-being. In the second part of this chapter, a somewhat different perspective on the family will be adopted. Families are not merely 'backdrops for individuals'. Neither are they simply collections of individual people. A family is a unit in which 'the whole is greater than the sum of the parts'. A family unit, indeed, can be viewed as if it were an organism in which the individual family members are constituent elements. The organism metaphor can be a fruitful one, for it leads to a number of interesting questions. What are the anatomical features of this type of organism? What is known of its physiology? What is known of the life cycle? What variations are there between different organisms (families)? And what forms of pathology are found?

Like organisms, families pass through a developmental sequence or 'career'. They are 'formed', they undergo changes, and in the end they 'die'. Some analysts divide the 'family life cycle' into a number of stages. Duvall (1977), for example, formulated eight stages, starting with the married couple who have no children and ending with the ageing family – a stage that lasts from retirement until death. Such models are clearly oversimplified, but they can be useful in mapping broad patterns of change and identifying common problems at particular stages of development. Thus the pressures typically experienced by 'young families' are somewhat different from those faced by families with adolescent children.

Families (like organisms) must adapt in response to both internal and external changes. The birth of a first child, for example, presents the couple with many new tasks and gives them new roles as parents. The family boundary becomes extended to include the infant, and there are marked changes in the nature of the couple's interactions. The original two-person ('dyadic') relationship (i.e. the couple) is replaced by three dyadic relationships (mother–father, mother–infant and father–infant) and one 'triadic' relationship. Even with this simple arrangement we can begin to get some idea of the 'reverberations' that occur within families. For example, a change in an infant's behaviour or health is likely to bring changes to the mother–infant relationship. These

changes may then affect the relationship between the parents, and the changed interparental relationship is then likely to affect the infant. This provides an example of the reverberations that occur constantly throughout the family system.

The elements within a family system are not just the individual family members but also the relationships between them, and any change in one individual or one relationship will be likely to have effects on all other elements and on the 'tone' or 'atmosphere' of the family as a whole. Another metaphor which may be useful at this point is that of the family as a 'hanging mobile'. Such a mobile consists of a frame, the various suspended items (or 'elements'), and the strings by which these elements are suspended from the frame. Any change in one element will affect every other element as well as the position and movement of the mobile as a whole. It is impossible to move any element without having a global effect on the mobile. Furthermore, it is impossible to move any one element without affecting all of the other elements and the resulting movements will reverberate back to affect the element that was originally moved.

Within a family system, any change such as an 'entrance' (a child being born; an elderly relative coming to live in the home) or an 'exit' (the death of a family member; an adolescent leaving) will have profound effects on individual family members. It will also affect the relationships between them and may completely transform the family interaction patterns. Thus in a family in which there is normally a good deal of hostility and open conflict, the knowledge that one family member is seriously ill may bring a period of apparent harmony and a cessation of hostilities. A family member who has previously appeared selfish and unhelpful may suddenly change to become cooperative and helpful. Such changes will affect the overall 'family atmosphere'. A crisis, such as that precipitated by a serious illness, inevitably brings many changes to the family. Some families become stronger, more united, and function better than ever before, whereas others become disorganized and lose their ability to function effectively. Any family can be expected to experience several 'entrances' and 'exits' throughout a lifetime, and many other changes will also alter the pattern of family relationships. Over a 30–40-year span there may be a complete reversal in roles, as the once-helpless infants grow towards middle-age and perhaps eventually taking on the care of their aged parents. The normal processes of family development demand major changes in interaction patterns. But in addition to such expected, or 'normative' changes, many families also experience exceptional circumstances such as the birth of a disabled child or the sudden death of a young parent that require extraordinary adaptations.

STRUCTURAL DIFFERENCES BETWEEN FAMILIES

There are many different ways of classifying families. One obvious variation is that of structure. Some families are single-parent units while others are two-parent families. Some families are childless, some have a single child, some have two children, etc. Families also differ in terms of their stage of development. Thus there are new partnerships without children, families with young children, families with adolescent children, and 'empty nest' families in which all of the children have grown to adulthood and left home. Working out a comprehensive system for classifying families, even in such concrete structural terms, is not easy because we would have to include families that include three or even four generations, step-families (sometimes known as 'reconstituted families') and homosexual partnerships with and without children living in the home. There has been a notable broadening of 'family configurations' in recent decades, and only a minority of families now fit into the traditional 'married couple with their children' category.

DIFFERENCES IN FAMILY INTERACTION STYLES

There are many contexts in which it is useful to group families in terms of their structural characteristics (for example, when addressing social policy issues). However, families that share a common structural characteristic may differ markedly in terms of the interactions between family members. Psychologists are typically less interested in structural aspects than in interactional and relationship characteristics and therefore tend to differentiate families in terms of their 'character' or 'interactive style'. Thus psychologists may differentiate between 'harmonious' and 'conflictual' families or between 'depressed families' and 'non-depressed families'.

There are of course many thousands of characteristics such as these that might be used to distinguish families, although it is likely that some of them will be far more useful than others. Thankfully, a wealth of research evidence, as well as clinical experience, points to two dimensions that are particularly useful in differentiating family interaction styles. The two dimensions that emerge consistently as providing a useful basis for classification are 'adaptability' and 'cohesion'. 'Adaptability' refers to the family's ability to change its structure, roles and rules when adjustment is called for. 'Cohesion' relates to the degree of emotional bonding between family members and to their independence and autonomy.

According to the 'Circumplex Model' devised by Olson and his colleagues (Olson 2000, Olson et al 1979), families can be classified into one of four 'types' on each of the two key dimensions. On the 'adaptability' dimension, the classification proceeds from one extreme – 'rigid' – through 'structured' and then 'flexible' to the other extreme – 'chaotic'. On the 'cohesion' dimension, the classification proceeds from one extreme – 'enmeshed' – through 'connected' and then 'separated' to the other extreme – 'disengaged'. The labels used for the extremes of each dimension were chosen to convey the belief that all extreme positions are relatively 'unhealthy'. Thus families at either end of the adaptability dimension (i.e. either rigid or chaotic) are likely to experience special problems, particularly when they face a need to change. Families classified in terms of the middle positions on the adaptability dimension (i.e. structured and flexible families) would be expected to respond to change more effectively.

In 'rigid' families each member maintains fixed roles and rarely strays into another person's allocated role. The family has set ways of doing things. The power structure within such families is inflexible, leadership is authoritarian, and discipline is managed in an autocratic way. 'Rules are rules' and compromise is rare. At the other extreme, chaotic families have few clear rules. Lacking established patterns of action and inter-action, they are constantly having to work out how to do things. Because there is no clear alloca-tion of special roles or responsibilities between members, for example, discussion will be needed (and conflict may result) whenever a chore needs to be done. The power structure within such fam-ilies is unstable, and there is no reliable mutual support between family members. The lack of rules is likely to lead to frequent confusion and, in the face of erratic and inconsistent parental discipline, children are likely to lack guidance.

The other dimension in the Circumplex Model is 'cohesion'. Families that are very low in terms of cohesion are said to be 'disengaged' while those that have extremely high cohesion are described as 'enmeshed'. Families classified in positions between these extremes are described either as 'separated' or as 'connected'. The two mid-positions on the cohesion dimension are associ-ated with relatively good family functioning. Connected and separated families, in their differ-ent ways, avoid the lack of family unity and fam-ily feeling typical of disengaged families, while also avoiding the suffocating closeness found in enmeshed families. Members of enmeshed fami-lies identify with the family so closely, and the bonds between members are so tight, that indi-viduals have little sense of personal identity (Amerikaner et al 1994).

DYSFUNCTIONAL FAMILIES

Many families can be identified as occupying an extreme position on one of the two dimensions of adaptability and cohesion. Some families, indeed, occupy extreme positions on both dimensions (they may be rigid–disengaged, rigid–enmeshed, chaotic–disengaged or chaotic–enmeshed). A fam-ily placed at an extreme on one or both dimen-sions is likely to have difficulty in maintaining a good level of functioning and in providing for the needs and personal growth of family members.

Dysfunctional families may well develop prob-lems even without external pressures, and they are certainly unlikely to function well in the face of severe stress. Such families are likely to experi-ence a crisis when they are under pressure and the health of family members may suffer as a result (Schulz et al 1996).

Dysfunctional families provide a major chal-lenge for the health professional. Enmeshed fam-ilies tend to be 'closed' to the outside world and are so used to keeping themselves to themselves that they are likely to regard all agencies and pro-fessionals with suspicion and disdain. The tight-knit nature of enmeshed families may mean that when one person becomes seriously ill, every other family member feels personally stricken. At the other extreme, in a disengaged family, there is little family feeling. When one member becomes ill, the others may resent the inconvenience and may attempt to carry on their own lives regard-less of their relative's illness or disability. The professional cannot rely on such families to offer significant emotional and practical support to the patient. If a child or adult from a disengaged family is hospitalized, for example, the other family members may prefer the patient to remain in hospital until completely recovered.

The two extremes on the adaptability dimension are labelled 'rigid' and 'chaotic'. Faced with the ill-ness of one family member, a rigid family will find it difficult, or even impossible, to make appropriate adaptations. If the father is incapacitated, for exam-ple, his routine tasks will be left undone. No-one will attempt, temporarily, to 'step into his shoes'. The family will find it very difficult to make allowances for the new situation and to evolve ways of dealing with new demands. Eventually, family life may become untenable. The challenge for the health professional is to help such a family to modify its rules and interactional patterns so that the patient is protected from undue pressure to 'carry on as normal'. At the other extreme, chaotic families present a different kind of chal-lenge. The fact that they have very few established patterns of interaction, or problem solving, means that they are unlikely to be effective in dealing with a crisis such as a serious illness. Such families are unable to 'get their act together' even in normal circumstances and are likely to be completely thrown when a threatening situation arises. There may be a willingness to help the patient, but because family members hardly ever consult one another or engage in forward planning, their attempts to adapt to a changed situation are unlikely to be effective (Kashani et al 1995). To assist such families in providing patient care, it may be necessary for professionals to make highly specific suggestions concerning the timetabling and allocation of tasks. The normal assumption that a family will work out its own routines and devise strategies for handing over responsibility, etc. does not apply to families that are extremely chaotic in their organization.

Some families that manage to adapt fairly well to a patient's illness have difficulty in readjusting when the patient is recovering. Thus a patient in a family of this type may be maintained in the patient role long after they have returned to health. In some cases an individual's recovery from a physical or psychiatric illness threatens to disturb a precarious and convenient equilibrium within the family, and the family as a whole may then have a 'vested interest' in the patient remaining unwell. Family therapists have long recognized the fact that an illness may be 'useful' to a family (for example, by postponing serious long-term arguments that threaten to destroy the family). Family therapy addresses such issues by dealing with the family system as a whole (Carr 2000, Dallos & Draper 2000). All families maintain certain 'myths', most of which are harmless and some of which are constructive. When a family member is seriously ill, for example, many families develop positive myths about the quality of service they are receiving. They may regard their general practitioner as a leading authority in a highly specialized field, for instance, or imagine that the local clinic is internationally renowned for its treatment of the illness from which their relative is suffering. For the most part, such myths instil hope, alleviate anxiety, and contribute to good relations between the family and professionals. However, some families subscribe to a 'rescue myth' which can encourage passivity. Families that subscribe to this myth might believe that they only have to wait and maintain a 'helpless' stance and someone will come to provide all the necessary help, to rescue them from their predicament, and to solve all of their problems. Any professional who comes into contact with the family may therefore be considered as a candidate for the role of 'saviour'. Family members may believe that there is little point in actively seeking to improve the current situation before the 'saviour' arrives on the scene and takes over (McDaniel et al 1999).

Other families develop more hostile myths about the professionals involved in the patient's care and the quality of service being provided. Services and professionals are 'demonized' and blamed for any problems or deterioration in the patient's health. Such myths may jeopardize the patient's recovery in a number of ways, for example by lowering family morale, or reducing compliance with medical advice. It is important to recognize that some families have well-established suspicions about all aspects of health care and that these may lead to one or more professionals being unfairly 'scapegoated' by the family.

HEALTHY FAMILIES

Well-functioning, or 'healthy', families occupy the middle ground in terms of both adaptability and cohesion. They are neither rigid nor chaotic, neither disengaged nor enmeshed. Family members have reasonably warm and close relationships with one another, each identifying with the family as a whole and having some sense of 'family pride'. Within such families, members share common goals. There is a general air of solidarity, but each person is also allowed to be an individual. Healthy families act as 'open' systems and are willing to accept help and advice from external sources. They interact with neighbours and feel integrated within the wider social community. They welcome professional help but are appropriately assertive when they feel that the level of service being provided falls short of the ideal. They do not regard professionals as 'saviours' and maintain an active role in the patient's care.

Healthy families share power fairly, and everyone is encouraged to share their opinions and feelings. Such a sharing of power, however, does not mean that all members are treated as equals. The parents work together as a unit in the care and control of their children. Roles within the family are clearly differentiated and are complementary. Tasks are assigned fairly and appropriately to particular individuals, but some degree of flexibility is maintained so that when one person is unavailable another person is able to take on some of his or her responsibilities. Family 'rules' are understood and supported by all family members, and infringements of these rules are confronted openly. Appropriate sanctions are applied firmly but without hostility or vindictiveness. Family rules are changed when necessary (for example as children get older) and such changes are brought about through a process of negotiation (Carr 2000).

Communication within healthy families is open and effective. Questions are clearly asked and plainly answered, and all transactions have a clear beginning, middle and end (in that order!). Family members are able to disclose their opinions, hopes and fears without anxiety and there is also a healthy respect for an individual's (or the couple's) privacy. Any conflicts that arise are usually resolved by negotiation and compromise. Healthy families are able to deal effectively with a wide range of challenges, for they have at their disposal a wide repertoire of effective coping strategies and are able to respond flexibly.

CONCLUSION

Although many families are devastated by serious troubles, in many cases both individuals and family units manage to endure the most formidable upsets and tragedies. Families often adapt to severe misfortune with remarkable resilience and resourcefulness. Thus despite the fact that family life often produces extreme anxiety, fear or depression, and despite the fact that many families break down in disarray, the majority display an impressive array of strategies for coping with changing circumstances. But when a family faces a sudden major change, or significant adversity, the inner resources of the system may not be

sufficient to maintain the equilibrium, and support from other sources – from relatives, neighbours, community organizations, and from professionals – can make a substantial contribution to the well-being of the family system and of the individuals who constitute the family group.

SUMMARY

- Family relationships are important determinants of an individual's physical health and psychological well-being.

- Families bring costs and benefits to the individual, but, on the whole, close relationships are seen as beneficial.

- There is a correlation between major adverse life changes and physical or psychological illness.

- The family should not be seen merely as a group of individuals, but as a unit in its own right, with events 'reverberating' around family members rather than affecting them on an individual basis.

- Families should be identified less by their structure and more by their 'adaptability' and 'cohesion'.

DISCUSSION POINTS

1. To what extent, and in what ways, does nursing practice (as you have experienced it) involve a consideration of family interactions, family influences and family styles?

2. Consider two women aged in their 30s. One is single (never married, with no children). The other is married with two young children. Discuss how their lifestyles might compare in terms of such factors as stress and social support.

3. How convinced are you that good relationships (especially with an adult partner) promote physical and psychological health – explain your answer?

4. Taking an example from a caseload, use the metaphor of 'the family as an organism' to explore some key aspects of family life.

5. Compare the interactional styles (and 'family atmospheres') of two contrasting families that you know reasonably well (either professionally or personally). Try to make use of the concepts from the 'Circumplex Model' in your account.

REFERENCES

Amerikaner M, Monks G, Wolfe P, Thomas S 1994 Family interaction and individual psychological health. Journal of Counseling and Development 72: 614–620

Argyle M, Henderson M 1985 The anatomy of relationships. Penguin, Harmondsworth

Bebbington P, Brugha T, Meltzer H, Farrell M, Ceresa C, Jenkins R, Lewis G 2000 Psychiatric disorder and dysfunction in the UK National Survey of Psychiatric Morbidity. Social Psychiatry and Psychiatric Epidemiology 35: 191–197

Ben-Shlomo Y, Smith GD, Shipley M, Marmot MG 1993 Magnitude and causes of mortality differences between married and unmarried men. Journal of Epidemiology and Community Health 47: 200–205

Bernard J 1973 The future of marriage. Bantam, New York

Bloom BL, Asher SR, White SW 1979 Marital disruption as a stressor. Psychological Bulletin 85: 867–894

Brown GW, Harris T 1978 The social origins of depression. Tavistock, London

Carr A 2000 Family therapy. Wiley, Chichester

Cohen S, Syme SL (eds) 1985 Social support and health. Academic Press, New York

Dallos R, Draper R 2000 An introduction to family therapy. Open University Press, Milton Keynes

Duvall E 1977 Marriage and family development. JB Lippincott, Philadelphia

Freedman JL 1978 Happy people. Harcourt Brace Jovanovich, New York

Frude NJ 1991 Understanding family problems: A psychological approach. Wiley, Chichester

Goldman N, Koreman S, Weinstein R 1995 Marital status and health among the elderly. Social Science and Medicine 40: 1717–1730

Griffith J 1985 Social support providers: Who are they? Where are they met? And the relationship of network characteristics to psychological distress. Basic and Applied Social Psychology 6: 41–49

Harper JM, Schaalje BG, Sandberg JG 2000 Daily hassles, intimacy, and marital quality in later life marriages. American Journal of Family Therapy 28: 1–18

Holmes TH, Rahe RH 1967 The social readjustment rating scales. Journal of Psychosomatic Research 11: 213–218

Kashani JH, Allan WD, Dahlmeier JM, Rezvani M 1995 An examination of family functioning utilizing the circumplex model in psychiatrically hospitalized children with depression. Journal of Affective Disorders 35: 65–73

Lillard LA, Waite LJ 1995 'Til death do us part: Marital disruption and mortality. American Journal of Sociology 100: 1131–1156

Maybery DJ, Graham D 2001 Hassles and uplifts: Including interpersonal events. Stress and Health 17: 91–104

McDaniel SH, Hepworth J, Doherty WJ 1999 The shared emotional themes of illness. Journal of Family Psychotherapy 10: 1–8

Nye FI 1982 Family relationships: Rewards and costs. Sage, Beverly Hills, CA

Nye FI, McLaughlin S 1982 Role competence and marital satisfaction. In: Nye FI (ed) Family relationships: Rewards and costs. Sage, Beverly Hills, CA

Olson DH 2000 Circumplex model of marital and family systems. Journal of Family Therapy 22: 144–167

Olson DH, Russell CS, Sprenkle DH 1979 Circumplex model of marital and family systems II: Empirical studies and clinical intervention. In: Vincent J (ed) Advances in family intervention, assessment and theory. JAI, Greenwich, CT

Richter V, Guthke J 1993 Life events as indicator of change in life and as risk factor for cardiovascular heart disease. In: Schroeder H, Reschke K (eds) Health psychology: Potential in diversity. Roderer Verlag, Regensburg

Rigazio-DiGilio SA, Cramer BD 2000 Families with learning disabilities, physical disabilities, and other childhood challenges. In: Nichols WC, Pace-Nichols MA (eds) Handbook of family development and intervention. Wiley, New York, NY

Ruben DH 1998 Social exchange theory: Dynamics of a system governing the dysfunctional family and guide to assessment. Journal of Contemporary Psychotherapy 28: 307–325

Schulz KH, Schulz H, Schulz O, von Kerekjarto M 1996 Family structure and psychosocial stress in families of cancer patients. In: Baider L and Cooper CL (eds) Cancer and the family. Wiley, New York, NY

Tucker JS, Mueller JS 2000 Spouses' social control of health behaviors: Use and effectiveness of specific strategies. Personality and Social Psychology Bulletin 26: 1120–1130

Tucker JS, Schwartz JE, Clark KM, Friedman HS 1999 Age-related changes in the associations of social network ties with mortality risk. Psychology and Aging 14: 564–571

Veevers JE, Mitchell BA 1998 Intergenerational exchanges and perceptions of support within "boomerang kid" family environments. International Journal of Aging and Human Development 46: 91–108

Wood W, Rhodes N, Whelan M 1989 Sex differences in positive wellbeing: A consideration of emotional style and marital status. Psychological Bulletin 106: 249–264

FURTHER READING

Frude NJ 1991 Understanding family problems: a psychological approach. Wiley, Chichester

This book reviews a number of major family problems. It considers how and why these problems arise, how families attempt to cope with them and how professionals can best help families to deal with them. Four major areas are covered: illness and handicap, conflict and violence, separation and divorce, and dying and bereavement.

10

Violence within the family

N. Frude

KEY ISSUES

◆ Different forms and consequences of violence.

◆ Explanations of family violence.

◆ Women and children as long-term victims of family violence.

◆ Abuse of older people.

◆ Intervention and help.

INTRODUCTION

There are many forms of abuse within families, including physical (injurious) abuse, sexual abuse, emotional abuse, and neglect. Abuse may take place between members of the same generation (marital abuse or sibling abuse) or between different generations (e.g. child abuse by parents, or elder abuse).

Table 10.1 provides an overview of some forms of family-based abuse. The columns specify particular forms of abuse and the rows specify the family relationship between the victim and the perpetrator. It would not be difficult to quote cases which illustrate each of the 16 boxes in the grid in Table 10.1. Box 10 for example, would include marital rape, and Box 16 would include cases in which the needs of elderly people are neglected by other family members.

This chapter will begin with a discussion of violence within the family and will proceed to consider four types of family violence; marital violence, the physical and sexual abuse of children and abuse of older people.

Table 10.1 An overview of some forms of family-based abuse

	Physical	Sexual	Emotional	Neglect
Parent to child	1	2	3	4
Sibling	5	6	7	8
Marital	9	10	11	12
Elderly	13	14	15	16

VIOLENCE WITHIN THE FAMILY

The family is the setting for a substantial proportion of the violence that occurs within society. Most estimates agree that in any average week at least two children in the UK die as a result of a violent attack by a parent or caregiver; many more women are seriously injured as a result of marital battering than as a result of road accidents and street violence; and violence is a significant cause of bruising and more severe injuries among older people living with relatives. Estimates of the prevalence of the various forms of family violence depend to a great extent on the definitions used, and on diagnostic criteria, but it is clear from all of the available evidence that many forms of family violence are all too common.

EXPLANATIONS OF FAMILY VIOLENCE

The issue of how family violence is best explained is somewhat controversial. Some authorities consider violence in families to be a 'natural' effect of the kind of society in which we live, and a reflection of the attitudes that adults generally have towards children and that men generally have towards women. Others, while not denying the relevance of the cultural climate, suggest that acts of domestic violence are 'deviant' behaviours that are best explained as aggressive responses to interpersonal conflict. Such 'interactional' explanations account for physical abuse by focusing on the relationships and interactions between the assailant and the victim, particularly in conflict and disciplinary situations, and attribute the violence to the assailant's high level of anger and low level of inhibition regarding the aggressive assault.

In trying to understand particular incidents of family violence it is useful to bear in mind the distinction between hostile and instrumental violence. Hostile violence is driven by anger and the principal motive for the action is that of hurting the victim. Instrumental violence is driven principally by a desire for certain 'gains', with aggression being used merely as a means to this end. Thus the 'mugger' is aggressive not because

he wishes to hurt his victim but because he believes that his attack will enable him to steal money. Some incidents of family violence are best explained as examples of instrumental aggression. A husband may be violent towards his wife, for example, because he believes that violence will enable him to 'get his own way' or that violence will help to maintain 'a reign of terror' that will allow him to dominate his wife. Instrumental violence may also be used strategically to 'teach' the wife that a beating will follow if she criticizes, makes claims on resources, or refuses any demand.

On the other hand, most incidents of marital violence, physical child abuse, and elder abuse are probably best understood as examples of hostile aggression. Typically, one person does something which makes another person very angry and, in the absence of sufficient inhibitions, the angry person then assaults the victim. This simple model suggests that in order to understand the nature of family violence we need to understand anger triggers, the way in which individuals judge (or 'appraise') other people's behaviour, the dynamics of anger, and inhibitions against physical violence. The model also suggests that effective interventions might involve strategies for reducing anger, for increasing inhibitions, and for maintaining self-control (Frude 1991).

The interactional model will form the basis for much of the analysis provided in this chapter, and the discussion will focus, for the most part, on hostile rather than on instrumental violence. Four types of family violence will be examined – marital violence, physical child abuse, child sexual abuse and elder abuse. But first we will consider the general issue of why violent assaults occur so frequently in so many families.

WHY IS THERE SO MUCH VIOLENCE WITHIN THE FAMILY?

One reason why family violence may be considerably more common than street violence, or violence towards neighbours, friends and work colleagues, is that contact between family members is prolonged and is often intense. People who live together, eat together, sleep together and play together will be in close proximity for so much of the time that strong emotions, including anger, are likely to be generated at least occasionally. In addition, family members are locked into the family situation. It is possible to avoid or to walk away from an annoying stranger, but a demanding child, or a crying baby, cannot be avoided or ignored.

Irritating behaviours such as constant 'complaints' or 'nags' by one partner about the other, a child's persistent attention seeking, or a baby's continual 'grizzling', are likely to lead to extreme annoyance. Family members are interdependent, and the behaviour of one of them can affect everyone else. A person who invests a lot of time and energy in helping or caring for others is likely to feel aggrieved if there is no appreciation of the effort involved. Babies, children and the elderly infirm, especially, demand a great deal of attention and their care involves considerable 'costs' to carers in terms of time, effort and money. In such circumstances it is not difficult to appreciate that a carer might become angry in response to an apparent lack of gratitude or when additional demands are made. Thus a parent who is finding it difficult to cope with a demanding child may become angry if an infant soils a nappy immediately following a change, or if a child refuses to eat food that has taken a long time to prepare.

Anger may also result when there is a conflict over the allocation of space, money or other resources, and such disputes may be especially bitter if the relevant resources are very limited (for example, if the family is poor). Thus some marital fights concern money, with one partner being accused of wasting money (for example, on drink or gambling). Other conflicts focus on the allocation of duties, responsibilities and household chores. Those who feel that they are being exploited or are being 'taken for granted' are likely to object, and their complaint will often generate an angry response. Conflicts on such matters may escalate, with accusations being made and insults thrown, until one person becomes physically violent and attacks the other.

Anger is often preceded by the judgement that someone has behaved badly or has 'broken a rule'. Family life is governed by so many unwritten 'rules' that these are likely to be broken frequently even in families that function well. Thus accusations of rule-breaking (or 'transgressions') are likely to feature prominently in family interactions. Such accusations are usually expressed in terms of what a person 'should' or 'should not' have done. The person being accused in this way is likely to defend himself or herself and may make a protestation of innocence or a counter-accusation. Real or supposed transgressions frequently initiate an episode that ultimately results in violence. Some parents even judge that very young babies are guilty of rule-breaking and regard certain aspects of the infant's behaviour as 'naughty' and 'blameworthy'.

Family violence is not simply a reflection of the fact that family situations frequently generate anger, but also reflects the fact that people have relatively few inhibitions in the home situation. In most other contexts expressions of anger are regularly inhibited, or at least 'toned down', but people often have few reservations about expressing their disagreement with other members of the family, making complaints to them, or even threatening them. In contrast to a disagreement arising in a work situation, for example, or a dispute with a neighbour, family conflicts may involve little verbal sparring before a rapid onslaught of insults and disparagements focuses on particularly sensitive areas. Family members know about each other's vulnerabilities and therefore have the 'advantage' of being able to inflict maximum hurt.

Furthermore, inhibitions against physical aggression are often particularly low in family situations, and many people feel justified in behaving aggressively towards family members within the home. Parents may believe that it is their right to physically discipline children by smacking them, and some men maintain that they have a right to physically abuse a wife who has 'misbehaved'. If pushing, pulling or slapping a relative is regarded as acceptable, and becomes habitual, then regular low-level physical aggression may occasionally escalate to a dangerous level to include punches, kicks and the use of weapons. In addition, many other constraints which normally inhibit violence towards strangers, may be absent in the family situation. For example, a man may assume that, if he were to attack his wife, his child, or his aged mother, his actions would not come to the attention of the police. In addition, his physical size and strength may eliminate any fear of physical reprisal by his victim. If previous assaults have passed without serious repercussions, then inhibitions about a further assault may be particularly low.

Thus it appears that family aggression is relatively common because a good deal of anger is generated in family situations and because there are relatively few inhibitions that prevent this anger from being expressed in the form of physical aggression.

MARITAL VIOLENCE

There is enormous variation in the estimates of the incidence of marital violence, largely as a result of the different criteria used to define 'violence'. According to national US surveys, when 'violence' is defined to include slapping, pushing and more serious forms of attack, around a sixth of all couples experience violence within any given 12 month period (Straus & Gelles 1986). Such surveys suggest that 30% of women will be victims of intimate-partner violence during their lifetime and that over 50% of these will suffer some form of physical injury as a result of an assault by their partner (Centers for Disease Control 1998). The rate of 'marital' abuse is significantly higher for cohabiting couples than for married couples (Brownridge & Halli 2000), perhaps because cohabiting relationships are less well defined and may generate frequent confrontations regarding the issue of commitment. Although some women do attack their male partners, it is clear that many more women than men are injured as a result of marital violence. Aggressive behaviour by a woman against her partner will rarely lead to serious injury, and female aggression is often retaliatory (Hamberger et al 1994). It has been estimated that marital violence is the single most common source of serious injury to women, being responsible for more injuries than road accidents, muggings and rape combined (Stark & Flitcraft 1988).

Two principal models are used to explain marital violence. The sociological model suggests that wife battering is a socially approved strategy that reflects patriarchy and is used to maintain women in an inferior position in society (Dobash & Dobash 1979). The psychological interaction model regards marital abuse as a hostile aggressive attack by an assailant on a victim, usually following a conflictual encounter between the two (Frude 1994). It is important to recognize that although the interactional model attempts to explain violent attacks as the outcome of the behaviour of both the aggressor and the victim, the blame for the violence is attributed solely to the assailant.

THE INTERACTIONAL EXPLANATION

Psychological accounts of marital violence suggest that the majority of cases of wife beating arise out of marital conflict and that most violent marriages are generally difficult and quarrelsome. Many men who beat their wives have extreme and objectionable views about how a wife should behave and judge many of the woman's actions as 'out of order'. If a man judges his wife to be unsupportive, or believes that she is failing to provide him with due attention, consideration, power, or privileges, the extreme hostility that he feels may lead to physical aggression. The issue of power is clearly central to this analysis, and a wide status difference between the partners is associated with a higher frequency of violence, particularly if the man has lower status than his wife (Holtzworth-Munroe et al 1997).

The marriages of assailant–victim couples are generally tense and conflict-ridden, and aggressive attacks usually arise out of conflicts and arguments (Goldsmith 1990). There is generally little powersharing within such relationships, and little discussion or negotiation. Studies have shown that even in those arguments that do not end in violence, physically abusive husbands are likely to be hostile and offensive in their manner and to accuse their wives of many misdemeanours. Conflicts between at-risk couples tend to escalate rapidly, and both partners may fight 'unfairly', each attacking their partner's self-esteem and making serious assertions about the other person's conduct or personality. Many abusive husbands are aggressive not only to their wives but also to their children, to neighbours, and to relatives and strangers (Holtzworth-Munroe et al 1997). They are likely to be jealous (sexual jealousy often features in dangerous conflicts), and they are typically low in self-esteem (Holtzworth-Munroe & Anglin 1991). Such men also have a high 'need for power' (Mason & Blankenship 1987, Rosenbaum & O'Leary 1981) and they usually hold strong traditional ('sexist') attitudes regarding women and marriage (Frieze & McHugh 1992).

THE VIOLENT INCIDENT

Gelles (1987) maintains that an assailant's attack is almost always 'spontaneous' (i.e. not planned), 'justified' from the abuser's perspective, and 'interactional' (a reaction to some aspect of the victim's behaviour). (This last characteristic, which suggests that the victim's behaviour plays a key role in precipitating the attack, does *not* mean that the victim is responsible for the violence.) Marital abuse frequently results from conflicts over such issues as child discipline, meals, chores, and alcohol, sexual conduct or performance and money (Dobash & Dobash 1979; Pahl 1985).

Gelles found that physical attacks were often precipitated by some aspect of the victim's verbal behaviour (including criticizing, name-calling, or gibes about sexual performance) and that these usually reflected the victim's own extreme anger. Partners become experts at identifying each other's weaknesses, and when one decides to 'go for the jugular' or to 'hit below the belt', then the other is likely to regard the allegations as outrageous and highly offensive. A man who feels that his wife's verbal attacks against him are vicious will often, in his rage, feel that he is fully justified in beating her.

Alcohol is often implicated in marital violence. Drunkenness may be a cause for complaint, and alcohol tends to reduce inhibitions, so that a person who is both angry and intoxicated is likely to attack in a violent and uncontrolled way. The abuse of alcohol is often a key factor in marital abuse and efforts to control the drink problem may be highly effective in preventing further attacks on the partner (O'Farrell & Murphy 1995).

THE FORM OF VIOLENCE

Marital abuse may involve slaps, kicks, hair-pulling, punches to the limbs or abdomen, or blows to the head. Although extreme anger may lead to an 'all out' attack in which the woman is badly beaten by her partner who is totally out of control, some men modulate their attack so that they 'only go so far' and inflict injuries that are less severe or inflicted only on some parts of the body. Thus some men avoid inflicting injuries, such as a black eye, that will later draw attention to their brutality. Assailants typically maintain idiosyncratic guidelines regarding 'legitimate' and 'illegitimate' forms of aggression (examples of personal 'rules' regarding violence against wives include: 'a woman should never be hit in the stomach or face' or 'it's ok to punch or kick but you should never use a knife').

INTERVENTION

The physical and psychological effects of marital abuse are often extremely severe, and once a relationship has become violent there is a high probability of recurrent attacks. The availability of shelters or refuges is a major contribution to the safety of women and children, but around half of those who enter a shelter eventually return to live with the man who attacked them. Various forms of 'treatment' have been developed, some of which focus principally on the violent husband (e.g. anger control training) and some of which focus on the victim's need to develop an effective 'personal safety plan'. A number of extensive couple-based intervention programmes aim to modify the couple's conflict interactions, to teach the assaultive husband anger-control techniques, and to help the victim to promote her own safety (Heyman & Neidig 1997). Changes in social policy and law enforcement practices in recent decades (for example, the setting up of police domestic violence units and the widespread adoption of a 'zero tolerance' philosophy) may have gone some way to reducing the extreme danger that so many women face within their own home, but this effect has been minimal. There is clearly a great deal more that needs to be done.

PHYSICAL CHILD ABUSE

DEFINITION AND PREVALENCE

Most estimates of the prevalence of the physical abuse of children are based on extrapolations from injuries that are known to have been deliberately inflicted. Such methods, however, may lead to a serious underestimation, since only a proportion of injuries to children are ever reported, and some which are said to be accidental probably do result from a parental attack. Some people maintain that any assault on a child which leaves a bruise should count as a case of physical child abuse, while others go further and insist that any form of physical disciplining constitutes physical abuse (in which case over 90% of parents in the UK might be described as 'abusive' – Nobes & Smith 1997, Nobes et al 1999). Physical methods of discipline are used in the majority of homes and the average child is subjected to hundreds or maybe thousands of slaps before he or she reaches adolescence. The definition of physical child abuse is therefore a matter of some controversy. Some people equate abuse with any physical disciplining method while others maintain a sharp distinction between such 'ordinary' behaviours and those which cause serious injury to a child.

DEMOGRAPHIC PATTERNS

Focusing on serious assaults (those which result in some degree of injury to a child), roughly equal numbers of boys and girls are victims of attacks made by a parent or caregiver, and the attacker is equally likely to be a man or a woman. Babies and young children are much more likely to be injured by their parents than older children (hence the term 'baby battering' originally used to describe physical child abuse), partly because the very young are physically more vulnerable, but also because babies are very demanding and need continuous care. They cry a lot, the reason for their crying is not always easy to judge, and it is impossible to 'reason' with them or to cajole, beg or threaten them in order to gain compliance. Factors associated with a relatively high risk of physical abuse include poor accommodation, poverty, marital instability and social isolation. At one stage it was hoped that information about such correlates (or 'risk identifiers') would permit the 'high-risk' families to be recognized before any damage had been done to the child, but attempts at formulating a useful 'risk index' in this way have proved impractical (Browne & Saqi 1988).

AN EXPLANATION OF PHYSICAL CHILD ABUSE

According to the interactional model of physical child abuse (Frude 1980, 1991, Kadushin & Martin 1981) physical abuse is best understood as a form of aggression, a hostile attack made by an angry parent who has been intensely annoyed, usually by some action of the child victim. The child's behaviour triggers a high degree of parental anger so that, in the absence of effective inhibitions against attacking the child, an assault will occur. The suggestion that the victim's behaviour plays an important role in the events leading up to an attack does not mean, of course, that children are to be held responsible for the injuries that they suffer. Certain children, however, are more vulnerable to attack than others by virtue of their physical characteristics, their behavioural style, and their response to the parents' attempts at discipline (Martin 1976). Parents who are at high risk of abusing a child include those with an aggressive personality, those who have poor child-care and disciplining skills, those whose beliefs about children are inappropriate, and those who generally lack self control (Frude 1991).

Briefly, the interactional model of physical child abuse suggests that a poor parent–child relationship is likely to lead to disciplinary problems, and that frequent and badly handled disciplinary encounters are likely to escalate in seriousness and may lead to habitual low-level aggression. Against such a background, it is suggested, it is likely that on one or more occasions the aggressive parent will lose control and attack the child so severely that the child is injured. A fuller account of this model has been provided elsewhere (Frude 1989a, 1991).

THE EFFECTS OF PHYSICAL ABUSE ON THE VICTIM

Some physically abused children die as a result of a parental attack, others are permanently scarred, and some sustain serious brain damage. Even where there are no external injuries, an action such as the parent shaking the child severely may lead to neurological damage (Shepherd & Sampson 2000, Showers 1992). Blows to the head can also result in permanent visual impairments, and intraocular bleeding can lead to retinal scarring, squints and a loss in visual acuity (Lynch 1988).

Abused children show a higher incidence of various types of behavioural disturbance, although some of these may predate the abuse (a child's high level of aggressiveness, for example, may be the result of abuse or may have been a contributing factor leading up to the abusive incident). Compared to nonabused children, for example, abused children show relatively high rates of bedwetting, tantrums, aggression, 'oppositional behaviour', social withdrawal, disturbed attachment to parents, depression, low self-esteem, self-destructive behaviour, and suicide attempts (Cicchetti & Toth 1995).

However, no psychological symptom or syndrome inevitably follows abuse, and some children who are abused, including some who suffer serious injuries, appear not to show any significant psychological effects. As Wolfe (1987) notes: '…a remarkable number of children seem capable of adapting successfully to extremely traumatic and stressful situations'. The degree of disturbance caused by physical abuse depends on such factors as the number and severity of attacks, the age of the child, and the quality of the

everyday relationship between the parents and the child. Protracted legal proceedings and a history of frequent placement changes are associated with a relatively poor outcome (Lynch 1988), while factors associated with a positive outcome include the child's retention of a basic sense of 'trust' in adults and the presence of supportive relatives (Wolfe 1987).

Many victims of physical child abuse show evidence of delinquency during adolescence and, in adulthood, victims as a group have a relatively high rate of convictions for violent crimes (including murder and rape) as well as an increased rate of suicide (Briere 1992, Malinosky-Rummell & Hansen 1993, Stevenson 1999). However, although victims are over-represented in these troubled and troublesome groups, it needs to be stressed that only a minority of abused children go on to lead a life of crime or violence. It is therefore very important to avoid the suggestion that an abused child is somehow destined to lead a life of assaultive lawbreaking. Although victims may be at greater risk than nonvictims of becoming perpetrators of family assaults, most abused children do not grow up to become abusive parents or abusive partners.

THERAPY FOR ABUSIVE FAMILIES

Some parents confide to a professional that they are under considerable stress and that their child may be at risk, and many different types of treatment can be offered to such high-risk families. Parents who frequently use severe and dangerous methods of disciplining, for example, can be guided towards the use of more refined techniques that are not only more appropriate but are also much more effective. Parents may also be helped to develop effective childcare skills, to manage their anger, and to formulate a range of 'escape tactics' for emergency use when they feel that they might attack the child (Browne & Herbert 1997, Stevenson 1999, Veltkamp & Miller 1994). Some parents have strong propunishment attitudes and these may need to be challenged directly by parent education programmes (Cowen 2001).

Various techniques, including behavioural, cognitive, counselling and family therapy techniques, have been incorporated into intervention pro-grammes. Although such programmes are often successful in bringing about positive change, it is often considered necessary for the child to be removed from the home, at least temporarily. While it is judged that there is a continuing risk of injury, the child may need to be accommo-dated elsewhere until it is judged that it is safe for the parents to resume their role as the principal caregivers (Dale et al 1986). The issue of removal is not easy, however, for there is evidence that this carries its own risk of adverse psychosocial effects on the child (Drach & Devoe 2000). (Other issues surrounding child protection, in the con-text of community nursing, are dealt with in more detail in Chapter 11.)

CHILD SEXUAL ABUSE

Sexual interference with a child is a crime which sickens, angers or frightens most people, includ-ing those who deal professionally with victims and perpetrators. However, perpetrators are less likely to reoffend, and child victims are more likely to receive the protection and help they need, if the professionals who deal with them have an understanding of the problem that is based on accurate information rather than on moral outrage.

Whatever criteria are employed to define sexual abuse, it is clear from prevalence estimates that sexual abuse is much more common than was imagined until recent times. It is also clear that inappropriate sexual attention leads many chil-dren to suffer greatly both during childhood and in the longer term (Haugaard & Repucci 1988, Stevenson 1999, Oddone-Paolucci et al 2001).

Most victims of sexual abuse are aged between 8 and 14 years, and girls are at somewhat greater risk than boys. It has always been understood that most perpetrators of sexual abuse are male, although it is now recognized that sexual abuse by females is by no means rare (Elliot 1996, Saradjian & Hanks 1996). Whereas physical abuse is an aggressive act carried out in anger and intended to hurt the victim, sexual abuse is

essentially self-gratificatory behaviour in which there are few, if any, hostile feelings towards the victim. Sexual abuse is sometimes, but by no means always, perpetrated by a member of the victim's family (in which case it is referred to as 'intrafamilial abuse'). The victim's older brothers are the relatives most likely to be perpetrators of intrafamilial sexual abuse, but other perpetrators include the father, an uncle, a grandfather or a female relative.

Most cases of sexual abuse do not involve sex-ual intercourse. Most involve other abusive actions including oral–genital contact, masturba-tion, fondling, exposure to pornography, and indecent exposure. The term 'incest' is best used in the legal sense (in which case it refers to inter-course between two people who have a close blood relationship – neither need be a child). Once a child has become a victim of intrafamilial sexual abuse, the victimization is likely to con-tinue for some time; incidents may be numbered in hundreds, and the abuse may extend over several years (Frude 1985).

Abusive adults use a variety of strategies to overcome their own inhibitions and those of their victims. They may insist that the victim is 'old for her years' or play upon the positive and loving nature of their relationship. The sexual approach will typically be very gradual, and may begin with the perpetrator conversing on sexual topics with the child, or indulging in various kissing, touching or tickling games.

EXPLAINING SEXUALLY ABUSIVE BEHAVIOUR

Why do adults interfere sexually with children? The idea that those who sexually abuse children are all 'psychopathic', 'psychotic', or 'criminal types' can safely be dismissed. Evidence has shown that the vast majority of perpetrators of sexual abuse do not engage in other forms of ser-ious crime and are not suffering from any psychi-atric condition.

Neither is it true that all or most sexual abusers are 'paedophiles' in the true sense of that term. Paedophilia is a well-defined psychiatric dis-order in which the person's sexual interests are focused exclusively on young children. Although it is true that active paedophiles abuse children, and are thus responsible for a proportion of cases of sexual abuse, the majority of those who commit sexual offences (especially perpetrators of intrafamilial abuse) are not paedophiles. Typically their sexual desires are not restricted to children.

One model portrays sexual abuse as a variation of a 'normal' seduction pattern in which the age of the seduction 'target', the victim's inability to give informed consent, and the relationship between the victim and the 'seducer' make the sexual approach aberrant and unacceptable (Frude 1982, 1989b). The model suggests that, either because they develop an inappropriate romantic passion for a particular child, or because they have unmet sexual urges, certain adults come to find a child sexually attractive. Some of these adults (the majority of whom are men) attempt to engage the child in sexual practices, usually through persuasion and the subtle exertion of power rather than through physical force. Power is a central feature of the model, since the adult is seen to misuse his power (his adult status, his 'rights' as a trusted family member, and his greater sophistication) to gain sexual access to the child. However, power is regarded as a means rather than an end, and the principal motive for sexual abuse, it is suggested, is not the acquisition of power but the pursuit of sexual gratification.

In an earlier section of this chapter we considered the issue of why the family context is the setting for so much violence. We can ask a similar question about sexual abuse, and suggest a number of reasons why sexual abuse is so often perpetrated against young family members. A child is likely to be trusting and compliant with a close relative, and some adults take advantage of their loving relationship with the child and regard the child as a legitimate target for a sexual advance. Family members generally have little suspicion that a child might be at risk from one of their number, and a potential perpetrator is therefore likely to have many opportunities to be alone with the child. Such opportunities can be used initially to implement gradual and subtle strategies that initiate the seduction process (these are

labelled 'grooming strategies'). A child who has been initiated into abusive activities may then be especially susceptible to threats and bribes and may thus continue to comply with the perpetrator's wishes. The adult's position and power within the family may persuade him that even if the child were to disclose to other family members his denials would be believed and that, even if his protestations of innocence were not accepted, his secret would remain safely hidden within the family.

It is likely that many adults who recognize that they have sexual feelings towards a young child, are encouraged by the victim's apparent lack of rejection or distress. Some children do protest and struggle when approached sexually but the majority behave in a compliant way (Meiselman 1978, Kaufman et al 2001). The victim's acquiescence may allow the perpetrator to tell himself that 'she is enjoying it', 'she doesn't mind' or 'she won't be harmed'. Perpetrators generally act as 'careful seducers' rather than as 'rapists', partly because they have no desire to hurt the victim and partly because they realize that an aggressive attack would be likely to lead to disclosure.

CONSEQUENCES FOR THE VICTIM

Sexual abuse may lead to physical injury. Attempts at intercourse with young children (or anal intercourse with a child at any age) may lead to bruising or to more severe injuries. Some victims contract a sexually transmitted disease and older girls who are subjected to intercourse run the additional risk of pregnancy. In the majority of cases, however, the abuse takes the form of masturbation, fondling or indecent exposure and does not leave any physical damage or any forensic evidence. In terms of psychological effects, there is no 'post-sexual abuse syndrome' and symptom patterns vary greatly in nature and degree. Immediate effects are sometimes, but not always, traumatic and may include extreme anxiety, depression, various forms of behaviour disturbance and an abnormal interest in sexual matters (Haugaard & Repucci 1988, Oddone-Paolucci et al 2001). Some abused children continue to show symptoms into adulthood, and some victims who appear to be relatively unscathed during childhood develop symptoms much later in life.

It is unfortunate that many people believe psychological trauma to be an inevitable consequence of sexual abuse, for the relevant research has consistently shown that a significant proportion of abused children are resilient and cope relatively well following sexual abuse (Himelein & McElrath 1996, Powell & Chalkley 1981). There is a danger that professionals who simply assume a traumatic consequence of abuse will communicate this assumption to the children in their care. Hunting for 'latent trauma' in children who present as healthy and well-adjusted is rarely helpful and may do considerable harm. The resilience shown by many children following sexual interference should be appreciated and enhanced rather than disregarded or undermined. In many cases, of course, the child *will* be in need of specialist psychological help, and any child who has been sexually abused needs to be carefully assessed. Following this, appropriate forms of intervention may be used, for example, to alleviate any feelings of guilt or depression, to promote self-esteem, to deal with any outstanding sexual issues and to foster relationship-building skills (Edgeworth & Carr 2000). Traumatic effects are more likely when the child is young at the time of abuse and in the relatively rare cases in which force is used. Needless to say, sexual abuse is an appalling infringement of a child's rights and any such interference runs the risk that the child victim may suffer severe acute and chronic psychological problems. Even when such effects are not apparent, however, the grievous nature of such abuse is clear.

Difficulties of adult survivors of childhood sexual abuse include mood disturbances (feelings of guilt, low self-esteem and depression), interpersonal difficulties (isolation, insecurity, discord and inadequacy) and sexual difficulties (sexual phobias and aversion, and sexual dissatisfaction) (Jehu 1988). Early sexual abuse also appears to be a risk factor for a variety of psychiatric disorders, including eating disorders. In recent years various therapeutic strategies have been developed to help survivors, and these are offered both by professional agencies and through voluntary and self-help groups (Ainscough & Toon 2000, Hall and Lloyd 1993, Stevenson 1999). Unfortunately, the sexual abuse of children is by no means rare, and any professional who comes into regular contact with families should be vigilant for evidence of such abuse. Child protection policies and practices in this field have developed rapidly and most relevant agencies have established guidelines for any professional (including teachers, nurses, general practitioners and youth leaders) who has reason to suspect that a child may have been subjected to sexual victimization.

ABUSE OF OLDER MEMBERS OF THE FAMILY

The frailty, illness and deterioration of function that are often features of older age demand various adaptations in the family structure and functioning. For an elderly couple, old age may mean major changes in responsibilities and the allocation of chores, for example, as one partner becomes dependent upon the other for help with feeding and toileting. In well-established three-generational households, the increasing dependency of an elderly person may require gradual changes in family organization. In other families, an older person's health may mean that he or she can no longer live independently and needs to move in with younger relatives, and this means that family life for all of them will be subject to sudden and radical changes.

Although the presence of an elderly person in the household with younger relatives often proves agreeable and successful, this arrangement frequently leads to tension, and the atmosphere often becomes fraught and conflictual. In many cases the family is subjected to increasing stress as the care demands increase due to progressive illness or disability, or as the cognitive and emotional health of the older person deteriorates. Family life may be severely disrupted as the consequences of the elderly person's condition reverberate around the family, affecting the relationships between other family members. If a general atmosphere of tension and hostility develops, even minor setbacks and annoyances may generate very strong emotional responses. These often take the form of depression or anxiety, but in some cases (especially those in which the elderly person becomes highly critical and demanding), family members feel a good deal of resentment and anger. Physical attacks on elderly people by their younger relatives are almost always driven by such anger, very few assaults being 'cold-blooded' (Gordon & Brill 2001, Zdorkowski & Galbraith 1985).

Only a minority of cases of elder abuse ever come to light, mostly because neither the perpetrators nor the victims are likely to disclose information about an attack. Perpetrators may be profoundly ashamed of the way they have treated their elderly relative and fear the possible legal consequences. Victims may be unable or reluctant to report incidents because of their isolation, their sense of shame, fear of possible reprisal, and the fact that, even if they have been seriously assaulted within the home, they may dread the thought of being admitted to a residential institution.

FAMILY DYNAMICS AND THE BURDEN OF CARE

We know from the cases that do come to light that an attack is rarely an isolated occurrence, and that many elderly people are subjected to prolonged emotional and physical cruelty. Many victims are made to feel that they are a burden to the family and are held responsible for all manner of family difficulties. Sometimes the needs of the older relative are totally neglected. He or she may be confined to a small part of the house or may be exploited financially. Such cruelty or neglect usually reflects a chronic breakdown of relationships, whereas the aggressive attacks made on old people by their caregivers usually reflect acute stress and annoyance. Such feelings may be a direct response to the elderly person's demands for care, or critical behaviour, but the high level of stress experienced by a younger relative may also reflect wider family factors such as marital instability or financial hardship (Gordon & Brill 2001, Steinmetz 1984).

When an elderly person comes to live with the family because of ill-health or infirmity, customary patterns of interaction will need to change. There may be considerable tension about the older person's role in the family, the extent to which they have power and a 'voice' in family decisions, and the nature and extent of their rights and duties. When the elderly person has been living with the family for a number of years, any deterioration in their health or psychological functioning will demand changes, but the family (and, especially, the old person) may struggle to preserve established patterns for as long as possible. Changes, and resistance to change, may gradually add to the tension so that it eventually reaches a breaking point.

Several aspects of the older person's behaviour may prove especially irritating. Memory problems may lead to endless repetition, for example, and items may be constantly mislaid. Hearing difficulties may require family members to shout, and the high volume necessary for the person to enjoy radio and television programmes may be intrusive and annoying. Constant 'aimless' wandering, and prolonged periods of silent sitting, may also prove very annoying, and erratic patterns of sleep and waking may disturb normal family interaction.

The presence of an older person may also impose very high 'costs' on other family members. As well as any 'burden of care' (which often falls unevenly on the shoulders of particular family members), considerable demands may be made on the family's financial resources. Susceptibility to the cold may lead to increased heating bills, and special mobility, dietary and toileting needs may affect the family's budget. Such costs may be resented, particularly if the family is relatively poor and if some members feel deprived as a result of the expenditure on the elderly person. Family members may also resent any loss of space and privacy consequent on the arrival of the elderly relative.

Certain actions by the elderly person may be experienced as 'interfering', or as 'careless', and the person may be accused of such 'offences' as withholding finances, or of attempting to impose outdated views about such matters as child discipline, the 'manners' of adolescent children, or the preparation of meals. The neurological effects of certain disorders lead to certain personality changes, so that some older people become especially cantankerous, uninhibited, or 'childish'. Intense resentment may be generated if no allowance is made for the disorder and if critical and disruptive behaviours are judged to be 'deliberate' attempts to undermine the family.

It needs to be emphasized that the picture of family life with an elderly person presented above emphasizes those aspects that are potentially problematic. Such circumstances are by no means universal, and may be far from typical. Many families care for their elderly relatives without undue hardship or stress, and in many cases such an arrangement proves highly successful and mutually gratifying. It also needs to be emphasized that however stressful the circumstances may become, there can never be any justification or excuse for the psychological or physical mistreatment of an older relative. But we do need to appreciate the stresses, costs and irritations in order to understand how people who are normally kindly and supportive can behave violently towards a vulnerable person in their charge (Pillemer & Suitor 1988).

ESCALATION AND INTERVENTION

Acute anger on one occasion may lead to a push or a fretful slap, and once such a threshold has been passed then inhibitions about hitting the elderly person may gradually erode. An understanding of elder abuse demands an understanding of why anger arises and why the normally powerful inhibitions against physical aggression towards an elderly person may be overcome. Violence towards older people frequently reflects a misunderstanding by the assailant of the nature and causes of the victim's annoying behaviour. Those who abuse elderly people may regard certain behaviour as deliberately provocative or 'careless', for example, when it really reflects some difficulty such as a memory lapse or a hearing impairment, or when it is 'symptomatic' of some physical or psychological disorder. Furthermore, those who assault elderly relatives often lack skills in managing difficult situations and gaining the compliance of the person they are attempting to care for.

Other relatives, friends, and (especially) professionals, may be able to help caregivers to understand why an older person is behaving oddly, or disruptively, or in a challenging fashion. If the caregiver comes to realize that the person's medical condition may lead to certain psychological problems (including changes of mood, difficulties of memory, confusion and disorientation) which then give rise to awkwardness or a quarrelsome attitude, the difficult behaviour may be judged more charitably. Health professionals can often advise the family on effective ways of dealing with disruptive behaviour and, through their own interaction with the elderly person, can provide a model of skillful and tolerant care.

CONCLUSION

Family violence takes on many different forms and is alarmingly common, marital (or spousal) violence occurring in a relatively high proportion of relationships. The intimate nature and social context of family life contribute to some explanations of violence, while other explanations focus on attitudes in society to women and children or to an absence of inhibition when angry. The physical abuse of children is probably best understood as an act of aggression by an angry parent, while sexually abusive adults use a variety of strategies to overcome both their own and their victim's inhibitions. The evidence suggests that interventions with regard to marital violence have only limited effectiveness and, where child protection and the protection of older people is concerned, health professionals need to be aware of the issues and to maintain vigilance, following local policies and procedures in the face of high-risk situations or evidence of abuse.

SUMMARY

◆ Abuse within the family comes in many forms and involves diverse relationships including marital, child and elder abuse.

◆ Violence can be either 'hostile' or instrumental.

◆ Figures for abuse are unclear as, for example, in the case of physical child abuse, some measure this as any physical disciplining of children, whereas others only include physical discipline which results in serious injury. The numbers affected are significant with, for example, more women seriously injured through marital violence than in road traffic accidents, street violence and rape combined.

◆ In general, assaults, especially marital and child sexual abuse, are carried out by men, although some assailants are women.

DISCUSSION POINTS

1. Why is there so much violence within the family?

2. What are some of the immediate and longer-term psychological effects of child physical abuse?

3. Is any form of physical punishment (e.g. slapping) acceptable in the context of a parent disciplining a young child – explain the reasons for your answer?

4. Why do so many women stay in relationships in which they are subjected to physical abuse by their partner?

5. Why are some children who are subjected to child sexual abuse able to shrug off the experience while many are devastated by the assault?

REFERENCES

Ainscough C, Toon K 2000 Breaking Free. Sheldon Press, London

Baker AW, Duncan SP 1985 Child sexual abuse: a study of prevalence in Great Britain. Child Abuse and Neglect 9: 457–467

Briere JN 1992 Child abuse trauma: theory and treatment of the lasting effects. Sage Publications, Thousand Oaks, CA

Browne K, Herbert M 1997 Preventing family violence. Wiley, Chichester

Browne K, Saqi S 1988 Approaches to screening for child abuse and neglect. In: Browne K, Davies C, Stratton P (eds) Early prediction and prevention of child abuse. Wiley, Chichester

Brownridge DA, Halli SS 2000 'Living in sin' and sinful living: toward filling a gap in the explanation of violence against women. Aggression and Violent Behaviour 5(6): 565–583

Centers for Disease Control 1998 Lifetime and annual incidence of intimate partner violence and resulting injuries – Georgia, 1995. Morbidity and Mortality Weekly Report 47: 849–853

Cicchetti D, Toth J 1995 A developmental psychopathology perspective on child abuse and neglect. Journal of the American Academy of Child and Adolescent Psychiatry 34: 451–565

Cowen PS 2001 Effectiveness of a parent education intervention for at-risk families. Journal of the Society of Pediatric Nurses 6: 73–82

Dale P, Davies M, Morrison A, Waters J 1986 Dangerous families: assessment and treatment of child abuse. Tavistock, London

Dobash RE, Dobash R 1979 Violence against wives. Free Press, New York

Drach KM, Devoe L 2000 Initial psychosocial treatment of the physically abused child: The issue of removal. In: Reece RM (ed) Treatment of child abuse: Common ground for mental health, medical, and legal practitioners. The Johns Hopkins University Press, Baltimore, MD

Edgeworth J, Carr A 2000 Child abuse. In: Carr A (ed) What works with children and adolescents? A critical review of psychological interventions with children, adolescents and their families. Routledge, London

Elliot M 1996 Female sexual abuse of children. Wiley, Chichester

Frieze IH, McHugh MC 1992 Power and influence strategies in violent and nonviolent marriages. Psychology of Women Quarterly 16: 449–465

Frude NJ 1980 Child abuse as aggression. In: Frude N (ed) Psychological approaches to child abuse. Batsford Academic, London

Frude NJ 1982 The sexual nature of sexual abuse: A review of the literature. Child Abuse and Neglect 6: 211–215

Frude NJ 1985 The sexual abuse of children within the family. Medicine and Law 4: 463–469

Frude NJ 1989a The physical abuse of children. In: Howells K, Hollin C (eds) Clinical approaches to violence. Wiley, Chichester

Frude NJ 1989b Sexual abuse: An overview. Educational and Child Psychology 6: 34–41

Frude NJ 1991 Understanding family problems: A psychological approach. Wiley, Chichester

Frude NJ 1994 Marital violence. In: Archer J (ed) Male violence. Routledge, London

Gelles RJ 1987 The violent home: Updated edition. Sage, Beverly Hills, CA

Goldsmith HR 1990 Men who abuse their spouses: An approach to assessing future risk. Journal of Offender Counseling, Services and Rehabilitation 15: 45–57

Gordon RM, Brill D 2001 The abuse and neglect of the elderly. International Journal of Law and Psychiatry 24: 183–197

Hall L, Lloyd S 1993 Surviving child sexual abuse: A handbook for helping women challenge their past (2nd edn). Falmer Press, London

Hamberger LK, Lohr JM, Bonge D 1994 The intended function of domestic violence is different in male and female arrested perpetrators. Journal of Family Violence and Sexual Assault 10: 40–44

Haugaard JJ, Repucci ND 1988 The sexual abuse of children. Jossey-Bass, San Francisco

Heyman RE, Neidig PH 1997 Physical aggression couples treatment. In: Halford WK, Markman HJ (eds) Clinical handbook of marriage and couples intervention. Wiley, Chichester

Himelein MJ, McElrath JV 1996 Resilient child sexual abuse survivors: Coping and illusion. Child Abuse and Neglect 20: 747–758

Holtzworth-Munroe A, Anglin K 1991 The competency of responses given by maritally violent versus non-violent men to problematic marital situations. Violence and Victims 6: 257–269

Holtzworth-Munroe A, Smutzler N, Bates L, Sandin E 1997 Husband violence: Basic facts and clinical implications. In: Halford WK, Markman HJ (eds) Clinical handbook of marriage and couples intervention. Wiley, Chichester

Jehu D 1988 Beyond sexual abuse: Therapy with women who were childhood victims. Wiley, Chichester

Kadushin A, Martin JA 1981 Child abuse: An interactional event. Columbia University Press, New York

Kaufman KL, Hilliker DR, Dalieden EL 2001 Subgroup differences in the modus operandi of adolescent sexual offenders. Child Maltreatment 1: 17–24

Kessler DB 1985 Pediatric assessment and differential diagnosis of child abuse. In: Newberger EH, Bourne R (eds) Unhappy families: Clinical and research perspectives on family violence. PSG Publishing Co, Littleton, MA

Lynch M 1988 The consequences of child abuse. In: Browne K, Davies C, Stratton P (eds) Early prediction and prevention of child abuse. Wiley, Chichester

Malinosky-Rummell R, Hansen H 1993 Long-term consequences of childhood physical abuse. Psychological Bulletin 114: 68–79

Martin HP 1976 Which children get abused: High risk factors in the child. In: Martin HP (ed) The abused child: A multidisciplinary approach to developmental issues and treatment. Ballinger, Cambridge

Mason A, Blankenship V 1987 Power and affiliation motivation, stress and abuse in intimate relationships. Journal of Personality and Social Psychology 52: 203–210

Meiselman K 1978 Incest: A psychological study of causes and effects. Jossey-Bass, San Francisco

Nobes G, Smith M 1997 Physical punishment of children in two-parent families. Clinical Child Psychology and Psychiatry 2: 271–281

Nobes G, Smith M, Upton P, Heverin A 1999 Physical punishment by mothers and fathers in British homes. Journal of Interpersonal Violence 14: 887–902

O'Farrell TJ, Murphy CM 1995 Marital violence before and after alcoholism treatment. Journal of Consulting and Clinical Psychology 63: 256–262

Oddone-Paolucci E, Genuis ML, Violata C 2001 A meta-analysis of the published research on the effects of child sexual abuse. Journal of Psychology 135: 17–36

Pahl J (ed) 1985 Private violence and public policy: The needs of battered women and the response of the public services. Routledge and Kegan Paul, London

Pillemer K, Suitor JJ 1988 Elder abuse. In: Van Hasselt VB, Morrison RL, Bellack AS, Hersen M (eds) Handbook of family violence. Plenum, New York

Powell GE, Chalkley AJ 1981 The effects of paedophile attention on the child. In: Taylor B (ed) Perspectives on paedophilia. Batsford Academic, London

Rosenbaum A, O'Leary KD 1981 Marital violence: Characteristics of abusive couples. Journal of Consulting and Clinical Psychology 49: 63–75

Saradjian J, Hanks H 1996 Women who sexually abuse children. Wiley, Chichester

Shepherd J, Sampson A 2000 'Don't shake the baby': Towards a prevention strategy. British Journal of Social Work 30: 721–735

Showers J 1992 'Don't Shake the Baby': The effectiveness of a prevention program. Child Abuse and Neglect 16: 11–18

Stark E, Flitcraft A 1988 Violence among intimates: An epidemiological review. In: Van Hasselt VB, Morrison RL, Bellack AS, Hersen M (eds) Handbook of family violence. Plenum, New York

Steinmetz SK 1984 Family violence towards elders. In: Saunders S, Anderson A, Hart C, Rubenstein G (eds) Violent individuals and families: A handbook for practitioners. Charles C Thomas, Springfield, IL

Stevenson J 1999 The treatment of the long-term sequelae of child abuse. Journal of Child Psychology and Psychiatry and Allied Disciplines 40: 89–111

Straus MA, Gelles RJ 1986 Societal change and family violence from 1975 to 1985 as revealed by two national surveys. Journal of Marriage and the Family 48: 465–479

Veltkamp LJ, Miller TW 1994 Clinical handbook of child abuse and neglect. International Universities Press, Madison, CT

Wolfe DA 1987 Child abuse: Implications for child development and psychopathology. Sage, Beverly Hills, CA

Zdorkowski RT, Galbraith MW 1985 An inductive approach to the investigation of elder abuse. Ageing and Society 5: 413–423

FURTHER READING

Ainscough C, Toon K 2000 Breaking free. Sheldon Press, London

A practical self-help guide for adult survivors of child sexual abuse based on many years of experience in helping survivors. It investigates the persistent effects of child sexual abuse including guilt and shame, depression, fear of relationships and sexual problems. The book draws on accounts of survivors and offers a positive and optimistic approach to help survivors break free from the past.

Browne K, Herbert M 1997 Preventing family violence. Wiley, Chichester

An evidence-based review of the facts, theories and intervention strategies relating to spouse abuse, child abuse and maltreatment of the elderly within the family setting. Discusses the nature and causes of abuse as well as treatment and prevention measures.

Carr A 1999 The handbook of child and adolescent clinical psychology. Routledge, London

Covers a wide range of concerns within the field of child psychology, including emotional problems, learning disabilities, child protection, depression, drug abuse, divorce, foster care and bereavement.

11

Theories and prevention of child physical abuse

D. Watkins

INTRODUCTION

Society's focus on child abuse as a uniquely contemporary issue, both in terms of numerical prevalence and social/moral intolerance is an erroneous one. Recent history indicates that recognition of child abuse has only proved an embarrassment to society over the last 40 years. This interest was initiated by an American, Henry Kempe, who first diagnosed the 'Battered Baby Syndrome' in the 1960s (Kempe et al 1962). Since this time there has been a growing realization that children are meaningfully abused by their parents and others in society.

Statistics demonstrate that child abuse is a major public health issue, with 160 000 children a year at risk of deliberate harm in the United Kingdom (National Commission 1996). In England there were 26 800 children on children protection registers in 2001, which represents 24 children per 10 000 of the population aged under 18 years (DoH 2002). Whilst in the United States of America more than three children die per day as a result of child abuse in the home (US Department of Health and Human Services 2000). Numerous theories are proposed which attempt to explain the reasons why child abuse occurs, the majority of which are based on findings of research performed over the previous two decades. Although many of these studies are retrospective and may lack the rigour associated with randomized control studies, there is agreement amongst eminent researchers that the causes of child abuse are multifaceted, and in most instances can not be isolated to one determinant (Barnett et al 1997,

Bethea 1999, Brown et al 1998, Browne & Saqi 1988, Frude 1991, Parton et al 1985, 1997). Studies in the 1980s tended to focus on a positivist approach which blamed the perpetrator, placing child abuse within a medical framework (Parton 1985). However more recent literature reflects a paradigm shift away from a 'cause and effect' model, towards an 'ecological' model, which incorporates a complexity of interactions between the individual, family, community and society (Bethea 1999).

This chapter will begin by defining child abuse and exploring macrotheoretical and microtheoretical perspectives, which attempt to explain the possible contributing factors to physical abuse of children. Macrotheory includes reference to cultural and sociological reasons, structural characteristics of the family and stress attributed to the environment. Microtheory incorporates parental biological and lifestyle factors, biological differences in the child, the socialization experience of parents, and interaction between family members. The chapter will conclude with the development of a framework that will guide and inform ·primary preventive nursing practice in the field of child maltreatment.

DEFINING CHILD ABUSE

Child abuse statistics are obtained from the numbers of children placed on 'Child Protection Registers' in England and Wales. Each social service department in the United Kingdom holds a central 'Child Protection Register' and children's names are placed on the register as the result of a child protection conference, where a decision is made that the child is at risk of significant harm and therefore in need of an interagency child protection plan. The primary purpose of the 'Child Protection Register' is to assist in the protection of children, and the statistics it generates are of a secondary benefit. Figures collated from the register should be viewed with caution, as under-reporting is a constant feature discussed in literature pertaining to child abuse (Browne & Saqi 1988, Cloke & Naish 1992, DoH 2002, National Commission 1996). A child's name is only added to the child protection register when certain criteria have been met, or child abuse has been diagnosed. This system of reporting prevents the inclusion of children who may be vulnerable, until substantial evidence proves a child is at risk of abuse. Omitted from statistics are those children unidentified who continue to suffer in silence. Numerical data do not always serve as an accurate representation of the problem (Naidoo & Wills 2000) and child abuse statistics may well present only the 'tip of the iceberg'.

There is an obvious need for consistency in definition when diagnosing and recording a particular health issue (Naidoo & Wills 2000). Any differences in terminology and criteria present problems in collating meaningful statistics on the incidence and prevalence of children abused, and lead to lack of clarity in referrals and interagency working. For this reason the National Commission of Inquiry into the Prevention of Child Abuse (1996, p. 10) adopted the following definition: 'Child abuse consists of anything which individuals, institutions, or processes do or fail to do which directly or indirectly harms children, or damages their prospects of safe and healthy development into adulthood'.

This definition is seen to encompass all types of abuse, however ambiguity is likely when professionals begin to unravel the subjective nature of 'indirect harm' or the damage to emotional or psychological development, which is often unseen in very young children. O'Hagan (1993) writes of the difficulties in proving that a child's emotional and psychological development has been adversely affected through abuse.

Definitions of child abuse have varied across time and continue to differ in countries and cultures throughout the world (Cloke & Naish 1992). Creighton (1988, p. 32) discusses child abuse as 'incorporating a wide range of activities which may include neglect, sexual abuse, emotional abuse, physically inflicted injuries, and physical abuse without physical injuries'. To allow for more accurate recording, the Home Office (1991, p. 48) categorized child abuse into four distinct areas and offers the following definitions:

1. 'Neglect: The persistent or severe neglect of a child, or the failure to protect a child from exposure to any kind of danger, including cold or starvation, or extreme failure to carry out important aspects of care, resulting in the significant impairment of the child's health or development, including non-organic failure to thrive.

2. Physical Injury: Actual or likely physical injury to a child, or failure to prevent physical injury (or suffering) to a child including deliberate poisoning, suffocation and Munchausen's syndrome by proxy.

3. Sexual Abuse: Actual or likely sexual exploitation of a child or adolescent. The child may be dependent and/or developmentally immature.

4. Emotional Abuse: Actual or likely severe adverse effect on the emotional and behavioural development of a child caused by persistent or severe emotional ill-treatment or rejection. All abuse involves some emotional ill-treatment. This category should be used where it is the main or sole form of abuse'.

For a child's name to be added to the 'register', a conference would need to decide whether the child has been subjected to 'significant harm' or whether there is a likelihood of 'significant harm' to the child. In cases of unsubstantiated abuse, that is no identifiable incidents, the judgement of the professionals involved is called upon to decide whether the child is at risk of 'significant harm'. Differences of opinion may prevail between professionals, as each presents their case of working with the child and family/carer. When there is divergence in professional experience and opinion, then it can become problematic proving to the conference committee that a child is at risk of 'significant harm'.

Physical injury to children would appear to be a category more easy to define than emotional abuse or neglect. However the difference between 'normal patterns of child rearing', physical discipline and physical abuse are not clearly defined, and to 'smack or not to smack' has, and continues to be, a subject of great debate in the United Kingdom (Cook et al 1991, Leach 1998).

Sociocultural factors determine child rearing, as does sociological, family characteristics and environmental stressors. These issues will now be explored as macrotheoretical perspectives on the causation of 'child physical abuse'. It is beyond the realms of this chapter to discuss the other categories of abuse previously defined.

A MACROTHEORETICAL PERSPECTIVE ON CHILD PHYSICAL ABUSE AND NEGLECT

CULTURAL FACTORS

Historically physical punishment of children has been an accepted cultural norm in British society (Cloke & Naish 1992), and continues to influence child-rearing patterns in many families in the 21st century. The link between punishment of children and physical child abuse is well established (End Physical Punishment of Children (EPOCH) 1990) and in instances where parents are questioned and asked to explain why they have injured their child, many openly admit their punishment sometimes 'went too far' (Health Visitor Association (HVA) 1994). Social services departments also comment on over chastisement and loss of control resulting in serious injuries to children (EPOCH 1990).

Authors discuss cultural norms as a possible theory to explain violence in families, and punitive patterns of discipline (Barnett et al 1997, Bethea 1999). Society appears to accept violence within the home, particularly the chastisement of children, who are considered the property of parents. Intertwined with this is the 'privacy' of the family regarded as a cultural value in Britain, which often inhibits society from becoming involved in family affairs. This acceptance of physical punishment as a method of discipline contributes to the formation of accepted cultural norms and values. Whilst much discipline may not be regarded as a deliberate act of cruelty, it becomes difficult to differentiate between that which is considered 'tolerable' and that which is 'abusive' (Frude 1991, p. 176).

Research in Britain funded by the Department of Health (Smith 1995) confirms that 91% of children are hit by their parents (this equates to 97% of 4-year-old children), and 16% having suffered a severe blow which fits the criteria for physical abuse (25% of 4-year-olds). The data for this study, collected via interviews with 400 families, highlighted the behaviour of mothers with younger children in relation to physical discipline. A total of 75% of children under the age of 1 year had been smacked, and 38% of the total children in the study were hit more than once a week.

Cultural theorists argue society's view of violence, and an individual's decision to commit an act of violence against a family member, is condoned by the attitude of the law towards domestic violence, and the lax penalties associated with such acts. The law enforces greater punishments for violence outside the family than it does against family members with just 2% of men in reported incidents arrested and charged (James-Hanman 1998). A view based on 'deterrence theory' attempts to explain why family violence is common in British and American societies. The belief is that if the consequence of an action results in high social or legal costs, then an individual may be deterred from performing it (Barnett et al 1997). The low costs associated with family violence does little to deter individuals from committing these offences. Although this theory relates primarily to violence between men and women, evidence suggests children who witness these situations may be psychologically abused (O'Hagan 1993), and marital abuse is more likely to lead to child abuse (Browne & Saqi 1988, Frude 1991). Research indicates that 90% of children are in the same room as their parents when abusive attacks take place and that at least one third of these children are injured when trying to protect their mothers (Mullender & Morley 1994). (See Chapters 9 and 10 for further discussion on the family and family violence.)

Authors who support the cultural explanation comment on the contribution of the media to an acceptance of violence by society (Bee 1997). Television portrays continual aggressive and violent behaviour, and there is a body of evidence which proves a correlation between regular observed television violence and aggression as a child (Paik & Combstock 1994) and violent aggressive behaviour in adult life (Eron et al 1994). Although no one study has proved a direct correlation between television violence and child abuse, evidence suggests that frequent television viewing of violence leads to an 'emotional desensitization of violence', and to a learned belief that aggressive behaviour is a successful method of problem solving (Donnerstein et al 1994). This latter view could contribute to our understanding of parental patterns of discipline and punitive behaviour towards children.

Feminism also informs the cultural theory of child abuse, and maintains that violence by men against women and children in the family reaffirms the male position of power in society. This patriarchal view stems from a belief that men are of a higher order, which allows them greater power and control over women, who are lower in the social hierarchy (Barnett et al 1997). It thus becomes acceptable for men to abuse women, and this may even be seen as a normal expression of the male identity. Feminists maintain that society condones these attitudes, whilst Cooper (1993) argues society is changing its views about patriarchy based on our recent knowledge of child abuse and wife battering. He points out that feminist theories lack reliable research, in similar ways to all other theories, which try to identify a causal relationship in the abuse of children.

The link between domestic violence and child abuse is clear, with a substantial number of male domestic abusers also portraying violence towards children in the family (Welsh Office 1999). This, combined with the negative effects of them witnessing violence towards mothers, leads to a hidden epidemic of children suffering anxiety, depression, emotional and behavioural problems (Sudderman & Jaffe 1999) and even post-traumatic stress syndrome (Lehmann 1995). The way in which society ignores family violence, particularly abuse towards women, may well perpetuate the cycle of family violence. (See Chapter 10 for further discussion on family violence.)

SOCIOLOGICAL FACTORS

Social and economic factors play a crucial role in child abuse, and are closely related to degrees of poverty, in that the more extreme poverty families are subjected to, the greater the likelihood of child abuse occurring (Egan-Sage & Carpenter 1999, Parton 1985, Sedlak & Broadhurst 1996). Supporting evidence to justify this statement is upheld through child protection statistics, which highlight the large number of injuries sustained to children from lower socioeconomic groups (National Commission 1996, US Department of Health and Human Services 2000). In the USA figures suggest that children from families with annual incomes below US$15 000 as compared to children from families with annual incomes above US$30 000 were over 22 times more likely to experience maltreatment (US Department of Health and Human Services 2000).

Although it is known that the most severe injuries to children occur in the poorest families (Browne & Saqi 1988, US Department of Health and Human Services 2000), the research base to support a single cause and effect relationship in the absence of other factors is sparse. Some studies have found a positive correlation between factors such as poverty, unemployment, poor housing, low educational levels, lower social class and the abuse of children (Browne & Saqi 1988, Parton 1985, Sedlak & Broadhurst 1996), however other authors suggest the relationship between socioeconomic status and child maltreatment is inconclusive (Brown et al 1998).

Early work discusses a relationship between poverty and family violence, attributed to individuals enduring structural difficulties and economic problems, leading to frustration and consequently aggression. Gelles (1973) suggests that violence may be a response to structural or situational stress and hardship, usually faced by families from lower socioeconomic groups. This, combined with the unequal distribution of opportunities can create frustration, which may result in aggression, known as the frustration–aggression hypothesis (Frude 1991). This theory may partially explain the large number of perpetrators from lower social groups who direct their aggression at innocent victims such as children (Barnett et al 1997, Frude 1991, Parton 1985).

Frude (1991, p. 196) outlines the possible association between social class and child abuse, as what he terms a 'distal causal factor'. This is described in the following manner; an individual's attitude, perceptions and behavioural patterns will be formed as a result of the situational stresses placed upon them. For example being raised in a poor household, exposed to aggressive behaviour that is considered acceptable, surrounded by relatives and friends who share the same value systems, lack of exposure to the media or education which challenges these views, may well affect the child's perceptions of child rearing as an adult. As Frude points out this person may be authoritarian and their childhood experience may increase the risk of them abusing their children. This explanation portrays the complex nature of child abuse, and its association with social class. (See Chapter 10 for further information on theories of family violence.)

Others dispute this explanation and comment on a 'subculture of violence' which maintains there is greater acceptance of violence and aggression in the lower classes, which leads to violence being considered a 'way of life' (Barnett et al 1997). There is no empirical evidence to support either the frustration–aggression hypothesis, or the subculture of violence.

A multitude of other social factors has also been found to be associated with an increased vulnerability to child maltreatment. Young parents have been found to be at considerable risk of abusing their children (Bethea 1999, Brown et al 1998, Browne & Saqi 1988, Egan-Sage & Carpenter 1999). This is a consistent feature found in perpetrators, and may well be linked with immaturity and unrealistic expectations of the child, as well as lack of social support (Brown et al 1998). Some young parents may expect comfort and dependency from the child, and feel unable to cope with the huge emotional and physical demands of a normal child. Young parents may also be living in poverty, and therefore subjected to greater stresses as discussed earlier.

There appears to be a relationship between marital instability and conflict, marital violence, abusive relationships and child abuse. Browne and Saqi (1988) found marital discord to be a feature of abusing parents, and Frude (1991) comments on the lack of warmth between couples where there is abuse. Cummings (1997) has extensively studied the relationship between martial conflict and emotional abuse in children. In an overall review of nine studies completed by himself and colleagues he emphatically links marital discord with emotional abuse and the development of psychopathology in children, and the increased likelihood of physical abuse and injuries, particularly when interspousal abuse is present.

Abuse is also more common by step-parents, particularly fatal abuse, with an increase in abuse by step-fathers, compared with that of natural parents. The work of Egan-Sage and Carpenter (1999) cites step-fathers as being responsible for abuse of the child in 14% of referrals to social services where families are giving cause for concern, and 16% of those entered onto the Child Protection Register. The reason for this may relate to an inability to form an attachment relationship with the step-child (Olds 1997).

Social isolation and lack of a supportive network have been recognized as risk factors and the nuclear isolated family identified as being at greater risk of abusing their children (Egan-Sage & Carpenter 1999). The 'quality' of social support is probably more important than the quantity, as a protective factor for parents. Social isolation may be more common in single female parents, who tend to be at greater risk of abusing their children, with over 40% of single parents represented in British studies of abused children (Browne & Saqi 1988, Roberts 1988) and a quarter of children in an American longitudinal study by Brown et al (1998). However in a more recent review of family characteristics in cases of alleged child abuse and neglect in an English social services department, it was found that less than one third of a sample of 2069 children referred lived with a lone or unmarried mother (Egan-Sage & Carpenter 1999). Figures from the US conflict with this low percentage, in that children of single parents have a 77% greater chance of being harmed by physical abuse, an 87% greater risk of physical neglect, and an 80%

greater chance of being seriously injured or harmed by abuse, than children living with both parents (US Department of Health and Human Services 2000). The evidence on abuse being more common in mothers who live alone with their child is inconsistent, although the young age of abusers, that is under the age of 21 years, is universally proven as a risk factor for abuse (Brown et al 1998, Browne & Saqi 1988, Egan-Sage & Carpenter 1999, Olds et al 1997).

Poverty also has an effect on people's scope to participate in society. Naidoo and Wills (2000) discuss how choices are constrained for people on a low income, which in turn reduces opportunities for social contact. This can result in social isolation and poor social contacts for families who live on the 'bread line', and as previously discussed increases a family's vulnerability to child abuse (Brown et al 1998). (See Chapter 6 for discussion on structural issues related to poverty and health.)

In conclusion, evidence links wider socioeconomic factors with child abuse, with a strong association between poverty and neglect (Brown et al 1998, US Department of Health and Human Services 2000). Although overall, poverty environments tend to be chaotic, more highly stressed, and lack resources (Bee 1997), an assumption cannot be made, that all children from lower socioeconomic groups will be abused. These families are probably subjected to greater scrutiny by health professionals leading to increased detection rates in lower socioeconomic groups, however there are so many confounding variables present in families living in poverty, it becomes almost impossible to isolate a direct causal link.

A MICROTHEORETICAL PERSPECTIVE

PARENTAL BIOLOGICAL FACTORS: THE PSYCHOPATHIC MODEL AND ITS RELATIONSHIP TO CHILD ABUSE

This approach to determining the cause of child abuse explains it in terms of psychological malfunction or psychiatric illness in the abusing parent, and it ignores socioeconomic factors, or other possible causes of stress in the family, as contributing factors. It concentrates on psychopathology, that is abnormal behaviour or a mental disorder as the cause of child abuse (Barnett et al 1997). This follows a 'disease model' where the abusing parent is considered to have certain personality or character types, which predispose them to violent behaviour (Browne & Saqi 1988). This predisposition may be genetic or acquired through personal socialization, such as experience of being abused or neglected as a child itself, continually observing violence, or through experience of being involved in aggressive interactions (Barnett et al 1997, Bee 1997).

Bird (1999) is positive regarding the ability of a number of mothers with a mental health problem to care adequately for their children. However she acknowledges there are those who will be unable to cope, and at the extreme those who are capable of killing their children. An enquiry into homicides by the Royal College of Psychiatrists (1996) established that 30% of perpetrators were female, 40% of those were diagnosed as schizophrenic, and in 85% the victims were their own children. These figures suggest a causal link between mental illness and fatal child abuse, but Bird (1999) disputes this and argues that people suffering from severe mental illness are no more likely to physically abuse their children than the rest of the population.

In contrast with this view others believe parents with chronic mental health problems may well overtly affect their children's health. Parents who delude become a concern, as some may include the child in their delusions, or expect the child to behave in such a way that is compatible with their thoughts. This can lead to confusion, and fear with 'children becoming involved in a mad world where reality and unreality become confused and uncertain' (Parker 1999, p. 26). Psychological abuse in these instances may be unwittingly administered by a parent with a mental health disorder, resulting in possible psychological disturbances for the child.

Kaplan (1999) points out that in the vast majority of cases where a parent has a psychiatric

illness, an acute risk to the child is not usually an issue. It tends to be an accumulative chronic problem, which develops over time. In cases where there is a supportive partner the risk to the child may be minimal. However it should be emphasized that socioeconomic disadvantage such as poverty, unemployment, poor housing, marital discord, etc. are often associated with mental health problems. As discussed previously these issues also contribute to child abuse, and thus must be considered in the context of parents with mental health disorders. (See Chapter 6 for a detailed account of the effects of poverty on health and Chapter 20 for further discussion on mental health.)

When considering the effects of parents with mental illness on the health of children, other outcomes other than physical abuse of the child need to be examined. Depression in the parent can lead to 'apathy, to emotional instability, irritability and disinterest in the child' (Beck-Sander 1999, p. 75). This can in turn affect the normal development of the child, and mothers may experience particular difficulties in coping with distressed children. This has been described in mothers with postnatal depression, where chaotic meal times, inconsistent parenting patterns and children who fail to thrive, become examples of the difficulties faced by children of depressed mothers (Cox 1988, 1999). The result can be developmental delay in children, and later behaviour problems and it may also interfere with the parent/child attachment process (Cox 1988, 1999).

The development of a 'secure' attachment between mother and child is extremely important, as it is predictive of the mother's behaviour with the child. Research indicates in instances where a secure attachment is not formed, the child is more at risk of abuse from the mother (George 1996, Gutterman 1997). Several factors may prevent the development of a secure attachment between the mother and child and these relate to factors that prevent physical or emotional proximity between both parties, or the mother lacking the skills to be able to demonstrate affection and respond appropriately to the needs of the child. An inability to form a secure attachment has been linked to the mother's own experience of childhood, where a secure attachment between herself and her mother (or another carer) has failed to develop. This can form the grounding for 'transgenerational child abuse', that frequently occurs between mother and child across generations. It is beyond the realms of this chapter to explore attachment theory in great detail, but it is worthy of further exploration (see George 1996 cited in the Further Reading section).

What must be considered when assessing risk for child abuse is a combination of a mental disorder and use of elicit drugs, as this significantly increases the risk of violence (Mulvey 1994) and therefore constitutes a risk of physical abuse directed at children. The view of Sayce (1996) is that carers who are alcoholics or misuse drugs pose a significant risk to children, which probably exceeds that associated with mental health problems.

PARENTAL LIFESTYLE FACTORS: DRUG AND ALCOHOL DEPENDENCY AND THE RISKS OF CHILD ABUSE

Narcotic dependence in parents and potential antisocial lifestyle patterns to support the habit are of concern when children are involved, and numerous studies prove a clear association between these variables (Miller et al 1999, Wasserman & Leventhal 1993).

The study by Wasserman and Leventhal (1993) set out to identify whether women who were cocaine dependent were more likely to physically abuse their children. A cocaine-dependent group were matched with a control group and the results demonstrated that by 2 years of age, 23% of children in the cocaine-dependent group sustained physical abuse compared with 4% in the control group. There was no documented evidence of neglect in the control group, whilst 11% suffered neglect in the cocaine-dependent group. Another more recent study supports these findings (Miller et al 1999).

Mothers with alcohol and drug problems (AOD) and their punitiveness towards their children has been researched in an attempt to determine the relationship between AOD and physical

child abuse (Miller et al 1999). The findings from this study demonstrated that a history of AOD was consistently found to be associated with verbal aggression towards children, and this was strongly influenced by a history of parental violence and partner violence. Other important findings confirm that the mother's experience of 'childhood severe violence predicted higher levels of moderate violence, and partner severe violence predicted higher levels of verbal aggression and higher scores on a child abuse scale' (Miller et al 1999, p. 638). Other work confirms the association between social learning theory and modelling of violence observed in childhood, and subsequent violence directed by the parent towards their own child (Frude 1991).

In relation to alcohol and drug misuse and its association with punitive patterns of discipline, the authors comment that the study does not prove a direct 'causal link' between AOD problems and punitive punishment, although the presence of alcohol or drugs may well increase the mother's hostility towards the child, and decrease inhibitions regarding physical punishment. The study confirms this point in that it found a mother's hostility towards her child is increased in the presence of AOD resulting in significantly increased levels of punitive punishment (Miller et al 1999).

In conclusion, there are numerous studies confirming an association between alcohol and drug misuse and child abuse. Although a direct causal link cannot be confirmed, the diminishing inhibitory effect of these drugs; the lifestyle associated with addiction and the chaotic environment associated with drug and alcohol abuse, probably places these children at greater risk of abuse. These factors combined with an increased exposure to violence in childhood and violence by partners outlined in the study by Miller and colleagues, places these children at considerable risk of abuse.

CHILD BIOLOGICAL FACTORS AND THEIR RELATIONSHIP TO CHILD ABUSE

Biological factors are thought to increase the potential for child abuse. Browne and Saqi (1988) and Kaplan (1999) discuss low birth weight and the premature infant as possible risk factors, in relation to the increased difficulties associated with feeding and handling small infants.

Biologically, children are probably born different, and according to the early work of Thomas and Chess (1977) they quickly exhibit different temperaments. The authors outline three distinct categories of temperament; the first category includes children who cope with changes easily, are placid by nature, adaptable and contented. These children quickly establish good routines in relation to eating and sleeping and are termed the 'easy' child. The second category relates to children who are more 'difficult', react less positively to changes, and are slow to establish eating and sleeping routines. They are more irritable than the easy child and cry more often. Once these children have adapted to something new then they become positive, although the process of adaption may have been difficult for both the parents and the child (Thomas & Chess 1977). The third category of temperament identified by Thomas and Chess is that of the 'slow to warm up' child. These children often have a passive resistance or ambivalence to change, showing neither a negative nor a positive reaction.

Research indicates that children who fall into the 'difficult' category are criticized and physically punished more than those who fall into the other two categories (Bates 1989). This is not to say all difficult children are subjected to criticism and punishment by their parents; some skilled parents who regard the child's temperament as a 'quality' may handle the situations which arise in a positive manner. It is difficult to ascertain whether the temperament of a child is influenced by the parent's reaction to their behaviour, thereby reinforcing or counteracting negativity. However research suggests the reactions of mothers towards their children influence children's negative and positive behaviour (Bousha & Twentyman 1984).

The ill or disabled child is likely to make greater demands on parents, who may not be able to cope with the level of care required. It is recognized that children with longstanding physical or mental disabilities form a large proportion of children abused (Ammerman et al

1991), and that children born 'different' for whatever reason may be more susceptible to abuse by their parents (Roberts 1988). This is reiterated in the work of Browne and Saqi (1988) and their identification of vulnerability factors in children subjected to abuse.

The National Centre on Child Abuse and Neglect in America found the rate of physical abuse to be almost twice as high in disabled children compared to those without disabilities. The most common factors associated with abuse were 'physical health problems, a learning disability, emotional disturbance and delay or impairment in speech and language' (DHSS 1993 cited in Barnett et al 1997, p. 49).

Others comment that stress may occur when family members spend a disproportionate amount of time with one another, as can happen with an ill or handicapped child (Barnett et al 1997). If the exchange of emotions is one-sided, in that the child with a disability or illness is unable to return the affection, then this could result in the child being vulnerable to abuse. This scenario fits into 'social exchange theory' (Frude 1991, p. 17, Barnett et al 1997, p. 31) where people stay in relationships when they perceive the benefits to outweigh the costs. (See Chapters 10 and 12 for further work in this area).

SOCIALIZATION OF PARENTS AND THE RISKS ASSOCIATED WITH CHILD ABUSE

Interaction theory is based on the view that interactions between family members may result in conflict, aggressive behaviour and physical abuse of children (Barnett et al 1997, Bee 1997, Frude 1991). The manner in which the parent interacts with the child will be dependent on a variety of factors, both in the perpetrator and the victim.

Emotional and behavioural difficulties in the parent may adversely affect their interactions with the child. A number of American studies have found several adult characteristics to be associated with child physical abuse. These relate to 'anger control problems, low frustration tolerance, depression, low self-esteem and deficits in empathy and rigidity' (cited in Barnett et al 1997, p. 51). British researchers support these findings (Frude 1991).

There is an assumption that cases of child physical abuse occur as a result of an interaction between the perpetrator and the victim, which leads to an aggressive response and violence. Agreement with this theory implies there is an annoyance from the child, which triggers off a hostile reaction by the parent, who in the absence of effective inhibitions, assaults the child (Frude 1991). This is a rather oversimplistic view of physical abuse directed at children, for as we have seen from previous research reviewed a host of other factors may predispose the parent to react in this way. We are also aware that not all parents react to children's adverse behaviour with violence. It is probably an accumulation of factors present within the parent combined with the behaviour of the child, which results in some cases of abuse. Frude (1991) argues the role the victim plays must be considered; difficulty in controlling the child's behaviour may lead to exacerbations of extreme anger, which if controlled by harsh discipline, may mitigate into severe punishment termed as abuse.

Barnett et al (1997, p. 14) discuss the issue of abused children becoming abusive parents and imply there is some truth in this common generalization. Egeland (1991) confirms that those who abuse their children have consistently been exposed to violence themselves as a child. This is supported by the work of Miller et al (1999) who identify that mothers who engage in punitive discipline towards their children have often sustained a violent childhood, or live with abusive partners. However this, and other research, which identifies the relationship between cause and effect is usually retrospective, and fails to engage control groups. Barnett et al (1997) indicate that when the general population is surveyed the strength of this argument declines, compared with only studying violent groups of people. We do not know how many parents who were abused themselves go on to succeed as parents. Other confounding variables are also present in studies that explore transgenerational child abuse. It is known that women abused as

children are likely to have lower self-esteem, suffer greater stresses in life, are more socially isolated (George 1996, Roberts 1988) and engage in adverse lifestyle behaviour such as drug and alcohol misuse (Miller et al 1999).

Feelings of worthlessness have been observed in parents of abused children and cross-sectional and longitudinal studies report strong links between low self-esteem and child maltreatment, with at least seven studies reviewed by Milner and Dopke (1997) confirming this association. Worthlessness can be linked to a variety of circumstances, including an abusive childhood, which can lead to an inability to trust individuals. In some instances where the parent has been continually criticized or rejected by their own parents, they become apprehensive of trusting anyone. This is reflected in the parent's relationship with the child, where the parent fears forming a close relationship, in case the child should reject them (Milner & Dopke 1997).

Experience of observing violent behaviour, and then imitating this behaviour, has received some attention as a causative factor in family violence (Barnett et al 1997). Social learning theorists (Bandura 1973) suggest we learn through observing and then 'modelling' the behaviour of others, particularly those we hold in high esteem. Children who observe violent behaviour in the home, may learn this and model it in childhood and later adult life. There are numerous studies that support this theory, where exposure to violence as a child has resulted in adults who are abusive to partners and their children (Rodriguez and Sutherland 1999, Strauss et al 1980). The theory postulates that children exposed to parental violence as a method of resolving conflict, learn this mechanism for dealing with difficult situations. Unfortunately it is unlikely these children are provided with opportunities to learn non-violent assertive behaviour as an alternative resolution. (See Chapters 9 and 10 for further discussion on violence within families.)

Research by Rodriguez and Sutherland (1999) looked at predictors of parental physical disciplinary practices in an attempt to determine whether a history of physical punishment sustained as a child predicted an acceptance of harsh punishments perpetrated against children. Discipline scenarios were shown to the parents, which represented a range of situations depicting a child as deliberately naughty, for example aggravating a sibling, and instances where the child was blameless, such as a child accidentally dropping a dish. Criteria were set for mild (slap on the hand), moderate (spanking, pulling the child by the arm) and severe (hit with an object such as a belt or a wooden spoon) disciplinary actions attributed to the events and parents were asked to rate the level of discipline on likert scales. Parents were also later questioned as to whether the discipline observed had been administered to them as children, and if they implemented it with their own children.

The results illustrated that parents with a history of a particular childhood discipline were more likely to use this form of discipline with their own children. This confirms the cycle of violence theory in that a confirmed history of a particular discipline pattern can be perpetuated in the next generation, and this is seen as acceptable. Rodriguez and Sutherland (1999) also point out that personal experience of physical discipline results in the parents considering it as less severe, and they may well feel more justified in using it with their own children.

The other important finding from this study relates to the parent's perception of children deliberately misbehaving, and so deserving of physical punishment. Parents reported a history of punishment as a child for culpable behaviour and administered punishment to their own child for what they considered as deliberate naughty behaviour. This has implications for physical child abuse, as studies show abusing parents view their children negatively and problematic, and feel their children deliberately engage in naughty behaviour which results in physical discipline (Bauer & Twentyman 1985, Chilamkurti & Milner 1993, Larrance & Twentyman 1983).

Parental expectations of child behaviour have been studied in relation to child abuse, and this may be related to both ends of a continuum; high expectations of a child, and low expectations relating to the child behaving in a negative manner. Chilamkurti and Milner (1993) found that parents'

expectations varied according to the severity of the transgression. Of interest is the fact that mothers considered at high risk of abuse had higher expectations of their child in relation to minor instances of misbehaviour, and lower expectations from them in relation to serious misbehaviour, compared with a control group. This demonstrates perhaps unrealistic expectations of children.

Larrance and Twentyman (1983) set out to test the hypothesis that abusing and neglecting mothers had either low or unrealistic expectations of their child, and that they attributed blame for abuse and neglect on the child's behaviour. Photographs were taken of the parent's child and other children behaving in a variety of ways in different situations. Some portrayed children performing behaviour such as crayoning on the wall, whilst others depicted them behaving in a more positive manner. The mothers were shown six different pictures, and were asked to tell a story of how they thought their own child may behave in the sets of situations, and how other children may behave.

The results demonstrated that abusive mothers were more likely to see their child as behaving negatively in the situations portrayed, these findings reaching statistical significance when compared with a control group. Neglectful mothers also saw their children in a negative light, however abusive mothers demonstrated slightly more negativity.

The findings of the study support 'attribution theory', in that the dysfunctional groups of mothers attributed blame to their children for adverse behaviour, whilst parents in the control group felt their child's negative behaviour could have been caused by factors other than the child. The results also illustrate that abusive and neglectful parents felt their children encroached on their own needs. This suggests that abusing and neglectful mothers may view their children as competing for emotional attention, and regard them as taking up time and effort, which detracts from meeting their personal needs (Larrance & Twentyman 1983).

Bousha and Twentyman (1984) add to our understanding of mother–child interactions through studying abusive mothers, neglectful mothers and a control group. The results indicated abusive parents responded with aggressive verbal and physical behaviour, and this was markedly different from the two other groups. The neglectful parents had the least interaction with their child compared with the other groups, they were withdrawn, and their behaviour was indicative of socially isolating the child within the family. The dysfunctional groups also exhibited less verbal affection and played with their children less often than the control group.

The observed behaviour of the children and mothers from the neglectful group in this study provide tremendous insight into how these families interact. Neglected children demonstrated aggressive behaviour, probably in an attempt to gain attention, as their mothers were the least likely to socially interact with them and were found to be less inquisitive, and completely lacking in environmental stimulation (Bousha & Twentyman 1984). One can only surmise that in families where the child has little social interaction with the mother, and consequently finds interaction with others outside the family difficult, some neglected children live in a world of almost complete social isolation.

This study highlights opportunities for preventative strategies designed specifically to meet the differing needs of abusing and neglectful mothers. Interventions with neglecting mothers need to focus on increasing social interactions with the child, whilst interventions with mothers who physically abuse their children would need to be directed at reducing aggressive behaviour and increasing positive reinforcement. (See Chapter 12 for more information on how to work constructively with families.)

A FRAMEWORK FOR THE PREVENTION OF CHILD PHYSICAL ABUSE

An analysis of the many theories formulated to explain child abuse leave little doubt that it occurs as a result of a complex interaction of individual, social and environmental influences that requires an integrated approach to prevention. Browne and Saqi (1988) discuss the association between social factors and relationships to child abuse and build on the work of Gelles (1973). These two authors propose that violent behaviour is influenced by (Browne & Saqi 1988, p. 22):

1. Situational stressors – this may include difficult family relationships, unwanted or problem children, low self-esteem.
2. Structural stressors – this would incorporate poverty, poor housing, financial problems, unemployment, social isolation and health problems.

Browne and Saqi (1988) expand on the effects of structural and situational stressors and suggest that the 'chances of structural and situational stressors resulting in family violence depend on the interactive relationships within the family' (p. 22). Good secure relationships may well act as a 'buffer' even in circumstances where the structural and situational stressors would appear to be raised. These protective relationships may well lead to a reduction in stress, and result in coping, caring behaviour. When the opposite occurs and insecure relationships are present within the family, then the effects of structural and situational stressors may be heightened, resulting in an attack of violence against a family member. The effect of the 'buffering' process is then further reduced, resulting in a 'coercive spiral of violence' (Patterson 1976 cited in Browne & Saqi 1988, p. 22). The family may become overloaded, as each aggressive and violent attack further aggravates the situation, leading to an increase in situational stressors.

Table 11.1 summarizes the theoretical perspectives explored earlier in the chapter and categorizes them into situational and structural stressors.

Obviously any strategy aimed at the prevention of child physical abuse would need to incorporate the above stressors. Newman's model of nursing (Newman 1980) is one such framework which could be utilized in that it considers those elements that cause the individual/family and nurse concern (stressors), it encompasses a broad perspective and works within a health promotion framework. A similar systems model has been

Table 11.1 Situational and structural stressors of theoretical perspectives

Macrotheories	Microtheories
Society's view of child abuse	Individual differences in parent and child (to include physical, social and psychological)
Cultural norms and values	
The legal and political framework	Parent–child interaction
Socioeconomic factors	Relationships between parents and significant others
Structural characteristics of the family	Psychopathic states
Quality of social support	Socialization experience (to include acquired models of parenting and methods of conflict resolution)
↓	↓
Situational stressors	**Structural stressors**

Adapted from the work of Browne and Saqi (1988), Cooper (1993) and Barnett et al (1997).

proposed by Cooper (1993) that specifically relates to child abuse. This ecological model, originally based on the work of Bronfenbrenner (1979) seeks to encompass the macro- and microtheories mentioned previously and tries to address these within a framework based on human ecology, that values the importance of social contexts as influences on human development. Cooper and Ball's model consists of the following interrelated dimensions:

◆ the microsystem
◆ the mesosystem
◆ the exosytem
◆ the macrosystem.

The microsystem includes relationships, and the close 'day to day' experiences of an individual. In some instances this may only include the relationship between the child and parents, however in other situations, relationships with others, such as grandparents or siblings may be extremely influential. There may be someone else who is not part of the nuclear or extended family who would be included in the microsystem if they have a significant relationship with the child. The mesosystem refers to close relationships the child may have with the microsystem, for example nursery school or school. The child's

experiences in these settings may link closely to the microsystem. The exosystem is seen to incorporate 'others' involved with the family who are influential, but whom the family may have little control over, however they influence family functioning. For example the case conference child protection plan which may involve the social worker, health visitor, police, etc. The macrosystem includes the broader cultural, social and political perspectives regarding child abuse. It is inclusive of historical perspectives on child rearing, family norms and values, and legislation regarding child abuse, as society's view of abuse will influence all other systems (Cooper 1993).

This model attempts to incorporate the wider influences on child abuse, and prevents cause being attributed to one particular theory. It also highlights that child abuse is not static, but a dynamic changing situation, influenced by the interaction between the different systems. It should influence practitioners to move away from a narrow knowledge base and to look beyond the individual to the situational dynamics that influence child abuse. Table 11.2 links the theories reviewed to the ecological model discussed, outlining preventative strategies.

CONCLUSION

The theories reviewed assist our understanding of how child abuse can occur, however it is by no means inclusive, and does not account for all cases. The vicious unprovoked attack on a child, the deliberate affliction of burns, and the sexual abuse of children, are more difficult to explain and certain types of abuse could well be attributed to psychopathic tendencies. However some instances of physical abuse directed towards children may occur as a result of an accumulation of extrinsic and intrinsic factors.

In conclusion, it would appear that society's acceptance of violence may well lay the foundations for child abuse. Although as mentioned at the beginning of this chapter it is unlikely that cultural factors in isolation of other determinants would result in abuse of children, society's attitudes towards physical discipline most certainly

Table 11.2 Child abuse preventative strategies and ecological models

Ecological model	Preventative strategy
Macrosystem	i. Engage in political action to change legislation that bans 'smacking' and physical punishment of children ii. Work with the United Nations Convention on the Rights of the Child to protect children from all forms of physical punishment iii. Tackle domestic violence through developing a national strategy iv. Co-ordinate multiagency working in relation to protecting women and children from domestic abuse v. Work to change society's view of children and punitive discipline vi. Reduce the coverage of violence in the media as an accepted form of dealing with conflict situations vii. Tackle poverty through working at a national, local and community level to change policy and establish programmes to assist with financial hardship, e.g. food co-operatives
Mesosystem	i. Work collaboratively and in partnership with communities to identify health and social needs and establish community development programmes ii. Identify families in need of social support and establish community-based networks to help combat social isolation iii. Communicate effectively with nursery, school, general practitioner, paediatrician, etc.
Exosystem	i. Develop a multiagency team approach to working with families and children ii. Engage constructively with voluntary groups and services in the community iii. Perform accurate needs assessment and clarity in definition and reporting between agencies iv. Promote excellence in communication between agencies involved with the child and family v. Work in partnership with parents vi. Develop quality assurance mechanisms and measure the process and outcome of professional practice vii. Engage in multiagency collaborative policy development and research to further the evidence base on the prevention of child abuse
Microsystem	i. Identify mothers in the antenatal period who would benefit from parenting programmes ii. Identify those children who may be vulnerable to abuse because of prematurity, physical or mental health problems or disability and provide these families with multiagency support iii. Work in partnership with mothers to build self-esteem and confidence in child rearing iv. Establish home visiting programmes that concentrate on developing a relationship with the mother, reviewing their own child-rearing histories, and promoting sensitive, responsive and engaged care giving to the child (Olds et al 1997) v. Establish parenting programmes in the community and on a one/one basis that seek to build the mother's self efficacy (a belief in one's own ability to make life changes and succeed), promote the attributes of attachment between mother and child and provide education on appropriate modes of discipline vi. Diagnose postnatal depression quickly and treat as appropriate vii. Provide extra support to mothers and families with disabilities, physical or mental illness, or drug and alcohol misuse

contributes to child physical abuse and is an issue that must be addressed in the United Kingdom.

In the face of adversity, families living in poverty will be subjected to greater situational stress. Whilst the literature suggests no direct cause and effect, the distal causal relationship cannot be ignored, presenting opportunities for prevention. The solutions to inadequate housing, low educational levels and poverty lie in a more equitable distribution of income, a redistribution of power and resources and an involvement in political activities by nurses.

To ignore the social context in which child physical abuse occurs is an omission of the dangerous circumstances in which people live, and, against all odds, try to successfully rear their children. Whilst we know the distribution of abuse to children is higher in lower socioeconomic groups, it is important to pay due regard to the bias which may exist in the patterns of abuse seen amongst the lower social strata. It is time to address the social inequalities present in Britain today and remember that 'those with the best chance of reducing future inequalities in mental and physical health relate to parents, particularly present and future mothers, and children' (Acheson 1998, p. 9).

SUMMARY

◆ Child physical abuse is difficult to define within the realms of what might be considered 'normal discipline' of children.

◆ The predisposing factors are multifactorial and include the broader environmental issues and individual factors within the child and parent (or carer).

◆ Prevention needs to focus on an ecological framework that seeks to address the macro-, meso-, exo- and microsystems that exist within society today.

DISCUSSION POINTS

1. Consider factors that may predispose families to physically abuse their children?

2. What could be the contribution of policy makers and politicians to the prevention of child physical abuse and how could you work proactively to bring about this political change?

3. As a community nurse how could you work in a preventative manner with families, to help prevent physical abuse of children?

REFERENCES

Acheson D 1998 Independent inquiry into inequalities in health. The Stationary Office, London
Ammerman RT 1991 The role of the child in physical abuse: A reappraisal. Violence and Victims 6: 87–101
Bandura A 1973 Aggression: A social learning analysis. Prentice Hall, Upper Saddle River, NJ
Barnett OW, Miller-Perrin CL, Perrin RD 1997 Family violence across the lifespan. Sage Publications, California
Bates JE 1989 Applications of temperament concepts. In: Kohnstamm JE, Bates JE, Rothbart MK (eds) Temperament in childhood. Wiley, Chichester
Bauer WD, Twentyman CT 1985 Abusing, neglectful and comparison mothers' responses to child related and non-child related stressors. Journal of Consulting and Clinical Psychology 53: 335–343

Beck-Sander A 1999 Working with parents with mental health problems: management of the many risks. In: Weir A, Douglas A (eds) Child protection and adult mental health. Butterworth Heinemann, Oxford
Bee H 1997 The developing child, 8th edn. Addison-Wesley Educational Publishers Inc, New York
Bethea L 1999 Primary prevention of child abuse. American Family Physican 59(6): 1577–1585
Bird A 1999 Families coping with mental health problems: the role and perspective of the general adult psychiatrist. In: Weir A, Douglas A (eds) Child protection and adult mental health. Butterworth Heinemann, Oxford
Bousha DM, Twentyman CT 1984 Mother–child interactional style in abuse, neglect, and control groups: Naturalistic observations in the home. Journal of Abnormal Psychology 93(1): 106–114
Bronfenbrenner U 1979 The experimental ecology of human development. Harvard University Press, Cambridge
Brown J, Cohen P, Johnson J, Salzinger S 1998 A longitudinal analysis of risk factors for child maltreatment: findings of a 17 year prospective study of officially recorded and self reported child abuse and neglect. Child Abuse and Neglect 22(11): 1065–1078
Browne K 1995 Preventing child maltreatment through community nursing. Journal of Advanced Nursing 21: 57–63
Browne K, Saqi S 1988 Approaches to screening for child abuse and neglect. In: Browne K, Davies C, Stratton P (eds) Early prediction and prevention of child abuse. John Wiley and Sons, Chichester
Chilamkurti C, Milner J 1993 Perceptions and evaluations of child transgressions and disciplinary techniques in high and low risk mothers and their children. Child Development 64: 1801–1814
Cloke C, Naish J 1992 Key issues in child protection for health visitors and nurses. Longman, Harlow
Cook A, James J, Leach P 1991 Positively no smacking. Health Visitors' Association and End Physical Punishment of Children (EPOCH), London
Cooper D 1993 Child abuse revisited: Children, society and social work. OUP, Buckingham
Cox A 1988 Maternal depression and impact on children's development. Archives of Disease in Childhood 63: 90–95
Cox J 1999 Postnatal depression in the context of changing patterns of childcare: the implications for primary prevention. In: Weir A, Douglas A (eds) Child protection and adult mental health. Butterworth Heinemann, Oxford
Creighton S 1988 The incidence of child abuse and neglect. In: Browne K, Davies C, Stratton P (eds) Early prediction and prevention of child abuse. John Wiley and Sons, Chichester
Cummings EM 1997 Marital conflict, abuse, and adversity in the family and child adjustment. In: Wolfe D, McMahon R, Peters R (eds) Child abuse: New directions in prevention and treatment across the lifespan. Sage Publications, California
Department of Health 1995 Child protection: Messages from research. HMSO, London
Department of Health 2002 Children and young people on child protection registers – Year ending 31 March 2001, England. www.doh.gov.uk/public/cpr2001.htm

Donnerstein E, Slaby R, Eron L 1994 The mass media and youth aggression. In: Eron L, Gentry J, Schlegel P (eds) Reason to hope: A psychological perspective on violence and youth. American Psychological Association, Washington

Egan-Sage E and Carpenter J 1999 Family characteristics in cases of alleged abuse and neglect. Child Abuse Review 8(5): 301–313

Egeland B 1991 A longitudinal study of high risk families: Issues and findings. In: Starr RH, Wolfe DA (eds) The effects of child abuse and neglect: Issues and research, pp. 33–56. Guilford Press, London

EPOCH 1990 Child abuse and punishment: report of a survey of UK social services and social work departments on policies and practice regarding physical punishment and perceptions of its relationship to child abuse. EPOCH, London

Eron L, Gentry J, Schlegel P (eds) 1994 Reason to hope: A psychological perspective on violence and youth. American Psychological Association, Washington

Frude N 1991 Understanding family problems. Wiley, Chichester

Gelles R 1973 Child abuse as psychopathology: a sociological critique and reformulation. American Journal of Orthopsychiatry 43: 611–621

George C 1996 A representational perspective of child abuse and prevention: Internal working models of attachment and caregiving. Child Abuse and Neglect 20(5): 411–424

Guterman N 1997 Early prevention of physical child abuse and neglect: Existing evidence and future directions. Child Maltreatment 2(1): 12–34

Health Visitors Association 1994 The health visitors role in child protection. HVA, London

Home Office, Department of Health, Department of Education and Science, Welsh Office 1991 Working together under the Children Act 1989: A guide to arrangements for inter-agency cooperation for the protection of children from abuse. HMSO, London

James-Hanman D 1998 Domestic violence: breaking the silence. Community Practitioner 71(12): 404–407

Kaplan C 1999 The real risks children face: the role and perspective of the child psychiatrist. In: Weir A, Douglas A (eds) Child protection and adult mental health. Butterworth Heinemann, Oxford

Kempe C, Silverman F, Steele B, Dregemueller W, Silver H 1962 The battered child syndrome. Journal of the American Medical Association 181: 17–24

Kitzman H, Olds D, Henderson C, et al 1997 Effect of prenatal and infancy home visitation by nurse on pregnancy outcomes, childhood injuries, and repeated childbearing. Journal of the American Medical Association 278(8): 644–652

Larrance DT, Twentyman CT 1983 Maternal attributions and child abuse. Journal of Abnormal Psychiatry 92(4): 449–457

Leach P 1998 Positively no smacking. Community Practitioner 171(11): 355–357

Lehmann P 1995 cited in Sudderman M, Jaffe P 1997 Children and youth who witness violence: New directions in intervention and prevention. In: Wolfe D, McMahon R, Peters R (eds) Child abuse: New directions in prevention and treatment across the lifespan. Sage Publications, California

MacMillan H, MacMillan J, Offord D, Griffith L, MacMillan A 1994 Primary prevention of child physical abuse and neglect: A critical review, Part 1. Journal of Child Psychology 35(5): 835–856

Miller BA, Smyth NJ, Mudar PJ 1999 Mothers' alcohol and other drug problems and their punitiveness toward their children. Journal of Study of Alcohol 60(5): 632–642

Milner J, Dopke C 1997 Child physical abuse: Review of offender characteristics. In: Wolfe D, McMahon R, Peters R (eds) Child abuse: New directions in prevention and treatment across the lifespan. Sage Publications, California

Mullender A, Morley R 1994 Children living with domestic violence. Whiting and Birch, London

Mulvey E 1994 Assessing the evidence of a link between mental illness and violence. Hospital and Community Psychiatry 45(7): 663–668

Naidoo J, Wills J 2000 Health promotion foundations for practice (2nd edn.). Baillière Tindall, Edinburgh

National Commission of Inquiry into the Prevention of Child Abuse 1996 Childhood matters. NSPCC, London

Newman B 1980 The Betty Newman health care systems model. In: Riehl J, Roy C Conceptual models for nursing practice. Appleton Century Crofts, New York

O'Hagan K 1993 Emotional and psychological abuse of children. Open University Press, Buckingham

Olds D, Eckenrode J, Henderson C, Kitzman H 1997 Long term effects of home visitation on maternal life course and child abuse and neglect. Journal of the American Medical Association 278(8): 637–643

Olds D 1997 The Prenatal Early Infancy Project: Preventing child abuse and neglect in the context of promoting maternal and child health. In: Wolfe D, McMahon R, Peters R (eds) Child abuse: New directions in prevention and treatment across the lifespan. Sage Publications, California

Paik H, Comstock G 1994 The effects of television violence on anti-social behaviour: A meta-analysis. Communication Research 21: 516–546

Parker E 1999 Professional challenges and dilemmas. In: Weir A, Douglas A (eds) Child protection and adult mental health. Butterworth Heinemann, Oxford

Parton N 1985 The politics of child abuse. Macmillan Press, Houndsmills

Parton N, Thorpe D, Wattam C 1997 Child protection: Risk and the moral order. Macmillan Press, Houndmills

Roberts J 1988 Why are some families more vulnerable to child abuse. In: Browne K, Davies C, Stratton P Early prediction and prevention of child abuse. John Wiley and Sons, Chichester

Rodriguez C, Sutherland D 1999 Predictors of parents' physical disciplinary practices. Child Abuse and Neglect 23(7): 651–657

Royal College of Psychiatrists 1996 Confidential inquiry into homicides and suicides by mentally ill people. Royal College of Psychiatrists, London

Sayce L 1996 Women with children. In: Perkins R (ed) Women in context. Good Practices in Mental Health, London

Scholer S, Mitchel E, Ray W 1997 Predictors of injury mortality in early childhood. Paediatrics 100(3): 342–347

Sedlak AJ, Broadhurst D 1996 Executive summary of the third national incidence study of child abuse and neglect.

National Clearing House on Child Abuse and Neglect Information, Washington. www.calib.com/ncccanch/pubs/statinfo/nis3.cfm

Smith MA 1995 A community study of physical violence to children in the home and associated variables. Presented at the 5th European Conference: International Society for the Prevention of Child Abuse and Neglect

Strauss M, Gelles RJ, Steinmetz SK 1980 Behind closed doors: Violence in the American family. Doubleday, Anchor

Strauss M, Stewart JH 1998 Corporal punishment by American parents: national data on prevalence, chronicity, severity and duration in relation to child and family characteristics. Family Research Laboratory, University of New Hampshire, New Hampshire

Sudermann M, Jaffe P 1999 Children and youth who witness violence: New directions in intervention and prevention. In: Wolfe D, McMahon R, Peters R (eds) Child abuse: new directions in prevention and treatment across the lifespan. Sage Publications, California

Thomas A, Chess S 1977 Temperament and development. Brunner/Mazel, New York

US Department of Health and Human Services, Children's Bureau 2000 National Child Abuse Statistics. www.acf.dhhs.gov/programs/cb/index.htm

Wasserman DR, Leventhal JM 1993 Maltreatment of children born to cocaine dependent mothers. American Journal of the Disabled Child 147(12): 1324–1328

Weir A, Douglas A (eds) 1999 Child protection and adult mental health. Butterworth Heinemann, Oxford

Welsh Office 1999 Learning how to make children safer: An analysis for the Welsh Office of serious child abuse cases in Wales. Cardiff: University of Welsh Anglia and Welsh Office

FURTHER READING

Wolfe DA, McMahon RJ, Peters R DeV (eds) 1997 Child abuse: New directions in prevention and treatment across the lifespan. Sage, London

This is an excellent textbook which provides insight into new developments in the field of the prevention of child abuse.

Weir A, Douglas A (eds) 1999 Child protection and adult mental health. Butterworth Heinemann, Oxford

This book is a very good source of reference for community nurses who wish to learn more about mental health issues and child protection.

Frude N 1991 Understanding family problems. Wiley, Chichester

Although an older textbook, this book remains extremely valuable in describing some of the issues relating to family violence.

George C 1996 A representational perspective of child abuse and prevention: Internal working models of attachment and caregiving. Child Abuse and Neglect 20(5): 411–424

This article is extremely interesting to those community nurses who wish to learn more about attachment theory and its relationship with child abuse.

Family nursing

J. Edwards

INTRODUCTION

This chapter will explore the development and implications of a family nursing perspective, as well as some underlying theoretical issues. Examples from the family nursing literature, which have special relevance for the specialist practice of community nursing (see Section 5), will also be used to explore the potential benefits of adopting a family perspective.

Community nurses are in a better position than most, not only to observe and assess the impact of contextual and environmental influences on the physical, emotional and mental health of individuals and family groups, but also to identify and make optimum use of family strengths. Chapters 8 and 9 in this section explore the nature of these influences from sociological and psychological perspectives, the former drawing attention to the social and cultural changes which have affected the composition and structure of family groups or households.

During the last decade, there has been an increasing interest in developing research paradigms which focus particularly on the interaction between a nurse and the family (Barnfather & Lyon 1993, Duffy et al 1998, Friedman 1998, Gillis 1991, Parse 1998, Ward-Griffin & McKeever 2000). It is in the context of the community nurse's interest in partnership and empowerment, as well as her role in making a comprehensive assessment of priority health needs, that draws attention to the importance of recognizing the impact of family relationships. Friedemann (1995) for instance, sees the family as an evolutionary system, one that is constantly interacting with other systems in the surrounding environment and striving to maintain some kind of harmony, or balance in the face of different and changing pressures. From this perspective, the role of the nurse becomes that of helping to find acceptable ways to pursue goals of stability and control in the face of health-related problems which may/may not be affected by cultural beliefs, or socioeconomic factors.

In addition, various writers in the field of family nursing have underlined the importance of differentiating between the family as the context in which an assessment of an individual takes place, and the family itself as the focus of assessment, negotiation, participation and evaluation. Traditionally, nurses operating within a stated family-centred framework have tended to see the role of the family as essentially passive, supplementing or reinforcing their professional expertise in the care of an individual patient. Those who are presently working successfully in the community will already be accustomed to adopting a family framework for health needs assessment, for problem identification and a participative approach to the identification of priority goals. Taking time to explore further the meaning of 'family-centred' or 'family-focused' care, provides useful opportunities to consider some of the implications for practice. In summary, some of the reasons for making the family unit, rather than an individual, the focus for specialist community nursing activity include:

♦ in the context of the family unit, a clearer understanding of individual functioning can be achieved;

♦ illness, traumatic injury, or some other form of health related suffering by one family member affects other family members and by limiting the focus of care to the individual, important information for holistic assessment may be missed;

♦ since there is a strong link between family inter-relationships and the health status of individual family members, the family itself plays a crucial role in all aspects of health care from prevention and health promotion, through to involvement in treatment and rehabilitation; the family-centred nurse adopts a partnership approach to the identification of actual and potential health risks, making use of stages in the empowerment process to promote the family's confidence to explore the potential benefits of different coping strategies;

♦ the role of community nursing incorporates self care education, health promotion, family support and facilitating the development of family involvement in problem-solving strategies where appropriate – all of which would be likely to benefit from a family-oriented perspective;

♦ the family can be a vital support system in times of crisis and, when sustained by a community nursing service, can become an even more important healthcare resource for continuing care.

Earlier chapters point to the dynamic nature of family relationships and by asking particular kinds of questions, a reflective community nurse can broaden the framework for assessment in a family setting. For example, why and how does the arrival of a first baby, or a baby with a disabling condition, have such a significant effect on a marriage or co-habiting partnership? In what ways can the continuing care of someone with a chronic condition cause stress and influence interactions between individual family members? How can patterns of family behaviour influence recovery or rehabilitation processes? What kinds of coping mechanisms might be predicted in the face of specified family crises? In the face of health-related difficulties, community nursing interventions have the potential to be beneficial in a number of different ways. By adopting a two-pronged perspective that focuses on the family unit (where this is deemed to be most appropriate) and on partnership, intervention activities can aim to optimize the resources and health potential of the family as a whole, utilizing processes and resources within and outside the family, to restore health, normal functioning and equilibrium.

DEFINING A 'FAMILY'

Whether traditional or otherwise, families have some basic characteristics and structures which are uniquely expressed by each individual family unit. Where health or healthcare needs exist, Craft and Willadson (1992) provide a useful perspective by drawing attention to the social context of a 'family' and to the mutual attachment, long-term responsibility and commitment between the individuals concerned. Friedemann (1995) also reminds us that in all cultural settings, the family is the most important social context in which health and health-related problems occur and are resolved.

For the purpose of much of this discussion, a family is seen as a special group of individuals who engage in patterns of interaction that derive from the intimacy and expectations of their relationships. Such interactions are often characterized by reciprocity, intensity and frequency and by their potential influence on individual members of the group. For example, a particular consequence of disturbed family relationships is child abuse. Several studies suggest that abusive parents share a number of characteristics, particularly in terms of how a child's behaviour is interpreted: inability to conform to unrealistic expectations can be seen as wilful and deliberate for example; a belief that punishment is not only right and deserved but is also applied with a level of severity which is quite inappropriate. (See Chapters 10 and 11 for a more detailed examination of family violence and child protection issues.)

From a very different perspective, the relevant literature associated with pain seems to identify rather different perspectives when associated with family dynamics, such as pain as a symptom *caused by* family dynamics; pain as *an agent* that shapes family dynamics and pain as something which has the *power* to maintain and reinforce family group processes. Such findings make reference to patterns of 'excessive togetherness' or enmeshment, rigidity and overprotection, suggesting that the presenting individual and family characteristics may have developed as a consequence of, rather than an antecedent of, the pain (see Chapter 9 for further discussion of family dynamics).

Research of the kind just mentioned reinforces the interest in developing theoretical frameworks of explanatory interest to the practicing community nurse; these have included developmental, interactional, ecological, social exchange and systems-based theories. Systems theory, for example, provides a way to understand and analyse the complexities and dynamics of a healthcare situation; an interactional theory would seek to explain family relationships and nurse–family relationships, exploring notions of partnership and teamwork while a developmental family theory would seek to explain changing health needs in relation to life-stages, predictable transitions and major life events.

SO WHAT IS FAMILY NURSING?

Most people probably think of nursing as a one-to-one health-related service and many nurses may still consider the individual as the client even though reference can be found to the significance of the family as long ago as in the writings of Florence Nightingale (Whall & Fawcett 1991). The individualized problem-oriented approach has been a common and traditional nursing perspective, one that focuses on the abnormal, or things that have gone wrong. A family nursing perspective however, is one that seeks and values the strengths and competencies within the family, recognizes individual differences and resists the temptation to label or stigmatize a family that appears to lack the ability to resolve its own problems without professional help. On reflection, it can hardly be surprising that in some circumstances, families can feel alienated by 'experts' who appear to possess the solutions and resources perceived to be lacking within their own family.

Therefore an effective family nursing approach not only requires a philosophical shift to *partnership* but also the skills to search for competencies, capacities and resources around an individual within a family, as well as in the surrounding neighbourhood. So ideally, family nursing theory should help community nurses to understand and appreciate the complexities of family life, how they become interwoven and change across time and in relation to stressors in the surrounding environment. Repeated infections, dietary and other lifestyle habits likely to impact on health, such as smoking and misuse of drugs, domestic violence and decision-making during terminal care, are just a few of the more obvious health-related issues where focusing on the family as the unit of care becomes quite critical for achieving effective service provision. Perhaps more importantly, the values and beliefs held by the family – which give meaning to their lives – need to be taken into account by the community nurse, when negotiating priorities and reaching agreement about individual and family goals for improving or maintaining health/quality of life.

Families may perceive the community nursing service rather differently and each family member may have a different perspective with regard to a health problem that may be facing them. This, together with established patterns of relating to each other, can provide valuable information for the nurse, where the aim is to achieve partnership in the decision-making about priorities, about the possible need for other resources and about the need for openness concerning the limitations of the particular service. Each family has a right and a responsibility to make choices about matters which affect its health and welfare and it is the interaction between family members and between the community nurse and the family that forms the context in which such choices are made – the nurse having a particular responsibility to ensure that the choice is an adequately informed one.

Nurses, however, often use time constraints to explain why the family as a whole is not incorporated into community nursing practice. Wright and Leahey (1999) argue that a 15-minute interview can be 'purposeful, effective, informative and even healing', providing that it includes the following essential ingredients:

◆ courtesy, respect and kindness
◆ listening and therapeutic conversation – providing opportunities for patient/client/carers to be acknowledged and affirmed
◆ collating relevant contextual and background information including current beliefs about the health status of individual family members
◆ at least three therapeutic questions, e.g. about expectations of treatment or the role of a community nursing service; most pressing

concerns; or the least/most helpful aspect of recent visits to the health centre or clinic
◆ commending family and individual strengths.

The community nurse who recognizes the value of developing a working relationship with a family and who takes time to observe and analyse interactions between family members, is more likely to be in a position to develop the capacities of individuals, to promote attitude change and to help the family remove barriers or stumbling blocks to achieving optimum health and stability. Life cycle changes for instance, can place considerable stress on family members, as each one struggles to adapt to the entrances and exits that mark such events as marriage, birth, migration, unemployment, divorce, hospitalization or death.

The kinds of strengths that generally enable individuals or families to cope can lie in individual characteristics. Neil Frude for example, discusses *traits* such as resilience and optimism in some detail in Chapter 9. Other kinds of *assets* affecting family functioning include adequate finance, a supportive extended family and a safe comfortable home. Feeley and Gottlieb (2000) draw attention to the importance of identifying *capacities* and *potentials* as part of a family nursing assessment. The former might include the capacity to locate and utilize local community-based resources, or innovative approaches to resolving problems. A more transient but nonetheless valuable capacity would be motivation. *Potentials* are significant for effective community nursing because they represent 'precursors' that could, with support, be developed into strengths.

Resources of this kind are likely to vary considerably between families. The community nurse will have a number of opportunities to make the most appropriate use of both individual and family strengths by:

◆ using well-developed observational and listening skills, together with open-ended questions
◆ locating strengths and providing feedback to the family about their value
◆ recognizing potential strengths and 'calling them forth' at an appropriate time
◆ promoting the development of particular strengths in the face of the current situation.

Open-ended questions, questions specifically designed to help individuals identify their own strengths and finding out how the family managed previously during predictable examples of 'life crises', all help to develop rapport between the community nurse and the family, which in turn is likely to facilitate collaboration and partnership. Once strengths have been identified, they can be openly discussed in concrete terms, both as a means to provide feedback and to link strengths with effects. It is the openness of such discussion that can help to boost confidence and may provide a different or new perspective that contributes to moving the situation forward.

PRACTICAL USE OF THEORETICAL AND RESEARCH PERSPECTIVES

For the community nurse, it will be important to explore different perspectives as a means, for example, to understand how stressors such as unresolved chronic pain (or any other significant stressor), can impact on family functioning. As mentioned above, systems theory can provide a useful framework to reflect on the individual's attempts to cope with something like chronic pain in the context of family responses – or lack of them – as well as the strategies adopted by the family to maintain some kind of harmony and accord in the face of the particular distress of one member. One example that fits this theoretical perspective is the amount of energy used by families defined as *excessively connected*, to maintain and control the status quo. Exhausted by efforts to control internal family dynamics, they can become isolated from potential sources of help and support outside the immediate family (Smith & Friedemann 1999). This particular study reinforces the notion that health professionals who focus on the individual who presents with a health problem that fits the health service agenda, may well miss the health-related needs of those in the family who are finding the situation almost unbearable. It certainly highlights important aspects of assessment and draws attention to the importance of discussion with family members, as the basis for

their involvement in the planning of care strategies and the negotiation of both individual and family goals.

A basic outline of family systems theory is described below because its particular perspective has contributed significantly both to the social science and family nursing literature. Wright and Leahy (1999) were probably the first to present a detailed explanation of family systems theory as applied to the practice of nursing. It offered the means to explore a family group in terms of how each member relates to others and to the outside world; the underlying principle being that individual parts can be affected by the whole and the whole can be affected by an individual part. A positive and functioning family system for example, can be recognized by its rules, which are overt and negotiable, by the open seeking of adjustments in the face of stress and by the balance obtained between 'togetherness' and 'individualism'. Hanson and Boyd (1996) note the usefulness of using an essentially mechanical model to explore complex entities, while Baumann (2000) draws attention to the problems facing nurses who use this framework to make judgements about family functioning, particularly when used across different cultures. The use of a family system perspective does however, enable the community nurse to shift her thinking from mechanistic and outcome-oriented explanations of change, to a more holistic process-oriented explanation.

More recently, other researchers have focused on sociological concepts such as roles and role enactment to examine family functioning, as well as psychological concepts such as stress and communication and their impact on family functioning. Landry-Meyer (1999) for example, studied the modification of roles when grandparents took on the responsibilities of parenting. She interestingly explores the concept of 'role-fit' in families, together with problems of role commitment in the face of disconnection from age-related developmental tasks. The use of the term *impact* makes assumptions that illness and other health changes can be seen as stressors (Friedman 1998). Models of stress have been developed to show the relationship between events or situations and their consequences – and more particularly the role of intervening variables such as the presence of social support (McCubbin 1993), an important factor in any assessment process conducted by a community nurse. The impact of stress can be highlighted for example, in prolonged family caregiving, Nolan and Grant (1992) finding evidence that stress could be moderated for families (and individual clients/patients) by encouraging them to consider the benefits of making optimum use of opportunities for respite care.

Communication theory also frequently appears in discussions of family nursing – the exchange of, and openness in the giving of, information between family members and between the family and the health professionals involved, has been seen to be critical for the effective practice of family nursing. Dunst and Trivette (1996) for example found that feelings of confidence are increased in parents when they are actively involved in healthcare experiences. The view that the family should be in active partnership with healthcare professionals is clearly evident in recent policy discussion concerned with quality improvement (see Chapter 4) although nurses have been reminded that they often fall short of recognizing that it is the family itself that is the expert in defining what health and the family mean for them (Parse 1998).

The above family theories also appear in the literature concerning domestic violence and aspects of child abuse although most nurses are likely to find it difficult to maintain a family-focused perspective, given the way emotions can be generated in the face of the victim of assault. Chapter 11 provides more detailed discussion of protecting a child at risk of abuse but there is considerable literature concerning the impact of violence, as well as other forms of abuse on family life and family relationships. In a study of adolescents for instance, Paavilainen et al (2000) found that maltreatment and neglect not only resulted in physical injuries but was also linked to feelings of worthlessness, behaviour problems, depression and difficulties at school, while the family as a whole showed an absence of caring, aggressiveness and a lack of togetherness.

FAMILY EMPOWERMENT

As mentioned above and in Chapter 4, the NHS has placed an increased emphasis on quality improvement, the indicators of which include achieving greater participation from patients/clients and their families in the decision-making associated with interventions and goals. This suggests that community nurses should be looking more critically at their practice analysing their activities and forms of communication in terms of meeting both the expectations of patients/clients and the overall purpose of the service.

Many families are able to adapt and find the means to overcome, for example, the challenges of long-term health care, while others experience the kind of difficulty likely to threaten family functioning. In such circumstances, Hulme (1999) points to the potential benefits of interventions aimed at empowerment – that is to say, interventions which are based on assumptions that all individuals have existing strengths and competencies, with the potential to grow and develop. She argues that it is within the interactive processes involved in empowerment that the community nurse firstly develops a level of trust which subsequently enables family members to participate fully in the decision-making to resolve the two major challenges faced, for example, by parents who have a chronically sick child: (i) meeting the healthcare needs of the child and (ii) preserving normality in family life.

However, all community nurses who use the concept of empowerment, need to reflect on the underlying philosophy and critically review their own capacity to share power and control. As Skelton (1995) so aptly notes, empowerment could easily be seen as the means by which the expert health professional gets someone to come round to their way of thinking and behaving (i.e. the way the expert thought to be best for them) while at the same time, encouraging them to think it was their own idea in the first place. The key components of family empowerment are generally accepted as the gaining or regaining of control – this to be achieved by reflection, joint action of family members in the social context of neighbourhood life and the parameters of the current healthcare system.

Documentation of any community nursing activity requires consideration to be given to outcomes – the anticipated consequences of intervention activities, in this case, the processes of empowerment. The purpose of family empowerment is to facilitate a family's capacity to recognize and meet its own health needs, to explore options for solving health-related problems and to make optimum use of appropriate and available resources – all as a means to satisfy priority healthcare needs and to preserve the integrity of family functioning.

In a review of several studies, Dixon (1996) was able to identify four stages in the process of empowerment, which seemed to be quite consistent and to provide useful insights for community nurses:

1. an initial professionally dominated phase, marked by dependence and passive responses linked to placing trust in the expert;
2. a participatory stage triggered by curiosity and the persistence of a condition, carers beginning to see themselves as having an important role to play;
3. a challenging stage representing the beginning of a power shift, where mistrust and anger begin to appear and parents/carers question aspects of care, sometimes reflecting frustration and disillusionment;
4. a final stage where the development of confidence and advocacy becomes evident in more assertive and self-reliant behaviour, predicting collaboration and partnership, with the capacity to negotiate fully with health professionals.

Such stages in the process of empowerment should not be seen as linear one-way processes. They represent the nature of the interaction between the nurse and the family, frequently involving repetition and overlap (Gibson 1995).

The kind of outcomes that might be expected from empowerment activities with a family caring for a child with a chronic condition for example, are predictable by the final stage. They highlight the kind of information, strategies and social skills

likely to be critical for a productive relationship between a community nurse and a family:

◆ active involvement by parents/main carers in decision-making with health professionals
◆ family members working together to minimize the effects of the condition on the child, as well as on siblings
◆ parents responding appropriately to the emotional and developmental needs of individual children
◆ family members agreeing to modify roles and/or behaviour to regain, or maintain, optimum family functioning
◆ a reduction in home visits by the community nurse, or reduced hospital admissions.

FAMILY NURSING AND THE FUTURE

The expertise implicit in family nursing is likely to have an important place in the future as the findings of genetic research become more widely known. A guest editorial by Suzanne Feetham in the *Journal of Family Nursing* in 1999 went so far as to be entitled: *The Future in Family Nursing is Genetics and it is Now*. Not only does she draw attention to the important ethical, legal and social implications of current research in this field but to the predictable expectations that families will anticipate being able to discuss their concerns with a qualified specialist community nurse who will be sufficiently knowledgeable to help interpret literature in the public domain and more particularly to explain the meaning of what has been said to them in a clinical setting.

The implications of genetic advances are evident in the continuing priority given to cardiovascular disease as a leading cause of morbidity and mortality. Although there have been diagnostic, technological and surgical advances in the treatment of this disease, a more comprehensive understanding of its origins and aetiology is still needed if more effective approaches to dealing with the underlying abnormalities are to be achieved. Genetic advances are expected to enable health professionals of the future to treat the primary cause of the damage, or its progression, rather than focusing on the treatment of secondary signs and symptoms.

Public interest in genetic research is evident from newspaper and magazine headlines but the general public are not so likely to be well informed about the time-lag between the discovery of a gene and the development of related treatments. They are also not likely to grasp the significance of research findings that apply to a high-risk group rather than to the population at large and they are unlikely to be used to having their family examined in the systematic way necessary for such lines of enquiry. Changes in information regarding high and low risk, are also likely to result in uncertainty for both individuals and families so it will be particularly important for example, for a community nurse to be sufficiently knowledgeable to explain that a genetic test only provides information about susceptibility and does not predict the onset of, for instance, cancer (Wilfond et al 1997).

The need for research studies to go beyond the individual with a gene mutation, as a means to answer complex questions about the nature and extent of risk, means that whole families may need to be identified and agree to participate in longitudinal studies. There is the potential for such involvement to place undue stress on family relationships, particularly where there is significant variation in beliefs about 'need to know' or willingness to disclose health-related information. For the community nurse adopting a family perspective, ethical as well as clinical issues can arise where for example, the results of a son's or daughter's test reveal information about a parent. However, the nurse will only be able to provide adequate support for families with anxieties about genetically based risk, if she recognizes that family relationships can be affected by the process of risk assessment (Salkovskis & Rimes 1997) and she has sufficiently up-to-date knowledge to explain the implications of available literature. Helping individuals identify and explore the likely ways that either a positive or negative test result could affect relationships within the family,

is another way to promote involvement in the decision-making processes.

CONCLUSION

Family nursing theory and research attempts to help community nurses recognize the complex, changing and interwoven aspects of family relationships. They also focus attention on the potential benefits of adopting a family framework for assessment and partnership and point to the critical elements of nurse–family interaction. The concept of *family* needs to be understood as having different meanings and purpose for individuals and that family satisfaction is more likely when members sense that the meaning given to health and family life are in accord with, and respected by, other family members.

In shifting the emphasis from the individual to the family, the community nurse broadens the focus of care and in doing so creates opportunities to recognize and value actual and potential strengths within and around the family and to achieve a productive working relationship based on equity and openness. Successful outcomes may also be more to do with participation and partnership than modifications to behaviour, symptom control or a reduction in morbidity, which themselves may follow the initial stages of involvement and empowerment.

SUMMARY

- ◆ The community health nurse is ideally placed to ensure that a holistic approach to health needs is followed and to adopt a family-oriented perspective rather than simply focusing on an individual within the context of a family group.

- ◆ Effective family nursing requires recognition of the complex nature of family relationships as well as a philosophical shift towards partnership, recognizing and valuing family resources and capacities.

- ◆ Family empowerment is achieved by a staged approach enabling the family to gain / regain control of their health needs.

DISCUSSION POINTS

1. Consider the processes involved in the development of a productive relationship between the community nurse and a family. Explore how these processes could influence the capacity of the family to manage the care of: (a) a child in receipt of palliative care; (b) a family member exhibiting problem behaviour; or (c) a frail elderly parent.

2. In what ways can the family assessment process undertaken by a community nurse influence the involvement of the family in decision-making?

3. The need for different types of support varies during different stages of family life and during the care of a family member with a long-term chronic disease. Consider different types and sources of support and the implications of ineffective nurse communication about their potential benefit.

REFERENCES

Barnfather JS, Lyon BL 1993 Stress and coping: state of the science and implications for nursing theory, research and practice. Sigma Theta Tau, Indianapolis, IN

Baumann SL 2000 Family nursing: Theory – Anemic, nursing theory-deprived. Nursing Science Quarterly 13(4): 286–290

Craft MJ, Willadson JA 1992 Interventions related to family. Nursing Clinics of North America 27: 517–540

Dixon DM 1996 Unifying concepts in parents' experience with health care providers. Journal of Family Nursing 2: 111–132

Duffy ME, Vehvilainen-Julkunen K, Huber D, Varjoranta P 1998 Family nursing practice in public health: Finland and Utah. Public Health Nursing 15: 281–287

Dunst CJ, Trivette CM 1996 Empowerment, effective help-giving practices and family centred care. Paediatric Nursing 22: 334–343

Feeley N, Gottlieb LN 2000 Nursing approaches for working with family strengths and resources. Journal of Family Nursing 6(1): 9–24

Friedemann ML 1995 The framework of systems organisation – a conceptual approach to families and nursing. Sage, Newbury Park, CA

Friedman MM 1998 Family nursing: research, theory and practice, 4th edn. Appleton and Lange, Stamford, Connecticut

Gibson CH 1995 The process of empowerment in mothers of chronically ill children. Journal of Advanced Nursing 21: 1201–1210

Gillis CL 1991 Family nursing research theory and practice. Journal of Nursing Scholarship 23(1): 19–22

Hanson SM, Boyd ST 1996 Family nursing: an overview. In: Hanson SM, Boyd ST (eds) Family health care nursing: theory, practice and research, pp. 5–37. FA Davis, Philadelphia

Hulme PA 1999 Family empowerment: a nursing intervention with suggested outcomes for families of children with a chronic health condition. Journal of Family Nursing 5(1): 33–50

Landry-Meyer L 1999 Research into action: recommended intervention strategies for grandparent caregivers. Family Relations 48: 381–389

McCubbin MA 1993 Family stress theory and development of nursing knowledge about family adaptation. In: Feetham SL, Meister SB, Bell JM, Gilliss CL (eds) The nursing of families: theory, research, education and practice. Sage, Newbury Park, CA

Nolan MR, Grant G 1992 Respite care: challenging traditions. British Journal of Nursing 1(3): 129–133

Paavilainen E, Astedt-Kurki P, Paunonen M 2000 Adolescents' experiences of maltreatment within the family: challenges for family nursing. Primary Health Care Research and Development 1: 235–241

Parse RR 1998 The human becoming school of thought: a perspective for nurses and other health professionals. Sage, Thousand Oaks, CA

Salkovskis PM, Rimes KA 1997 Predictive genetic testing: psychological factors. Journal of Psychosomatic Research 43(5): 477–487

Skelton R 1995 Nursing and empowerment: concepts and strategies. Journal of Advanced Nursing 19: 415–423

Smith AA, Friedemann ML 1999 Perceived family dynamics of persons with chronic pain. Journal of Advanced Nursing 30(3): 543–551

Ward-Griffin C, McKeever P 2000 Relationships between nurses and family caregivers: Partners in care? Advances in Nursing Science 22: 89–103

Whall AL, Fawcett J (eds) 1991 Family theory development in nursing: state of the science and art. FA Davis, Philadelphia

Wilfond BS, Rothenberg KH, Thomson EJ, Lerman C 1997 Cancer genetic susceptibility testing: ethical and policy implications for future research and clinical practice. Journal of Law, Medicine and Ethics 25: 243–251

Wright LM, Leahey M 1999 Maximising time, minimising suffering: the 15 minute family interview. Journal of Family Nursing 5(3): 259–274

FURTHER READING

Hanson SM, Boyd ST 1996 Family health care nursing: theory, practice and research. FA Davis, Philadelphia

Friedman MM 1998 Family nursing: research, theory and practice, 4th edn. Appleton and Lange, Stamford, Connecticut

Journal of Family Nursing – *provides up-to-date opportunities to explore in-depth analyses of family nursing practice in both Western and non-Western cultures, addressing both theory development and research related to physical, social and mental health.*

Wright LM, Leahey M 1994 Nurses and families: a guide to family assessment and intervention, 2nd edn. FA Davis, Philadelphia

Professional frameworks for practice

This section outlines legal and ethical 'frameworks for practice' and draws the reader's attention to a range of professional issues that impact upon community nursing. The legal framework is of prime concern, particularly with the development of new nursing roles in primary care and advancements in nurse prescribing. Ethical issues remain pertinent to practice, particularly in the light of advanced technology and clients increased collaboration in care. Professional leadership and effective team working are also highlighted as pivotal in delivering the National Health Service agenda in a community setting.

Chapter 13 opens with a review of legal issues relevant to community nursing practice. It explores pertinent issues such as the Human Rights Act, professional conduct and accountability issues and the legal aspects of nurse prescribing. Against this backdrop Chapter 14 moves on to explore a range of ethical considerations of significance to practice, inclusive of advocacy and respect for autonomy.

Chapter 15 follows with an exploration of teamwork and team development. The chapter begins with an overview of the theories of teamwork and work groups, followed by a critical analysis of team development initiatives and their contribution to collective working. Case studies drawn from health and social care practice are used to provide examples of teamwork evaluation and a speculative discussion on the future of teamwork concludes this chapter.

The closing chapter in this section is concerned with professional leadership and the management of change. It discusses the differences between management and leadership and highlights transformational leadership in driving forward change. The key skills of effective leaders are identified and barriers associated with this role are explored. The chapter concludes with emphasizing the significance of strong nursing leadership in the new world of primary care organizations and presents a framework for community nursing leadership development.

Legal aspects of community health nursing

B. Dimond

INTRODUCTION

It is clear that recent years have seen an increasing pressure upon those health professionals who work in the community. Shorter length of stay in hospital, more patients being treated in primary and community care alone and an ever-increasing development of technical equipment being used in the community have required community nurses to develop their skills and cope with a very much more sickly group of patients than in the past. In such circumstances it is essential that the nurse has a good understanding of the law which applies to her practice.[1,2]

Note

The Vancouver style of referencing which is a variant on the number system has been used in this chapter. The editors considered this form of text referencing to be the most appropriate considering the subject matter and the references cited.

THE ENGLISH LEGAL SYSTEM AND HUMAN RIGHTS

The main source of our laws is twofold: statutes and the common law. Statutes, also known as Acts of Parliament, often give powers to a Minister of the Crown to draw up detailed regulations, which are placed before the Houses of Parliament in the form of Statutory Instruments. Increasingly since the United Kingdom is a member of the European

Community an increasing proportion of our legislation derives from regulations and directives emanating from the European Community. Common law supplements Acts of Parliament and statutory instruments as a source of law by the decisions of judges in decided cases. These decisions are known as 'judge made law', 'case law' or the 'common law'. There is a hierarchy of courts headed by the House of Lords and a decision by the House of Lords would be binding on other courts except itself. Decisions of the Court of Appeal would be binding upon those courts below it. Official reports of the decisions of the judges are used to determine the principles of law and the reasons supporting those principles.

The Human Rights Act 1998 was passed to bring into effect in this country the European Convention on Human Rights. This convention was signed by many European countries after the Second World War but this country, although a signatory, had not incorporated the articles in the law of this country. Citizens who alleged that their rights had been violated had to take their case to the European Court in Strasbourg for determination of their rights, unless that particular article overlapped with a right recognized by statute or the common law. The effect of the Human Rights Act was to enable a person to take action in the courts of this country if there was an alleged breach of the articles of the European Convention. A duty was also placed on all public authorities and organizations exercising functions of a public nature to implement the articles of the Convention. The Act came into force on 2 October 2000 in England and Wales and in Scotland on devolution (see further below).

CIVIL AND CRIMINAL PROCEEDINGS

The law recognizes a distinction between civil and criminal proceedings and the courts in which the proceedings take place. Civil proceedings arise where a person or organization alleges that another person or organization is liable for a civil wrong. These include negligence, nuisance, breach of statutory duty, trespass and breach of contract.

Criminal proceedings arise where there is an allegation that a person is guilty of a criminal offence, which may be defined by an Act of Parliament (e.g. the Theft Act) or be based on common law (e.g. murder). Some actions may constitute both a civil wrong and a criminal offence, e.g. driving dangerously is a criminal offence and if a person is injured, it may lead to civil proceedings to obtain compensation for negligence. Recent significant changes have been made to our system for civil proceedings known as the Woolf reforms which are designed to ensure that civil procedure is made speedier, cheaper and more effective in securing justice.[3]

STRUCTURAL CHANGES AFFECTING PRIMARY CARE

HEALTH AND SOCIAL SERVICES STATUTORY DUTIES

Under the National Health Act 1977 statutory duties are placed upon the Secretary of State to provide a comprehensive health service to such extent as considered necessary to meet all reasonable requirements. These statutory duties are in turn devolved to health authorities which have the responsibility of securing long-term agreements with NHS trusts for the provision of health services and also for arranging the provision of primary care services. As a result of the NHS and Community Care Act 1990 duties were placed upon local authorities to carry out assessments for community care services, to publish (in conjunction with the health and voluntary sector) an annual community care plan, and ensure that a complaints procedure was established. Where it appears that there are health or housing needs, the local authority can require health and housing authorities to take part in the assessment for community services.

PRIMARY CARE TRUSTS

The 1990 Act also saw the establishment of group fundholding practices, but these were abolished by the Health Act 1999. Instead, primary health groups/local health groups linking general practitioners and community health and social services, have been established, which have increasingly been obtaining trust status. These Primary Care Trusts have the responsibility for arranging the provision of family practitioner and other primary care services. Care Trusts which arrange for the provision of social services as well as health care are also being set up. The Health and Social Care Act 2001 and the NHS Reform and Health Care Professions Act 2002 strengthen the powers of the Secretary of State over Care Trusts and comparable partnerships.

ACCOUNTABILITY: CRIMINAL, CIVIL, PROFESSIONAL AND EMPLOYMENT

Where harm occurs then any community nurse involved could face various courts and tribunals where her/his accountability would be examined from different perspectives.

CRIMINAL LAW

Any unexpected death would be reported to the coroner, who may decide to hold an inquest if it was considered necessary to have an investigation into the death. The purpose of the inquest is to determine the identity of the deceased and how and why the deceased came to die. In matters of public importance, a jury will be summoned to decide upon the cause of death. At any stage of the inquest, the coroner can adjourn the proceedings and pass the papers to the Crown Prosecution Service in order for criminal investigations to be initiated. At the conclusion of the criminal proceedings, the inquest will be resumed. Criminal proceedings may be initiated against any health professional if there are grounds for considering that a criminal offence has been committed. Where a patient has died, a community nurse could face prosecution if her conduct has been so grossly reckless or negligent as to lead to the death of the patient. For example, an anaesthetist failed to realize that during an operation a tube had become

disconnected as a result of which the patient died. He was prosecuted in the criminal courts and convicted of manslaughter.[4] The House of Lords held that the jury could convict him of manslaughter if they were satisfied beyond reasonable doubt that he was guilty of such gross recklessness or negligence as to amount to a crime.

The Health and Safety Inspectorate could also commence criminal proceedings against any employee in respect of a health and safety offence (see below).

CIVIL PROCEEDINGS

Where a patient has been harmed as a result of negligence then it is possible for a claim to be brought for compensation against the employer of the negligent employee. This is because an employer is vicariously liable for the actions which took place during the course of employment. Whilst the employee is also personally liable, the compensation would be paid by the employer on the basis of its vicarious liability for the negligence of an employee whilst working in the course of employment. In order to obtain compensation, the claimant would have to establish that a duty of care was owed to her and that an employee was in breach of that duty and this breach caused reasonably foreseeable harm to the claimant. Whether or not there has been a breach of duty is ascertained by applying what is known as the Bolam Test. In the case from which the test took its name[5] the court laid down the following principle to determine the standard of care which should be followed:

The standard of care expected is the 'standard of the ordinary skilled man exercising and professing to have that special skill'.

Evidence would be given to court, by persons respected in the relevant field of community nursing to show what standard would have been expected of the nurse in the specific circumstances which arose. Examples are given in the specific situations discussed below of the application of the Bolam Test to community nursing.

As well as showing that there was a failure to follow a reasonable standard of care, the claimant must show that this failure caused the harm which occurred.[6] This requires both factual causation to be shown,[7] and also evidence that the type of harm which occurred was reasonably foreseeable. In addition there must be no intervening cause which breaks the chain of causation.[8] Each of these elements of negligence: duty, breach, causation and harm, must be shown to exist by the claimant on a balance of probabilities.

PROFESSIONAL CONDUCT PROCEEDINGS

Misconduct by a community nurse could also be followed by proceedings before the Conduct and Competency Committee of the NMC. The ultimate sanction is for the nurse to be removed from the Register.

DISCIPLINARY ACTION BY AN EMPLOYER

In addition any community nurse guilty of failures in his/her professional practice could face disciplinary action by her employer. Under her contract of employment she has a duty to obey the implied (unwritten and implied by law) terms in the contract which require her to work with reasonable care and skill and obey the reasonable instructions of the employer. The ultimate sanction is dismissal, but an employee can challenge this if she has the requisite length of continuous service (12 months at present) by an application to the employment tribunal.

NMC AND PROVISIONS FOR PROFESSIONAL MISCONDUCT

From April 2002 the Nursing and Midwifery Council has replaced the United Kingdom Central Council as the registration body for nurses, midwives and health visitors. There are fewer members of Council and the Order setting out the powers and procedures of the new Council and its Committees has significant differences from

the previous regime. In particular, the National Boards in the different constituent parts of the United Kingdom have been abolished and separate arrangements are made in each country for the quality control of education and assessment for nursing and midwifery. Under the Order for the constitution of the NMC and its committees, it is envisaged that four committees, known as the statutory committees, of the Council shall be set up:

◆ Investigating Committee
◆ Conduct and Competence Committee
◆ Health Committee
◆ Midwifery Committee.

The first three are also known as the 'Practice Committees'. The Council may establish other committees to discharge its functions and can delegate functions to them, other than any power to make rules. At the time of writing it is not known how the definition of misconduct (currently 'conduct unworthy of a nurse, midwife or health visitor') will be agreed and the extent to which procedures will differ from those under the UKCC and its Professional Conduct Committee. There is concern to ensure that the new provisions for professional conduct hearings comply with the requirements of the European Convention on Human Rights.

HEALTH ACT 1999

The Health Act 1999 makes provision for some of the initiatives envisaged in the NHS White Paper.[9]

DUTY OF QUALITY: CLINICAL GOVERNANCE

A new statutory duty of quality set out in section 18 of the Act is shown below:

It is the duty of each Health Authority, Primary Care Trust and NHS Trust to put and keep in place arrangements for the purpose of monitoring and improving the quality of health care which it provides to individuals.

This statutory duty is the foundation for clinical governance, which is defined as:

A framework through which NHS organisations are accountable for continuously improving the quality of their services and safeguarding high standards of care by creating an environment in which excellence in clinical care will flourish.[10]

(See Chapter 4 for further discussion of clinical governance issues.)

THE COMMISSION FOR HEALTH IMPROVEMENT

The Commission for Health Improvement (CHI) was established under Sections 19 to 24 of the Health Act 1999 which set out its functions and powers. It is a body corporate, i.e. it can sue and be sued on its own account. It is effectively a watchdog for the NHS with considerable powers of inspection.

One of the earliest tasks undertaken by the CHI on the day it was established was to visit Garlands Hospital in Carlisle run by the North Lakeland Healthcare NHS Trust in Cumbria. An independent investigation[11] had found that staff had physically and mentally abused patients. The Chairman of the NHS Trust was dismissed by the Secretary of State. The Secretary of State ordered CHI to visit the hospital.

The Secretary of State has also asked the CHI to pay particular attention to resuscitation decision-making processes as part of its rolling programme of reviews of clinical governance arrangements put in place by NHS organizations.

THE NATIONAL INSTITUTE FOR CLINICAL EXCELLENCE

The National Institute for Clinical Excellence (NICE) was set up to end postcode prescribing in the NHS by making recommendations on the medicines and services which should be available in the NHS on the basis of research. One of the first drugs it reviewed was Relenza, a drug developed by Glaxo Welcome for preventing 'flu'. NICE concluded that the evidence did not justify funding through the NHS, since it appeared to have little benefit for those groups most at risk: the elderly and asthma sufferers. NICE's recommendations were accepted by the Secretary of State. Subsequently – and following further research – it recommended the use of Relenza in the NHS.

NATIONAL SERVICE FRAMEWORKS (NSF)

National Service Frameworks (NSF) are also part of the attempt to define minimum standards which should be seen in the NHS in different patient groups. NSFs have been published in respect of mental health, cancer care and care of older people (see below). (See Chapter 4 for a further discussion on quality improvement.)

PATIENTS' RIGHTS; HUMAN RIGHTS ACT; CONSENT; CONFIDENTIALITY; ACCESS TO RECORDS; RIGHT TO COMPLAIN; RIGHTS OF CARERS

HUMAN RIGHTS

The Human Rights Act 1998 brought into force in England, Wales and N. Ireland (it came into force on devolution in Scotland) on 2 October 2000 the European Convention of Human Rights. This requires public authorities and those organizations undertaking functions of a public nature to recognize and implement the Articles of the European Convention which are set out in Schedule 1 to the Act. In addition instead of taking a case to Strasbourg an individual who considers that his or her rights have been violated can take a case to the courts of this country. The rights are set out in the author's book on rights and responsibilities of patients.[12]

Significant rights include:

◆ Article 2 and the right to life which was referred to in the case where the separation of conjoined twins was considered.[13] It was also considered in two cases where withholding artificial feeding from a patient in a persistent vegetative state was being discussed. In both cases there was held to be no violation of the right to life as there was no intention to deprive the person of life.[14]

◆ Article 3 and the right not to be treated with inhuman or degrading treatment or punishment. This article may be relied upon by a patient in the community who considers that they are not obtaining the resources, support and assistance to enable them to have a reasonable quality of life. For example, having to wait several years for a chair lift may be seen as inhuman and degrading treatment. Clearly much would depend upon the actual circumstances with which the patient had to cope.

◆ Article 5 and the right to have freedom and security of person.

◆ Article 6 and the right to a fair hearing could affect the community nurse if she faced disciplinary or professional conduct proceedings.

◆ Article 8 and the right to respect for privacy and family life.

◆ Article 14 requires all the Articles to be implemented without any discrimination and gives an extensive list of kinds of discrimination which is not exclusive.

THE RIGHT TO CONSENT

Any adult mentally competent person has a right to refuse consent to treatment.[15] This even applies to life-saving treatment. However, where the person lacks the mental capacity to make a decision, then action must be taken in the best interests of that mentally incapacitated adult.[16]

CONFIDENTIALITY

All health professionals owe a duty of confidentiality to the patient and must be certain that where confidential information is disclosed to others, then there are clear justifications recognized in law for such disclosure. The exceptions include:

◆ disclosure with the consent of the patient
◆ disclosure in the public interest
◆ disclosure required by the courts or in the course of civil or criminal proceedings (the only profession which is exempt from the duty to disclose to the judge is the legal profession)

◆ disclosure which is required by Act of Parliament (such as the Prevention of Terrorism Act and Road Traffic Act)

◆ disclosure in the public interest. The latter reason for exception to the duty of confidentiality would include those situations where disclosure is necessary to prevent serious harm to the patient or to another person.

Further information can be obtained from the author's work.[17] The Data Protection Act 1998 applies to all health records, both those in computerized form and also those kept manually. The Act lays down basic principles which should apply to the keeping of records. In each trust a Caldicott Guardian should be appointed with responsibilities for ensuring that confidentiality is maintained as appropriate across the organization.

ACCESS TO RECORDS

A patient can access his or her health records under the provisions of the Data Protection Act 1998 and subsequent statutory instruments. However the right of access is not absolute and access can be withheld if serious harm to the physical or mental health or condition of the patient, or another person, is feared. In addition, where a third person, not a health professional involved in the care of the patient, has requested that certain information provided by him or her should not be made available, then that request should be respected.

RIGHT TO COMPLAIN

Every patient has a right to complain under the Hospital Complaints Procedure Act and the Department of Health requires the recognized complaints procedure to be implemented and to apply across community as well as hospital activities. The present system is a three-tier system: local resolution, independent review panel and finally the Health Service Commissioner. At the time of writing the Department of Health is following up research which it had commissioned to investigate the need for major revisions to the existing scheme. It published a consultation paper in September 2001 asking people to respond to proposals for changing the present complaints procedure. Implementation of a new scheme is expected to take place in 2003.

RIGHTS OF CARERS

The rights of carers to be assessed are set out in the Carer's Recognition and Services Act 1995. This Act did not require local authorities to provide services to carers and this omission was covered by the Carers and Disabled Children Act 2000, where following an assessment, services can be provided to carers on a means-tested basis.

STATUTORY RIGHTS OF ENTRY; STATUTORY RIGHT TO REMOVE TO PLACE OF SAFETY

A community nurse may become concerned about the safety and well-being of a person who fails to answer her call. She does not herself have statutory rights of entry, but she should be able to contact those who are able to enter the premises to ensure that the person is safe. These rights of entry include powers under:

◆ Police and Criminal Evidence Act 1984 section 17(e) where the police can enter and search premises for the purpose of saving life or limb
◆ Mental Health Act 1983 Section 135(1) and 135(2)
◆ National Assistance Act 1948 Section 47 and the emergency provisions under the National Assistance (Amendment) Act 1951
◆ Common law powers. The House of Lords has recognized the power that exists at common law, (judge made law or case law) for action to be taken out of necessity to act in the best interests of a mentally incapacitated adult.[18]

There are considerable advantages in the community nurse contacting the police if there are concerns about the well-being of a patient, since not only is there a clear statutory right for admission by the police, but they would also have the best means of effecting entry.

SPECIFIC CLIENT GROUPS
Children

A young person of 16 and 17 has a statutory right to give consent to treatment under Section 8(1) of the Family Law Reform Act 1969. Treatment is widely defined under Section 8(2).[19] The refusal of a young person to have necessary or life-saving treatment could be over-ruled in exceptional circumstances.

A young person and child under 16 may have a right recognized at common law (judge made law or case law) if they are 'Gillick competent.'[20] Clearly the level of competence which is required would be related to the nature of the decision to be made.

Rules about confidentiality of information relating to the child follow the rules on competence and consent, subject to disclosure of information which would be in the best interests of the child. Further information is readily available on the law relating to children generally[21] and specifically for community nursing.[22]

Elderly patients

There are no special laws which apply to older people who have the same human rights as others. However community nurses must be aware of the possibility of any abusive situation existing and take the appropriate steps to ensure that an elderly person is protected. Some local authorities now have agreed procedures and protocols comparable with those under Child Protection provisions, for the protection of older people, or mentally incapable adults, from abuse and victimization.

A National Service Framework for Older People was published in March 2001.[23] It covers older people wherever they live and is designed:

◆ to root out age discrimination
◆ to provide person-centred care with older people treated as individuals with respect and dignity

◆ to promote older people's health and independence.

In order to achieve these objectives eight standards are identified. The community nurse who cares for elderly patients should ensure that she takes steps to identify the impact these standards are likely to have on community nursing care, as well as the action being followed in her own area and her own personal involvement in the implementation of local standards.

People suffering from mental illness

The vast majority of those suffering from mental illness are cared for in the community and/or hospital and do not come under the Mental Health Act. About 10% of the mentally ill in hospital are admitted compulsorily. Major changes are anticipated in the law relating to mental illness as the result of a report by an Expert Panel and a White Paper issued by the Department of Health. A draft Mental Health Bill was issued in 2002. At the time of writing legislation is awaited. One likely consequence of the new legislation will be compulsory powers to ensure that those who have been discharged from hospital continue to take their medication, by compelling them to attend a treatment centre.

Mentally incapacitated adults

At present there are no statutory provisions for decisions to be made on behalf of those with learning difficulties, except in Scotland. Even relatives of mentally incapable adults do not have the powers to give consent for them to have medical, surgical or nursing procedures. When an adult cannot make treatment decisions on their own account, then the carers, both professional and unpaid, must act in their best interests following the Bolam Test.[24] The Government has published proposals[25] for establishing procedures for such decisions to be made which are in line with the recommendations of the Law Commission.[26] At the time of writing legislation is awaited for their implementation. Scotland is covered by the Adult Incapacity (Scotland) Act 2000.

NURSING HOMES: CARE STANDARDS ACT 2000 AND PROVISIONS FOR REGISTRATION, REGULATION AND INSPECTION

The Registered Homes Act 1984 placed responsibilities for the registering and inspection of nursing homes upon health authorities and for the registering and inspection of residential care homes upon local authorities. Under the Care Standards Act 2000 a new independent regulatory body for social care and private and voluntary healthcare services has been established in England, known as the National Care Standards Commission. In Wales, the National Assembly for Wales will set up a department or agency to be the regulatory body in Wales. These regulatory bodies will also be responsible for the regulation of nursing agencies. Part II of the Care Standards Act 2000 sets out provisions in relation to registration, and right of appeals, and provisions for the regulations of establishments and standards, creating offences in respect of the regulations. National minimum standards have been issued for all homes. Local authority homes will have to comply with the same standards as those set for independent homes. Community nurses who are concerned at the standards in those residential care homes which they visit, can take their concerns to the National Care Standards Commission. For example, if they are concerned that the dependence level and nursing needs of residents in a care home is such that they should be placed in a nursing home, this is an issue which the National Care Standards Commission would investigate. There are plans to amalgamate the Commission for Health Improvement and the National Care Standards Commission.

HEALTH AND SAFETY: STATUTORY DUTIES; MANUAL HANDLING; VIOLENCE; STRESS; MEDICAL DEVICES

The main statute regulating health and safety, the Health and Safety at Work Act 1974, is enforced through the criminal courts. Whilst the main responsibilities under the Act are those owed by the employer to the employee and by the employee to the employer, under Section 3 a general duty is owed by the employer to the public at large to ensure that their health and safety are not affected by its enterprise.

Manual handling

Community nurses should be trained in the carrying out of risk assessments under the manual handling regulations and the ways of reducing the risk of harm arising from any manual handling which cannot be avoided. If a community nurse suffered a back injury through work and was able to show that her employer had failed to ensure that she had adequate training, or the resources to ensure that she was reasonably safe, then she would be able to claim compensation. If on the other hand, she had received the appropriate training, but because of her own failure to follow the correct procedures, or take the correct precautions, she was injured, it is unlikely that there would be any liability by the employer. Much would of course depend upon what facts could be established. Documentation is essential with reference to training, to risk assessment and to the implementation of the plan.

Violence

Violence is increasing against NHS staff both in hospitals and in the community. Employers have a responsibility to take reasonable care of the health and safety of their staff and this would include preventing them from being subjected to physical abuse from others. If an employer fails to take reasonable action and the employee is harmed, then the employee could seek compensation from the employer. It was reported in October 1998[27] for example, that North West Durham Health Care Trust would meet the full legal costs and provide emotional and professional support for all healthcare staff who take court action against an assailant, in cases where the Crown Prosecution Service fails to pursue the offender. A zero tolerance policy on violence should be adopted by employers. Reference should

be made to the guidance prepared by the Health and Safety Commission.[28] This gives practical advice for reducing the risk of violence in a variety of settings and emphasizes the importance of commitment from the highest levels of management. An Appendix provides a check list to ensure the safety of community staff.

Stress

In a High Court case a social worker won over £150 000 compensation because his employers, Northumberland County Council, knowing that he was at risk of mental harm from the pressures in his job, failed to provide reasonable support and were therefore liable for his consequential breakdown.[29] In order to obtain compensation in such circumstances a nurse would have to show that she is under unacceptable pressure which is causing mental distress to her, that the manager is aware of the situation, that there is reasonable action which the manager could take, but fails to take and as a consequence of such failure, she suffers a serious mental illness. The burden would be on the employee to provide the evidence to show all these facts.

Medical devices

The Medical Devices Agency (MDA) was established in September 1994 to promote the safe and effective use of devices. In particular its role is to ensure that whenever a medical device is used, it is:

♦ suitable for its intended purpose
♦ properly understood by the professional user
♦ maintained in a safe and reliable condition.

What is a medical device?

The definition used by the MDA is based upon the European Directive definition:[30]

'Any instrument, apparatus, material or other article, whether used alone or in combination, including the software necessary for its proper application, intended by the manufacturer to be used for human beings for the purpose of:

♦ diagnosis, prevention, monitoring, treatment or alleviation of disease

◆ diagnosis, monitoring, treatment, alleviation of or compensation for an injury or handicap
◆ investigation, replacement or modification of the anatomy or of a physiological process
◆ control of contraception

and which does not achieve its principal intended action in or on the human body by pharmacological, immunological or metabolic means, but which may be assisted in its function by such means.'

Much of the equipment used by a community nurse would come under the Medical Devices Regulations. The nurse would be required to ensure that any defects were made known to the appropriate officer within her trust so that the MDA was notified of them. The nurse should also ensure that she is kept up-to-date with any warnings about defective equipment. Failure to be alert to such warnings and to take the necessary action could result in the disciplining of the nurse, professional misconduct proceedings and, if the patient is harmed, negligence action against the trust.

RECORD KEEPING: STANDARDS; ELECTRONIC HEALTH RECORDS

STANDARDS

Maintaining a reasonable standard of record keeping is a professional duty under the Code of Professional Conduct and hence failure to achieve the reasonable standard could be followed by professional conduct proceedings. The guidance issued by the NMC[31] should be followed.

ELECTRONIC PATIENT RECORDS

There is increasing introduction of computerized health records and it is the present Government's stated aim that by March 2005 every patient will have their own electronic health record. The use of computerized records in the community should facilitate the recording of patient information and access to other records held in the hospital, without having to transport manual records across the country. Most patients in the community keep their records in their own homes. After the completion of treatment, or at the death of the patient, these records should be collected and stored securely by the NHS Trust according to the storage times suggested by the Department of Health.[32] There should also be regular audit, both internal and external, to ensure that a reasonable standard of documentation is being maintained.

MEDICINES; NURSE PRESCRIBING; PATIENT GROUP PROTOCOLS; RECEIVING INSTRUCTIONS BY WORD OF MOUTH

The statutory framework for the prescribing, supply and administration of medicines is set out in the Medicines Act 1968 and the Misuse of Drugs Act 1971. There have been recent amendments to enable health professionals other than doctors, dentists and midwives to prescribe. The legislation is enforced through the criminal courts but is supported by codes of professional conduct: serious misconduct could be followed by striking off from the register.

NURSE PRESCRIBING

The Medicinal Products (Prescription by Nurses) Act 1992 was passed to give specified practitioners the power to prescribe specified medicines. The legislation followed the recommendations of the report of the advisory group on nurse prescribing (known as the first Crown Report) to the Department of Health in December 1989. Health visitors and community nurses who have had the requisite training can prescribe in the community from a nursing formulary. In February 2000 prescribing powers were given to nurses employed by a doctor on the medical list (i.e. GP) and also to nurses working in Walk-in Centres, defined in the regulations as 'A Centre at which information and treatment for minor conditions is provided to the public under arrangements made by or on behalf of the Secretary of State.' (See Chapter 24 for further discussion on alternative ways of working.)

Nurses prescribe against a British Nursing Formulary and have their own prescription pads.

They are personally and professionally accountable for their actions, but in practice their employers would accept vicarious liability for the payment of any compensation which arose from any negligence by them, occurring in the course of their employment.

PATIENT GROUP PROTOCOLS

The Crown Committee first considered the arrangements for and legality of group protocols and reported in March 1998. It recommended legislation to ensure that their legal validity was clarified. New regulations came into force on 9 August 2000.[33] These provide for Patient Group Directions to be drawn up to make provision for the sale or supply of a prescription-only medicine, in hospitals in accordance with the written direction of a doctor or dentist. To be lawful, the Patient Group Direction must cover the particulars which are set out in Part 1 of Schedule 7 of the Statutory Instrument. The particulars are set out in Box 13.1.

RECEIVING INSTRUCTIONS BY WORD OF MOUTH

Community nurses may be in a dilemma as to whether it is in order for them to take instructions over the telephone. The UKCC guidelines[34] state:

Instruction by telephone to a practitioner to administer a previously unprescribed substance is not acceptable. In exceptional circumstances, where the medication has been previously prescribed and the prescriber is unable to issue a new prescription, but where changes to the dose are considered necessary, the use of information technology (such as fax or e-mail) is the preferred method. This should be followed up by a new prescription confirming the changes within a given time period. The UKCC suggests a maximum of 24 hours. In any event, the changes must have been authorised before the new dosage is administered.

DEATH AND PALLIATIVE CARE: EUTHANASIA; SUICIDE; MANSLAUGHTER

EUTHANASIA

The law in this country does not accept euthanasia. The law in the UK does not recognize any right to assist a person who wishes to die. Such an action could constitute murder, manslaughter or assistance in a suicide bid. For example, in the case of Dr Nigel Cox[35] who gave potassium chloride to a patient who suffered from rheumatoid arthritis and who was terminally ill and in great pain, there was a conviction. He was found guilty of causing

---

Box 13.1 Particulars for Patient Group Direction

a. The period during which the Direction shall have effect.
b. The description or class of prescription only medicines to which the Direction relates.
c. Whether there are any restrictions on the quantity of medicine which may be supplied on any one occasion, and if so, what restrictions.
d. The clinical situations which prescription only medicines of that description or class may be used to treat.
e. The clinical criteria under which a person shall be eligible for treatment.
f. Whether any class of person is excluded from treatment under the Direction, and if so, what class of person.
g. Whether there are circumstances in which further advice should be sought from a doctor or dentist and, if so, in what circumstances.
h. The pharmaceutical form or forms in which prescription only medicines of that description or class are to be administered.

i. The strength, or maximum strength, at which prescription only medicines of that description or class are to be administered.
j. The applicable dosage or maximum dosage.
k. The route of administration.
l. The frequency of administration.
m. Any minimum or maximum period of administration applicable to prescription only medicines of that description or class.
n. Whether there are any relevant warnings to note, and if so, what warnings.
o. Whether there is any follow up action to be taken in any circumstances, and if so, what action and in what circumstances.
p. Arrangements for referral for medical advice.
q. Details of the records to be kept of the supply or the administration of medicines under the Direction.

her death and was sentenced to a year's imprisonment which was suspended for a year. He also had to appear before disciplinary proceedings of the Regional Health Authority, his employers and before the General Medical Council. However, he kept both his post and his state registration.

SUICIDE

Even where a patient is asking a community nurse to help her to die, the nurse would be committing a criminal offence if she were to assist in any way. Assistance in a suicide bid is illegal under Section 2(1) of the Suicide Act 1961 which is shown in Box 13.2.

Under the Suicide Act 1961 it is no longer a criminal act to attempt to commit suicide, so anyone who failed in the attempt could not be prosecuted as used to happen before the Act was passed.

It does not follow that where a nurse is caring for a dying patient who is suffering from extreme pain, that the necessary medication cannot be given because it may incidentally and unintentionally shorten a patient's life by a few days.

Diane Pretty's application for an advance pardon for her husband to help her die failed.[36]

MANSLAUGHTER

In the case of Dr Bodkin Adams, who was tried for the murder of a resident in an Eastbourne nursing home, the trial judge, Mr Justice Patrick Devlin, directed the jury that:

There has been a good deal of discussion about the circumstances in which a doctor might be justified in giving drugs which would shorten life in cases of severe pain. It is my duty to tell you that the law knows of no special defence of this character. But that does not mean that a doctor aiding the sick or dying has to calculate in minutes or hours, or perhaps in days or weeks, the effect on a patient's life of the

---

medicines which he administers. If the first purpose of medicine, – the restoration of health – can no longer be achieved, there is still much for the doctor to do, and he is entitled to do all that is proper and necessary to relieve pain and suffering even if the measures he takes may incidentally shorten life … It remains a law, that no doctor has the right to cut off life deliberately … What counsel for the defence was saying, was that the treatment that was given by the Doctor was designed to promote comfort, and if it was the right and proper treatment of the case, the fact that incidentally it shortened life does not give any grounds for convicting him of murder.[37]

This ruling still applies today. What would be a reasonable dose for pain management would relate to the reasonable professionally approved practice for caring for a patient in those particular circumstances.

Where a patient refuses care and treatment, then such care cannot be forced upon the mentally competent person over 18 years. Miss B's application to allow her ventilator to be switched off succeeded because she was mentally competent.[38]

SPECIFIC SITUATIONS

EXPANDED ROLE – NEW TECHNOLOGY FOR USE IN COMMUNITY; PATIENT BEING DISCHARGED

It is increasingly likely that the community nurse will be caring for patients at a much earlier stage in their rehabilitation than was originally foreseen. For example the patient may still be receiving an intravenous infusion and bring with them, on discharge, complex equipment. Clearly in such circumstances it is preferable if the community nurse can visit the hospital predischarge and learn about the treatment the patient is receiving and the equipment they bring with them. The community nurse must ensure that she complies with the guidance from the NMC which has incorporated the principles relating to the scope of professional practice in its new Code of Professional Conduct[39] and always work within her sphere of competence.

Box 13.2 Assisting a person to commit suicide

A person who aids, abets, counsels or procures the suicide of another or an attempt by another to commit suicide, shall be liable on conviction on indictment to imprisonment (up to 14 years).

TRANSPORT

It is essential that the community nurse checks with her insurers that she is covered for using her car at work and if necessary using it for the transport of patients and equipment. The duty is placed upon the person to be insured, who is responsible for advising the insurers of the intended use of the vehicle. If the nurse fails to give full details of the proposed use, she may find that her cover is defective. Any person harmed in an accident may have to obtain compensation from the Motor Vehicles Bureau which provides compensation for personal injuries for those who are the victims of uninsured drivers or hit-and-run drivers.

EQUIPMENT

Arrangements for the allocation, maintenance and supervision of equipment in the community vary across the country: sometimes local authorities and health trusts share a common equipment resource; in other areas each organization is responsible for its own equipment. Guidance is available from the Department of Health on community equipment services.[40]

RE-USE OF EQUIPMENT – PROBLEMS ABOUT SAFETY AND CROSS INFECTION

Equipment should only be transferred for use by another patient if it has been thoroughly inspected, repaired if necessary and subjected to a systematic cleaning and disinfectant. If a patient were to be harmed as a result of the re-use of another patient's equipment which had not been properly inspected, then an action could be brought against the employer of the staff concerned.

AWARENESS OF NEW DEVELOPMENTS

Nurses are required to keep up to date with new developments and failure regularly to review a patient's condition could amount to professional misconduct and lead to litigation against the employer. For example, a patient may have a severe ulcer on her leg, and one nurse may spend many years visiting the patient each week to ensure that the wound is dressed. The nurse might then be transferred to another area and a new nurse be assigned to this patient. The new nurse may try an innovative treatment which heals the wound speedily. The patient may then argue that there was a failure by the original nurse to follow a reasonable standard of care. The first nurse may be able to defend herself on the grounds that at the time that she was caring for the patient she followed the reasonable standard of care and that the treatment used by the second nurse had only just been introduced into practice. If of course this is not correct and the successful treatment had been used as part of standard practice much earlier then there may well be evidence of a failure to follow a reasonable standard of care by the first nurse.

HOSPITAL-ACQUIRED INFECTION (HAI) AND PATIENT BEING DISCHARGED WITH INFECTION

A recent report by the National Audit Office[41] has raised major concerns about the level of hospital-acquired infection (HAI). The report suggested that HAI could be the main or a contributory cause in 20 000 or 4% of deaths a year in the UK and that there are at least about 100 000 cases of HAI with an estimated cost to the NHS of £1 billion. In the light of these figures it is inevitable that the community nurse will be caring for patients who have become infected during their stay in hospital. She must be sure that she takes all necessary precautions to prevent the spread of this infection to other patients she visits. She should also ensure that the carers of the patient are given an understanding of good infection control procedures.

CONCLUSIONS

There are major challenges ahead for the community nurse. The establishment of Primary Care Trusts will lead to community health services being separated from the acute trusts and many nurses will find that their contracts are transferred to new employers and they may well share a common employer with social workers. In addition there are no signs that litigation is decreasing. On the contrary the National Audit Office[42] announced in May 2001 that almost £3.9 billion must be set aside to meet known and foreseeable claims for compensation arising in health care. Community nurses must ensure that they follow the reasonable standard of care as defined in the Bolam Test and that they have a good understanding of the rights of the patient, particularly as the role of the nurse is likely to be expanded as more activities are undertaken by nurses rather than by doctors. Nurse prescribing is now well established in the community and intermediate care is being provided across the country, where community nurses are likely to have a major role to play in that provision. The Report of the Bristol inquiry[43] into heart surgery for children in Bristol, whilst it was only concerned with hospital care, is likely to have major significance for the NHS. The Report has made fundamental proposals which if implemented would have a revolutionary effect on health care. For example it is suggested that the patient must be at the centre of everything which the NHS does; that the commitment and dedication of staff in the NHS must be valued and acknowledged; that those caring for patients must themselves be supported and cared for; and that there must be openness and transparency in everything which the NHS does.

There are thus considerable challenges ahead for the community nurse and it is hoped that this brief introduction to the framework of law within which she works will be of assistance to her.

SUMMARY

◆ The background to the English Legal System, the law relating to Human Rights; the structure of NHS and LA; PCT's and Care Authorities; role of HA's, duty of LA's statutory functions; community care provisions; Health and Social Care Act 2001 are considered.

◆ The accountability of the community professional in criminal, civil, employment and professional proceedings is examined.

◆ Patients' rights including the right to consent, to confidentiality, to access records, to complain are discussed together with the rights of carers. The rights of specific client groups including children, the elderly, mentally ill and mentally incapacitated adults are explained.

◆ Health and Safety laws and record keeping standards are identified together with laws relating to medicines.

◆ Finally the laws relating to death and palliative care: euthanasia; suicide; manslaughter are outlined and special situations relevent to the community nurse examined.

DISCUSSION POINTS

1. Take a relevant example from the specific situations mentioned above and explore current practice in relation to legal aspects of community nursing care.

2. Debate the motion that increased openness and transparency in relation to patient care will inevitably increase workload.

REFERENCES

1. Dimond B 2001 Legal aspects of nursing, 3rd edn. Pearson Education, London
2. Dimond B 1997 The legal aspects of care in the community. Macmillan Publications, Basingstoke, Hampshire
3. Lord Woolf 1996 Final Report Access to Justice. HMSO, London
4. R. v. Adomako. House of Lords, The Times Law Report, 4 July 1994
5. Bolam v. Friern Hospital Management Committee (1957) 1 WLR 582
6. Wilsher v. Essex Health Authority (1986) 3 All ER 801
7. Barnett v. Chelsea HMC (1968) 1 All ER 1068
8. Hotson v. E. Berks Health Authority (1987) AC 750
9. NHS White Paper 1997 The new NHS modern and dependable. HMSO. London
10. Department of Health 1998 A first class service: Quality in the new NHS. DoH, London
11. North Lakeland Healthcare NHS Trust Report of Independent Inquiry into Garlands Hospital March 2000 North Lakeland Healthcare NHS Trust and North Cumbria Health Authority
12. Dimond B 1999 Patients' rights, responsibilities and the nurse, 2nd edn. Quay Publications, Dinton, Wiltshire
13. In re A (Minors) (Conjoined Twins: Medical Treatment) The Times Law Report, 10 October 2000

14. NHS Trust A v. Mrs M. NHS Trust B v Mrs H. Family Division 25 October 2000
15. Re MB (Adult Medical Treatment) (1997) 2 FLR 426
16. F. v. West Berkshire Health Authority (1989) 2 All ER 545
17. Dimond B (2002) Confidentiality and the law. Quay Books, Mark Allen Publications, Dinton, Wiltshire
18. Re F (mental patient: sterilisation) (1990) 2 AC
19. Dimond B 2001 Legal aspects of consent 7: Young persons of 16 and 17 years. British Journal of Nursing 10(11): 732–733
20. Gillick v. West Norfolk and Wisbech Area Health Authority and the DHSS (1985) 3 All ER 402
21. Dimond B 1996 The legal aspects of child health care. Mosby, London
22. Dimond B 2000 Legal aspects of the community care of the sick child. In: Muir J, Sidley A (eds) Textbook of community children's nursing. Baillière Tindall and Royal College of Nursing, London
23. Department of Health National Service Framework for Older People HSC 2001/007
24. Re F (mental patient: sterilisation) (1990) 2AC 1
25. Lord Chancellor's Office Making Decisions LCD 1999
26. Law Commission Report No. 231 Mental Incapacity HMSO 1995
27. Alexandra Frean Funds for Nurses who prosecute violent patients. The Times 1 October 1998
28. Health and Safety Commission 1997 Violence and aggression to staff in health services. HSE Books, London
29. Walker v. Northumberland County Council. Times Law Report 24 November 1994 Queens Bench Division
30. European Union Directive 93/42/EEC
31. UKCC 1998 Guidelines for records and record keeping. UKCC, London
32. NHS Executive HSC 1999/053 For the Record DoH 1999
33. Prescription only Medicines (Human Use) Amendment Order 2000 S1 2000 No. 1917
34. UKCC 2000 Guidelines for the administration of medicines, p. 5. UKCC, London
35. R. v. Cox (1993) 2 All ER 19
36. R (on the application of Pretty) v. DPP [2001] UKHL 61 [2001] 3 WLR 1598; Pretty v. UK ECHR Current Law 380, June 2002
37. Sybille Bedford 1961 The best we can do. Penguin Books, London
38. Re B (Consent to treatment: capacity) [2002] 2 All ER 449
39. NMC 2002 Code of Professional Conduct, NMC
40. Department of Health 2000 Community equipment services: guide to integrating community equipment services HSC (2000) 8: LAC (2000) 13
41. National Audit Office 2000 The management and control of hospital acquired infection in acute NHS Trusts in England. HMSO, London
42. National Audit Office 2001 Handling clinical negligence claims in England. Report of the Comptroller and Auditor General. House of Commons Session 2000–2001, 3 May 2001
43. Bristol Royal Infirmary 2001 Learning from Bristol: the report of the public inquiry into children's heart surgery at the Bristol Royal Infirmary 1984–1995, Command Paper CM 5207, July 2001; http://www.bristol-inquiry.org.uk/

FURTHER READING

Dimond B 2001 Legal aspects of nursing, 3rd edn. Pearson Education, London

Hinchliff S (ed) 1995 The really useful handbook for community nurses. Publishing Initiatives Books, Beckenham

Muir J, Sidley A (eds) 2000 Textbook of community childrens nursing. Baillière Tindall and Royal College of Nursing, London

Ethics in practice

G. Rumbold

INTRODUCTION

Within one chapter it is clearly not possible to discuss all the ethical issues which might confront a community nurse. Community nursing is complex, and encompasses a range of specialist roles. Consequently, issues that may be considered of primary concern to, for example, a health visitor, may be of lesser concern to a district nurse. According to Seedhouse (1988) the key question for health workers is 'How can I intervene to the highest moral degree?'. In order to answer this question nurses (and all health workers) need to understand something of the nature of moral or ethical reasoning. For, as Seedhouse points out, 'being moral is not simply a matter of "doing the right thing" where there is just one course of action and one wrong way. Ethics is complex.'

This chapter begins therefore with a discussion of ethical theories, in order to provide the reader with a basis on which to make ethical decisions in practice. Two theoretical perspectives have been selected, viz. deontology and utilitarianism. The chapter then goes on to explore a range of issues subsumed within four themes: respect for persons, consent, accountability and advocacy.

THE NATURE OF ETHICS

As already noted, ethics is complex. What it is concerned with is, on one level, 'understanding rather than decision ... It steps back from the immediately practical and attempts to discover some underlying pattern or order in the immense variety of moral decisions and practices both of individuals and societies.' (Baelz, 1977). However, it does have practical application, not least in health care. 'The study of ethics seeks to provide means of formulating answers to questions and so guide actions. It provides a framework for dealing with issues, problems and dilemmas. The study of ethics, while it may at first appear to be a largely theoretical exercise, does have practical application.' (Rumbold 1999). Community nurses, as all health professionals, are confronted with questions and problems within their day-to-day work, which have an ethical dimension. Therefore, it is important that they have an understanding of the nature of ethical reasoning, and a grasp of ethical frameworks on which to base their decisions.

DEONTOLOGY

The word deontology comes from the Greek deon, meaning duty. And, as the name suggests, this school of thought places emphasis on determining one's moral duty – what one should or ought to do. A major proponent of this way of thinking was the 18th century German philosopher, Immanuel Kant. The basis of deontology is that there exist moral laws, just as there are laws of physics. The question is, 'how do we know what the law is?'. Kant argued that moral laws can be deduced through a process of practical reasoning. Kant argued that to determine whether a principle was a moral law you need first to ask the question 'what if the antithesis were adopted as a law?'. He applied this test to two examples; truth telling and promise keeping. If we were to adopt as a law 'do not always tell the truth', what would be the result? Kant concludes that it would be chaos, for we would never know when someone was telling the truth. Kant argues that there is no justification for telling an untruth, and that there is a moral duty to tell the truth. Similarly, he concluded that one should only make promises, which one intends to keep, that, having made them, there is a duty to keep them. Furthermore,

Kant argued that for a moral principle to be binding on one as a duty, it must be universal, unconditional and imperative. This he called the categorical imperative, and stated it as follows:

Act only on the maxim through which you can at the same time will that it should become a universal law. Or, to put it in simple English, only act in a way which you would want everyone to do all the time.

A second principle derived by Kant was what he described as respect for persons. 'So act as to treat humanity whether in thine own person or that of any other, in every case as an end withal, never as a means only.' This is clearly consistent with the notion that whatever health professionals do to or with patients/clients should be for their benefit, and with the concept of respecting autonomy. 'Kant argues that respect for autonomy is a universal law, and is supported both by the categorical imperative, and the concept of respect for persons. However, he argued that respect for the autonomy of one individual had to be seen within the context of respect for the autonomy of others.' (Rumbold 1999).

UTILITARIANISM

Utilitarianism is sometimes referred to as consequentialism, for what is seen as justifying any action or nonaction are the outcomes. It is the rightness or wrongness of the outcomes, rather than of the act itself, which justifies the action. This is clearly at odds with deontological theories which would argue, for example, that to tell the truth is right, and to tell an untruth is wrong, whatever the outcomes. Utilitarians would argue that there may be occasions when not telling the truth is justified if the end result is for the good.

The two main proponents of this line of thinking were Jeremy Bentham (1748–1832) and John Stuart Mill (1806–73). While they differed over some finer points of the theory, both agreed that what has ultimate value is happiness. As Mill himself wrote:

The creed which accepts as the foundation of morals, Utility, or the Greatest Happiness Principle, holds that actions are right in proportion as they tend to produce happiness, wrong as they tend to produce the reverse of happiness. By happiness is intended pleasure, and the absence of pain, and by unhappiness, pain and the privation of pleasure. (cited in Warnock 1962, p. 257)

An important aspect to note is that it is not the happiness of the individual which morally justifies an action but that of either the majority or all. It is the greatest happiness or good for the greatest number, rather than the individuals involved, that have to be considered. This clearly conflicts both with Kant's principle of *Respect for persons,* and one of the fundamental principles of healthcare ethics that the needs and well-being of the individual patient/client are paramount. It is however, a principle adopted by policy makers when determining the allocation of resources. When resources are limited and demand infinite the principle of the greatest good for the greatest number provides a valuable guide, both at a macro and at a micro level, for determining how best to allocate those resources. It is too, of course, the principle that underlies many public health measures.

However, 'The questions which can be argued, and utilitarians have failed to answer satisfactorily are "How can we know what happiness is?" and "How can we determine the best way of achieving it?"' (Rumbold 1999). A further problem is that we cannot always know for certain what the consequences of our actions will be.

RESPECT FOR PERSONS

As we have already seen, the principle of *respect for persons* is integral to Kant's philosophy. It can be seen to underpin much ethical teaching, and 'For many modern thinkers it is close to the essence of ethics.' (Cribb 1995). It is also clearly related to two of the central principles of traditional medical ethics: *beneficence* and *non-maleficence.* Beneficence means to do good, in terms of what will benefit the patient, and non-maleficence means to do no harm.

Respect for persons is also an essential component of professional codes. The UKCC *Code of Conduct* (1992), for example, states that the nurse, midwife or health visitor 'must act always in such a manner as to promote and safeguard the interests and well-being of patients and clients'.

It also underpins much criminal and civil law. Within civil law, for example, it includes the laws relating to trespass, defamation and, of particular relevance in health care, the principle of duty of care and the law of negligence. It is a broad principle which gives rise to a number of subprinciples, of which three are of particular relevance here – *respect for autonomy, respect for privacy* and *respect for property.*

RESPECT FOR AUTONOMY

Autonomy has been defined as 'the capacity to think, decide, and act on the basis of such thought and decision freely and independently and without let or hindrance' (Gillon 1986). Therefore, respecting autonomy means allowing others to make decisions and act upon them. 'Within the context of health care this means allowing patients/clients to make decisions about their health behaviours, lifestyle and treatment.' (Rumbold 2000). However, it is important to recognize that in order to exercise autonomy a person requires a number of attributes:

Possession of: the physical wherewithal to carry out one's chosen tasks (the environmental circumstances must also be suitable); a degree of knowledge sufficient to pursue an end; an understanding of the routes open towards that end, the pitfalls, and the ways in which the knowledge can be employed to achieve that end; and the possession of an ability (sometimes referred to as the possession of rationality) to select ends appropriate for that person. (Seedhouse 1988)

It is also important to recognize that the right to exercise autonomy, as with all rights, is not absolute. One only has the right to exercise one's autonomy to the extent that it does not impinge upon the right of others to exercise their autonomy. This is perhaps of greater significance in caring for patients/clients in the community than in hospital. The community nurse, perhaps more than his/her hospital colleagues, interacts not just with the patient/client but with their family and informal carers. They too have the right to act autonomously and this can lead to conflict and difficult decisions for the nurse/health visitor. While the nurse/health visitor's first and over-riding responsibility is to the individual patient/client, they also owe an element of responsibility to the patient/client's carers. And, of course, in some instances it is the family who is the 'client'.

Consider the following case study.

Case Study 1

Vera is 72 years old and a widow. She lives on her own, and until recently has been fully independent. She has always had a very keen mind, preferring to watch Open University programmes rather than soaps, and attending debating societies rather than Bingo. She has never been slow in making her opinions known, and while she has long since ceased to tell her children how to live their lives, she equally has not allowed them to influence her decisions.

She has two children, a daughter, Susan (aged 48 years), who is divorced with a teenage son; and a son, Jason (aged 46 years), who is married with two school-aged children. Susan lives about 5 miles away, while Jason lives in the neighbouring county, about 40 miles away.

Vera was diagnosed as having dementia a year ago, and until recently has continued to cope reasonably independently with support from her family and the community nurse. Of late, her periods of lucidity have become more infrequent, and this is causing concern to her children. Furthermore, they have to spend greater periods of time with her. The major burden of care has fallen on Susan, who is beginning to find it too stressful, holding down a job in the local supermarket, caring for her son who has 'behavioural problems', and caring for her mother.

At Jason's request, the General Practitioner has obtained a place for Vera in a local nursing home. Initially, Susan wasn't happy with this, but now realizes that she cannot cope for much longer, and says that her mother must go into the home. Vera, however, is far from happy about it, and insists in her lucid moments, that she is quite capable of living in her own house, and anyway 'I've never been able to stand old people! They're all intellectually dead!' She insists that she has

the right to remain in her home as long as she wants to, and the right to have her wishes respected.

What are the issues here? First, Vera is asserting her right to have her autonomy respected. However, the question is whether she has a valid claim. Of Seedhouse's attributes it is probably the last that applies – the possession of an ability (rationality) to select ends appropriate for that person. There are clearly times when she does possess that ability, but there are also times when she does not. The problem is that during those times when she does, her lucid moments, she is unaware of the times when she is confused. Furthermore, in insisting on her right to exercise autonomy she is impinging upon Susan's right to exercise her autonomy, her duty towards her son and the rights of her son. Second, Susan is asserting her right to autonomy. She appears to possess all the faculties required for the exercising of autonomy. The major constraint on her being able to do so is Vera's demand on her time. On balance, then Vera's claim cannot be upheld.

RESPECT FOR PRIVACY

The right to privacy in health care implies that patients have the right to three things. First they have the right for their treatment to be carried out in private. Second, they have the right to have all information about their diagnosis, care and treatment held in confidence. Third, they have the same basic right, as do all, to be private; that is to have time and space to themselves and to have time alone with their significant others. (Rumbold 2000)

The first of these is often less of an issue in the community than in hospital. Much of the care carried out by community nurses is in the patient/client's own home, and therefore ensuring privacy is generally easier. However, some community nurses carry out care in other settings, e.g. health centres, residential homes, schools, where ensuring privacy can be more problematic. Care and/or treatment is taken to include not solely physical care but also advice giving, counselling, etc., and ensuring privacy is not simply a matter of being out of sight but also out of hearing.

Furthermore, there may be occasions when clients do not wish others to know that they are accessing the service, for example drop-in sessions run by a school nurse. Therefore it is important, as far as possible, to ensure that access to such facilities is discrete. The third aspect is also less of an issue in the community, where the majority of patients/clients live in their own homes, though, again, cognisance needs to be taken of the lack of privacy available to patients in residential care settings.

It is the second aspect that is of prime concern. The UKCC *Code of Conduct* (1992) states that each nurse must 'protect all confidential information concerning patients and clients that is obtained in the course of professional practice and make disclosures only with consent, where required by the order of a court, or where you can justify disclosure in the wider public interest' (clause 10). In 1987 the UKCC expanded discussion of the clause in which it stated: 'That practitioners recognise the fundamental right of their patients/clients to have information about them held in secure and private storage.' (UKCC 1987). This can pose a problem for some community nurses, particularly district nurses, when nursing notes are kept in a patient's own home. Such notes may be accessible to others who have no authority to read them, for example neighbours and other visitors to the home. This is particularly so when the patient/client may, due to their condition, not have total control over their environment. In which case the nurse should either make every effort to ensure that notes are stored in as secure a place as possible in the patient's home, or if this is not possible then to remove them from the home altogether.

Furthermore, because community nurses undertake a considerable amount of care in patients'/clients' homes they are privy to far more information about the patient/client, their family and their lifestyle than are nurses working in hospital. While not all this information might be considered strictly of a confidential nature, much of it, although not directly relevant to their care, can nevertheless be considered 'confidential'. The point is that 'the information is acquired by the nurse as a result of her privileged position and therefore must be treated with respect for the patient's and family's right to privacy.' (Rumbold 2000).

RESPECT FOR PROPERTY

Community nurses are 'guests' in the home of a patient/client. It follows therefore that they should respect, not only the patient's privacy, but also their property. 'Obviously nurses should not deliberately damage a patient's property, nor should they assume they have the right to handle anything without the patient's or their family's permission, even if they need to do so as part of the nursing care.' (Rumbold 2000).

CONSENT

The UKCC (1996) states that all health professionals must obtain consent before giving any treatment or care. But, it is not simply a matter of obtaining consent. Consent must be given on the basis of adequate information. The question then is 'what constitutes adequate information?'. The answer to this is not absolutely clear. The UKCC (1996) states that practitioners should share information freely, 'in an accessible way and in appropriate circumstances', and goes on to point out 'that it is not safe to assume that the patient or client has enough knowledge about even basic treatment, for them to make an informed choice without an explanation' and 'it is essential that you give the patient or client adequate information so that he or she can make a meaningful decision'. This means that the patient/client needs to know and understand the effects of the proposed treatment, both the benefits and risks, alternative treatments and their effects, and the consequences of not accepting treatment. The emphasis is on *understanding*. Obtaining consent is not simply a case of providing information, but of ensuring that the patient/client understands the information. But, what of those patients who may not be capable of understanding the information in order to give informed consent? Two groups of patients/clients who may genuinely not be capable of forming an informed opinion are those with severe learning disabilities and children.

PATIENTS/CLIENTS WITH SEVERE LEARNING DISABILITIES

The first thing to remember is that we must not make assumptions about the ability of any person to understand information. It is crucial that the nurse, or health professional, who has responsibility for obtaining consent from any patient, first assesses their level of competence. 'Competence refers to the individual's capacity to weigh the information in processing the decision.' (Bailey & Schwartzberg 1995). It may be that some patients/clients with severe learning disability do not have the capacity to weigh the information when being asked to make some decisions. Thus, while they may be able to do so when making decisions about aspects of daily living, such as what to eat, wear, etc., they may not be able to do so when faced with more complex decisions, in particular those related to treatment or care. The question then is 'who should make the decision?'.

'If the patient is considered unable to give valid consent it is considered good practice to discuss any proposed treatment with the next of kin.' (NHS Management Executive 1990). It is important to note, then, that what is considered good practice is to merely discuss the treatment with the next of kin; there is no requirement to obtain their consent. The decision in law rests with the doctor. This poses no problem if what is being proposed is in the patient's best interests. It does however in itself pose two further questions. First, how do we know what is in the patient's best interests? And, second, who is best able to assess what is in the patient's best interests? Consider the following case study, working on the assumption that the patient, Tommy, is not competent to give consent.

Case Study 2

Tommy is 32 years old, and suffers from Down syndrome. Until 3 years ago he lived at home with his parents, attending a Day Centre 5 days a week, with occasional periods of respite care. His parents had always coped very well, although at times they became clearly exhausted. Three years ago his mother died, aged 65. Tommy's father, then aged 70, felt unable to continue caring for Tommy at home, and reluctantly agreed to Tommy being admitted into long-term care. The residential home in which Tommy lives is within walking distance of the family home, and provides good-quality care. Tommy's father is very satisfied with the care Tommy receives, and Tommy appears to be happy there.

Recently, several of Tommy's teeth have become rotten, and the dentist, who has met Tommy for the first time, has advised that they are extracted, and that Tommy has dentures fitted. Despite the condition of Tommy's teeth, he has no difficulty eating, and enjoys his food.

On several occasions in the past Tommy has had dental treatment, including fillings and extractions. These have always been very traumatic events for both Tommy and his parents. Tommy had to be sedated in order to have treatment, and becomes very disorientated for several days following. At the mention of the word 'dentist', Tommy becomes very agitated.

Tommy's father feels that the proposed treatment is not in Tommy's best interest. Tommy has no problem with eating, and would probably continue to enjoy his food if the treatment was not carried out. Furthermore, Tommy's father is not convinced that having the teeth extracted and dentures fitted will improve the situation, and indeed may cause more problems. Tommy may find it more difficult to eat without his teeth, and is likely to loose the dentures. He feels that to put Tommy through the trauma of treatment is unnecessary and unfair.

The dentist considers that the treatment will be in Tommy's best interest in the longer term.

The community nurse, who has been involved in Tommy's care for several years, is inclined to support Tommy's father, though recognizing that the treatment may be inevitable in the long term.

Is it then in Tommy's best interests that the treatment goes ahead? In the long term it may be, since there is likely to come a time when through the course of nature the teeth will fall out anyway. However, in the short term it probably is not.

The treatment will cause him great trauma, and is not going to greatly improve his situation. He is managing quite well with the teeth in their present condition. So, who should make the decision? Tommy's father knows him better than the dentist, as does the community nurse. It would seem then that Tommy's father is in a better position than the dentist to judge what is in Tommy's best interest.

CHILDREN

While it is custom and practice in the United Kingdom to obtain the consent of a parent or guardian to carry out treatment on a minor, there is no reason in law in England and Wales (in Scotland a child under the age of 16 is not allowed to consent to treatment by law) why a minor may not give consent to treatment, and there are strong moral arguments that they should. Clearly a baby or young infant is not able to give informed consent. But, the question is at what age does a child develop the necessary attributes to do so? 'Moral development, as all other aspects of development (physical, mental, social and emotional), varies from one individual to another.' (Rumbold, 1999). Therefore, morally and legally there is no reason why a child considerably younger than 16 years may not give consent to treatment. The only determinate being that they possess the necessary attributes to do so. And, these attributes are the same as for an adult, that is that they are able to understand the information, and have the ability to reason and deliberate about choices. It follows then that the person obtaining consent needs to assure themselves that the child possesses these attributes. In the case of babies, young infants or children whom it is considered are incapable of understanding and reasoning it should be the parent/guardian who gives consent.

REFUSAL TO ACCEPT TREATMENT

It follows that if patients/clients have the right to consent to treatment based on information, then on the basis of that same information they have the right to refuse treatment. 'You must respect the patient's refusal just as much as their consent.' (UKCC 1992). The same, of course, applies in the case of infants, to parents and guardians. Frequently, health visitors will be faced with the problem of a parent who refuses to give consent for their child to be vaccinated against a particular disease, or they may prefer one form of vaccine to another, for example to have separate vaccines rather than the combined MMR vaccine. The role of the nurse, again, is to ensure that the patient's/client's decision to refuse treatment is based on all available factual information.

ACCOUNTABILITY

'Accountability means taking responsibility for one's decisions and actions and being held liable for the results of those decisions and actions. It can therefore be seen in ethical terms as exercising autonomy responsibly...' (Rumbold 2000). Here, two aspects of the proper exercise of professional accountability are discussed:

♦ team working and delegation
♦ the scope of practice, with particular reference to nurse prescribing.

TEAM WORKING AND DELEGATION

Community nurses, of whatever discipline, generally work within multidisciplinary teams. In the case of district nurses, health visitors and practice nurses this will be the primary health care team (PHCT), while community mental health, community learning disability, community paediatric and school nurses may work within other multidisciplinary team compilations. Some community nurses, in particular district nurses, are members, often leaders, of a nursing team. Working as a member of a multidisciplinary team can raise a number of ethical issues, while team leadership gives rise to further issues.

WORKING AS PART OF A MULTIDISCIPLINARY TEAM

Each individual nurse is accountable for his or her own decisions and actions. They are accountable to the patient/client, their professional body and their employer. The latter, in particular, can be a cause of possible conflict for nurses working within a multidisciplinary team, where not all members of the team share the same employer. District nurses and health visitors are usually employed by a NHS Trust and as such are part of a management structure outwith the PHCT. General practitioners (GPs) are independent practitioners and are themselves employers of, amongst others, receptionists and practice nurses. The Trust and the GPs may not always share the same priorities, and this can result in divided loyalties and conflict for the community nurse.

In determining priorities the nurse's prime responsibility is to the patient/client, as clauses 1 and 2 of the Code of Conduct make clear. However, there is potential conflict between these two clauses and clause 6 which states: 'Work in a collaborative and co-operative manner with health care professionals, and others involved in providing care, and recognise and respect their particular contributions within the care team.' (UKCC 1992). One possible cause of conflict might be when the nurse considers that the treatment prescribed by the doctor, while not inappropriate, is not the best possible. This is not to suggest that the treatment prescribed will be harmful to the patient, but possibly less effective. The decision about which treatment to prescribe, having not been made solely on clinical grounds but also on that of cost. Clearly the nurse is not in a position to alter the prescribed treatment, but should clearly discuss it fully with the GP with a view to persuading him/her to change their decision. Given the historical power relationship between medicine and nursing this is never easy, but 'Whatever the strength of the historical legacy and the dominating status of medicine, whenever a nurse faces a choice between obligation to a physician and obligation to a client she must recognise that her obligation to a client is primary.' (Benjamin & Curtis 1992). However, the nurse/health visitor needs also to consider the

effects that questioning the doctor's decision might have on the effectiveness of teamwork in the future. To damage the spirit of collaboration and co-operation that is essential to good team working may have a damaging effect on the care of other patients/clients. Thus, in addition to considering what is in the best interests of an individual, the nurse/health visitor needs also to consider the interests of the whole practice population, in other words, what will create the greatest good for the greatest number. (See Chapter 15 for further discussion about team functioning and team development.)

As already noted, another possible cause of conflict is when there is disparity between the policies of the Trust and the wishes of the GPs, other medical staff, or, in the case of school nurses, of the school or Education Authority. Frequently occurring issues are related to the scope of practice, where the employing authority may impose limitations on the tasks nurses are allowed to undertake, but which the doctor wants them to carry out. 'Even if a nurse feels competent and the GP regards her to be so, she may not perform the task, except in an emergency situation, without the employer's authorisation.' (Rumbold 2000). The same principle would apply when the request to perform a task is made by any person, or agency, other than the nurse's employer.

DELEGATION

Some community nurses are leaders of a team of nurses, and have responsibility for delegating care to more junior members of the team. While the nurse to whom the care has been delegated is individually accountable for her/his decisions and actions, the person who delegates the care is not absolved of their accountability. The UKCC in *The Scope of Professional Practice* (1992) states:

The registered nurse, midwife or health visitor must, in serving the interests of patients and clients and the wider interests of society, avoid any inappropriate delegation to others which would compromise those interests.

Equally, in accepting delegation a nurse should only do so if they are appropriately qualified and competent to do so. It is no defence, either morally or in law, to say that you were acting under the orders or requests of others.

THE SCOPE OF PRACTICE – NURSE PRESCRIBING

The introduction of nurse prescribing has increased the responsibility of those nurses who undertake this role. When prescribing was the sole responsibility of the doctor, they shared accountability with the nurse. The nurse was accountable for their own actions in administering the treatment. Now that nurses prescribe treatments, total accountability rests with them. This has at least two implications. First, it means that the nurse is responsible for ensuring that they have the necessary knowledge in order to prescribe the treatment. Second, it means that nurses may be subject to pressure from pharmaceutical companies to prescribe specific products. Recent years have seen increased advertising in nursing journals, particularly community nursing journals, for products included in the Nursing Formulary. While it is doubtful that pharmaceutical companies will offer nurses such lavish gifts as they have in the past offered doctors, they need to ensure that their clinical decisions are not influenced by advertising or other inducements.

ADVOCACY

According to the UKCC (1989):

Advocacy is concerned with promoting and safeguarding the well-being and interests of clients. It is not concerned with conflict for its own sake... Dictionaries define advocate as 'one who pleads the cause of another' or 'one who recommends or urges something' and this indicates that advocacy is a positive, constructive activity.

Nevertheless, it can be a cause of conflict, not only between nurse and doctor, but also between the nurse and their employer. The conflict with the doctor, 'is not so much a clinical one as an ethical one, for nurse and doctor often approach the situation from opposing ethical stances; the nurse from an ethical position which holds respect for autonomy as paramount and the doctor from one

which holds that paternalism is justified in serving the patient's best interests when he or she rather than the patient has defined what those best interests are.' (Rumbold 1999). Return to the case of Tommy (Case Study 2 above). In that situation the community nurse might feel that their role is that of advocate for both Tommy and his father. Tommy is not capable of arguing his own case, and his father may also feel intimidated by the health professional, in this case the dentist. The nurse, having considered all the arguments might feel justified in arguing the case that the treatment not be carried out.

Community nurses, health visitors in particular, have also a role as advocate on behalf of groups of people within the community. 'The notion of inequality in existing healthcare provision and availability of service provision has concerned health visitors for many years and one of the stated principles of health visiting is that individual practitioners should seek to influence policies affecting health (UKSC HVA 1992)' (Gastrell & Coles 1996). Exercising this role may bring them into conflict with their employers and other statutory agencies.

The crucial elements in exercising the role of advocate, whether for individual patients/clients or for groups are:

◆ that the nurse having assured herself of the accuracy of the facts acts only in the bests interests of the patient/client
◆ that the nurse ensures that she is acting as a truly independent agent.

The second point gives rise to the question as to whether the nurse is always the best person to undertake the role of advocate. It can be argued that she may not in every situation be the best person to do so. First, as a health professional she will have formed her own professional judgement as to what is in the patient's best interests and may be influenced by her own values when putting forward a case. Or, conversely, she may allow her relationship with the patient/client to blur her professional judgement. It can therefore be argued that in some circumstances another advocate, who is not a health professional, would be better placed to act on behalf of the patient.

The notion of advocacy is inexorably linked to the notions of empowerment and enabling others to exercise autonomy. The role of the advocate is not simply a matter of arguing a case for someone else, but is about enabling them to argue their own case and ensuring that *their* wishes are being heard. Thus, it is an integral element of the role of the advocate to ensure that the patient/client is provided with the necessary knowledge in order to make an informed choice.

CONCLUSION

As stated at the beginning, it has not been possible in one chapter to address the whole range of ethical issues which confront a community nurse. This chapter has therefore attempted to provide a theoretical basis for ethical decision making, and two major schools of thought – deontology and utilitarianism – have been discussed. A number of principles have also been explored, namely, respect for persons, autonomy, informed consent, accountability and advocacy.

What should be clear is that ethical theories do not always provide answers to ethical dilemmas; what they can do is provide a framework for arriving at a particular position. In most situations there is no one right answer, and individuals might arrive at different conclusions. What is essential is that the conclusion arrived at is based on rational argument.

SUMMARY

◆ The nature of the work carried out by a community health nurse means they must be aware of the ethical considerations including respect for the person and their autonomy, privacy, property and that wherever possible consent should be obtained for treatment (including the right to refuse treatment).

◆ Patients with learning disabilities, children and other groups may provide challenges in respect of an ethical approach to treatment and one of the duties of the community health nurse is to ensure their rights are maintained.

◆ As the community health nurse often works as part of a multidisciplinary team, they should also ensure that the members of the team are working in a manner which fully respects the rights of the patient.

DISCUSSION POINTS

1. Consider the ethical issues that may arise when a provider tries to increase a client's compliance.

2. Demographic changes and the introduction of expensive high-technology medicine means that the health service cannot hope to meet demand, hence 'rationing' some services to some groups may result in a 'postcode lottery'. How would you decide priorities?

3. Two women want to conceive as a result of in vitro fertilization using frozen embryos whose sperm was provided by their former partners who are now unwilling to give consent. What ethical issues would need to be explored here?

REFERENCES

Baelz P 1977 Ethics and belief. Sheldon Press, London
Bailey DM, Schwartzberg SL 1995 Ethical and legal dilemmas in occupational therapy. FA Davis, Philadelphia
Benjamin M, Curtis J 1992 Ethics in nursing, 3rd edn. Oxford University Press, New York
Cribb A 1995 The ethical dimension. In: Tingle J, Cribb A (eds) Nursing law and ethics, Ch 2. Blackwell Science, Oxford
Gastrell P, Coles L 1996 Ethics in practice. In: Gastrell P, Edwards J (eds) Community health nursing: Frameworks for practice. Baillière Tindall, London
Gillon R 1986 Philosophical medical ethics. John Wiley, Chichester
NHS Management Executive 1990 A guide to consent for examination or treatment. NHS Management Executive, London
Rumbold G 1999 Ethics in nursing practice, 3rd edn. Baillière Tindall, Edinburgh
Rumbold GC 2000 Ethical and legal issues. In: Lawton S et al (eds) District nursing, providing care in a supportive context, Ch 10. Churchill Livingstone, Edinburgh
Seedhouse D 1988 Ethics: The heart of health care. John Wiley & Sons, Chichester
UKCC 1987 Confidentiality, an elaboration of clause 9 of the second edition of the UKCC's Code of Professional

Conduct for the Nurse, Midwife and Health Visitor. UKCC, London

UKCC 1989 Exercising accountability. UKCC, London

UKCC 1992 Code of conduct for the nurse, midwife and health visitor, 3rd edn. UKCC, London

UKCC 1996 Guidelines for professional practice. UKCC, London

UKSC HVA 1992 The principles of health visiting: a re-examination. HVA, London

Warnock M (ed) 1962 Utilitarianism. Fontana Library, Glasgow

FURTHER READING

On deontology and utilitarianism
Fromer MJ 1981 Ethical issues in health care. Mosby, St Louis

Husted GL, Husted JH 1991 Ethical decision-making in nursing. Mosby, St Louis

See Chapter 5 – Theories and Standards and references to Autonomy.

Warnock M (ed) 1962 Utilitarianism. Fontana Library, Glasgow

On autonomy
Rumbold G 1999 Ethics in nursing practice, 3rd edn. Baillière Tindall, Edinburgh

See Chapter 14 – Beneficence, non-maleficence and autonomy.

On consent
Freedman B 1975 A moral theory of informed consent. Hastings Centre Report 5(4): 32–39

Gorovitz S et al (eds) 1976 Moral problems in medicine. Prentice-Hall, Englewood Cliffs, NJ

See collection of papers on 'Informed Consent'.

Rumbold G 1999 Ethics in nursing practice, 3rd edn. Baillière Tindall, Edinburgh

See Chapter 9 – Hospitals should do no harm.

On accountability
Lawton S, Cantrell J, Harris J (eds) District nursing, providing care in a supportive context. Churchill Livingstone, Edinburgh

See references to accountability.

Thompson IE, Melia KM, Boyd KM (eds) 1983 Nursing ethics. Churchill Livingstone, Edinburgh

See Chapter 3 – Responsibility and Accountability in Nursing.

Tingle J, Cribb A (eds) 1995 Nursing law and ethics. Blackwell Scientific, Oxford

See Chapters 5A and 5B.

On advocacy
Carpenter D 1992 Advocacy. Nursing Times 88(27): i–viii

Copp LA 1986 The nurse as advocate for vulnerable persons. Journal of Advanced Nursing 11: 255–256

Rumbold G 1999 Ethics in nursing practice, 3rd edn. Baillière Tindall, Edinburgh

See references to Advocacy.

Nursing and healthcare ethics

In addition to the above cited texts, the following provide useful discussion of the principles and issues of health care ethics.

Bandman EI, Bandman B 1990 Nursing ethics through the lifespan. Prentice-Hall, Englewood Cliffs, NJ

Gillon R 1994 Principles of health care ethics. J Wiley & Sons, Chichester

Seedhouse D 1988 Ethics: the heart of health care. J Wiley & Sons, Chichester

KEY ISSUES

◆ The nature of teams and work groups – theoretical perspectives.

◆ Teams within health and social care.

◆ A critical analysis of team development initiatives.

◆ Evaluating the effectiveness of team-work in health and social care.

◆ The future for team-work within changing healthcare organizations.

15

Team-work and team development in health and social care

B. Poulton

INTRODUCTION

A team approach to the delivery of health and social care has dominated the UK health policy agenda throughout the last decade. However, there is limited evidence as to what constitutes a health and social care team; the extent to which teams are effective, in terms of improved outcomes for service users; and the value of team development in improving team functioning. This chapter addresses these issues by firstly exploring the theories of team-work and work groups; secondly, examining the variety of teams within health and social care; thirdly, critically examining team development initiatives and their contribution to collaborative working; fourthly, providing examples of team-work evaluations, using case studies from health and social care practice; and, finally speculating on the future of team-work within the changing context of health and social care provision.

THE NATURE OF TEAMS AND TEAM-WORK

The study of work groups has been a dominant feature within organizational psychology for several decades. Early studies of groups from a social psychological perspective focused on the effect of the group on individual behaviours and attitudes. For an analysis of the consequences of group influences on individual behaviours see Hackman (1992). A different approach to group research examines groups as performing units in organizations (Guzzo & Shea 1992). Such an approach focuses on the task of the group and the effects of a collective performance of a work group in achieving task effectiveness.

For most people the word 'team' conjures up images of sports teams and the analogy would seem appropriate as it implies a group of individuals working towards a common goal. Carpenter presents a comprehensive definition of a team as:

> ... a group of people, each of whom possess particular expertise; each of whom is responsible for making individual decisions; who hold together a common purpose; who meet together to communicate, collaborate and consolidate knowledge, from which plans are made, actions determined and future decisions influenced.
> (Carpenter 1986, pp. 3–4)

This definition implies that 'group' and 'team' are descriptions of the same type of entity. Brown (1988) distinguishes between three sorts of groups: people who experience a common fate (Campbell 1958, Lewin 1948), e.g. Jews in Nazi Europe; a formal or implicit social structure, incorporating status and role relationships (Sherif & Sherif 1969), e.g. the family group; and people in face-to-face interactions with one another (Bales 1950, Homans 1950), e.g. work groups. As Brown points out the second and third categories only seem applicable in small groups of 20 or less, excluding large-scale categories, such as racial or ethnic groups.

Guzzo and Shea (1992) introduce the idea of group identity where team members perceive themselves to be members of the team and are perceived as such by nonmembers familiar with its members. This is an important point as in a large survey of primary care teams (Poulton 1995) there was a lack of consensus as to the size of the team and who was a member of the team.

The belief that teams are more effective in delivering high-quality patient care is based on the assumption that each team member brings specific knowledge and skills to the decision-making process. To some extent this is true but there is also evidence to show that teams often fall short of the quality of decisions made by their most capable members (Rogelberg et al 1992). Additionally, highly cohesive teams tend to develop a state of

'groupthink' (Janis 1989) whereby they are more concerned with achieving agreement than with the quality of decisions.

Multidisciplinary teams in health and social care are made up of a broad range of professionals. The diversity of professional groups within primary health and social care results in conflicting values and beliefs which impede mutual role understanding and valuing of contributions of professions not subscribing to the dominant (medical) model of care delivery. Poulton and West (1999) used a Team Climate Inventory (Anderson & West 1998) to measure team-working in primary care and related this to effectiveness of outcomes. The study surveyed 528 members of 68 primary care teams in England and demonstrated that clear, shared objectives was the biggest single predictor of primary care team effectiveness. However, many of the teams in the study met together infrequently and several were not located in the same building. Furthermore the multiplicity of management, accountability and reward structures in primary care perpetuated a hierarchical structure which militated against a team approach to care. In spite of health care reforms supporting new primary care structures (DoH 1997, DHSSPS 2000), which purport to include all primary care practitioners in the decision-making process, the retention of general practitioners as independent contractors supports the general practitioner as the leader of most local primary care groups.

Farrell et al (2001) suggest that to reach effective functioning teams pass through a sequence of developmental stages. Using Tuckman's (1965) stages of team development (forming, storming, norming and performing) a testable theory of group development was developed. In the forming stage Farrell et al propose that a team is in a state of anomie characterized by a state of ambiguity, confusion and alienation. Teams in this state lack clarity and consensus about the team's mission, their professional roles, when and how team meetings should be conducted and the decision-making process. In a state of high anomie team members may seek orientation and direction from a dominant, usually high status member. The development of the group will be influenced by the leadership qualities of this member (i.e. whether the leader is charismatic or oppressive). Other members may fulfil alternative roles. For example, where the leader is oppressive another member of the team seeks to diffuse anxiety by ingratiating themself with the leader.

In the storming phase subgroups of the team result in polarization and power struggles. Disagreements ensue about team goals, work organization and the control one member should have over another. At this stage an oppressive leader may be challenged. Other roles may emerge: peacemaker – listener and mediator; clown – dispels tension with wit and humour; party host – dispels conflict by bringing in cakes and arranging social outings; and, scapegoat – seen as incompetent and blamed for poor functioning of the team. As the team progresses to the performing stage team members begin to understand and respect each other's roles, which are now based on knowledge and skills of individuals. At this stage anomie is low, communication improves and teams tend to work towards common goals.

Farrell et al tested out this informal role structure using Bales and Cohen's (1979) SYMLOG – a 26-item rating scale used to measure each member's perception of other members on three dimensions: prominence, sociability and task orientation. High scores on prominence indicate a team member who is active, dominant and assertive; high sociability is characterized by warmth and friendliness and those scoring high on task orientation are seen as logical, rational and task focused. Team development was measured using the Team Anomie Scale (Farrell et al 1996). Results demonstrated that as teams develop from a high to a low stage of anomie, the interpersonal behaviour of team members becomes less differentiated in terms of prominence, sociability and task orientation. In general physicians scored high on prominence and task orientation and low on sociability.

TEAMS WITHIN HEALTH AND SOCIAL CARE

Much of the research into team-working in health care has focused on multidisciplinary primary care teams. However, not all commentators agree on what constitutes a primary care team and even the titles to be used. There is much debate as to the use of the terms primary health care and primary care. Purists would argue that primary health care includes not only medical and nursing care provided by general practice and community health services but also social and psychological care provided by an extended group of professionals including social services. In England, Scotland and Wales there is an artificial split between health and social care. Health services are administered through central government and funded from taxation whilst social care is administered and funded by local metropolitan and district councils.

Although there is an integrated model of Health and Social Services in Northern Ireland, integration exists at the administrative and managerial level rather than at practitioner level. For instance, evaluation of a project aimed at integrating health and social service personnel to better meet the needs of a deprived inner city population (Poulton 1999a) demonstrated that social workers did not identify with primary health care. This term was felt to be medically modelled and not reflecting the social care provided by social workers. To overcome these political barriers most recent government directives use the term primary care, which encompasses both health and social care in the community.

PRIMARY CARE TEAM STRUCTURES

Primary care structures are determined by three key factors:

◆ *The global perspective* of primary health care as articulated by the WHO (1978). Using this perspective primary care team structures are designed to meet people's needs and will therefore differ depending on the nature of the local community.

◆ *Government policy.* Successive UK governments have expressed commitment to primary care empowerment and this has stimulated wide debate about the future direction and development of services. Such debates have resulted in a spate of government White Papers (DoH 1996, 1997, Health Departments of Great Britain 1996, DHSSPS 2000) which send clear messages of a commitment to:

- the promotion of high-quality care;
- user-sensitive primary care services;
- the organization of services to meet local need;
- flexible employment opportunities.

Recently, GP fundholding has been abolished by all four countries of the UK. This has been replaced by primary care-centred locality commissioning, giving all practitioners who make prescribing and referral decisions the opportunity to participate in financial decision-making in the best interest of service users. Such commissioning is locally based involving GPs and other primary care professionals.

◆ *Local needs and arrangements.* Attachment of community nurses to general medical practices goes back to the 1960s but there has been no nationally agreed plan as to which practitioners should constitute the primary care team and how their specific roles are defined (Usherwood et al 1997).

The NHS Primary Care Act (1998), allowing more flexible use of general medical services funding, paved the way for innovations in primary care structures and delivery. These new arrangements meant that new teams could emerge not solely led by GPs, and that nurse-led initiatives could be developed (Gardner 1998, Russell & Mitchell 2000). (See Chapter 24 for further discussion on alternative ways of working.)

Traditionally, the primary care team has centred around a general practice population. However, there is not always a consensus as to the membership of the team. For example in an evaluation of a primary care team development initiative (Poulton & Lynch 2000), several of the general practitioners in the study referred to the core team as GP, practice nurse, practice manager and receptionists (i.e. those practitioners generally based in the surgery) and the attached team as Trust-employed community nurses, professions allied to medicine (PAMs) and social workers.

Numerous studies have shown interdisciplinary conflicts in primary care teams (Audit Commission 1992, Bond et al 1985, Poulton & West 1999) and for this reason other healthcare team configurations have been explored. These include teams dedicated to specific client needs (e.g. mental health teams), teams of specific professional disciplines (e.g. integrated nursing teams) and crossagency teams (e.g. extended health and social care teams).

Cook et al (2001) studied decision-making in a health and a social care team for people with enduring mental health needs. This study demonstrated that a team approach influenced decision-making by team members making client care more responsive and proactive.

Integrated nursing teams have been implemented in several areas of the UK (Burke 1997, Cook et al 2001, Hodder 1999, Owen 1998). A practice-based teams project in Cardiff involved 12 practices. In this project groups of district nurses, general practice nurses and health visitors were made practice exclusive and had their own devolved budgets to organize nursing care based on patient needs (Poulton 1997a).

Extended health and social care teams have been developed in an attempt to promote a multidisciplinary, multiagency approach to community care. For example, in an effort to develop teams which covered the whole perspective of health and social care a health authority in West London set up a Joint Ventures Initiative (JVI) to develop team-working in primary care (Poulton 1997b). It has been acknowledged that one of the barriers to team-work is the multiple lines of management and accountability structures that currently exist in primary care. By bringing together the key stakeholders in the primary care process at a strategic level it was hoped that there would be agreement across the health and social care divide and between primary and secondary care. Thus the JVI steering group included a representative from the health authority (the commissioners); a representative from both the community and hospital trusts as providers of primary and secondary services respectively; a general practitioner representative; social services and the community health council as a representative of user interests. A consultancy company was commissioned to run a team development programme with the teams, which had agreed to participate. The teams included not only the traditional primary care team of doctors, practice nurses, attached district nurses and health visitors and administrative staff, but an extended team including a social worker, physiotherapist, school nurse, chiropodist, midwife, community pharmacist, community mental health nurse and Macmillan nurse. An independent researcher was commissioned to evaluate the project not only in terms of benefits to team-working and more cost-efficient care but also in terms of benefits to service users.

A CRITICAL ANALYSIS OF TEAM DEVELOPMENT INITIATIVES

The belief in the value of team-working in health and social care, coupled with the realization that it is not yet a reality, has stimulated the growth in team development workshops. A variety of team-building techniques exist within the organization development literature but Iles and Auluck (1990) suggest that much of the research has been done with groups of like individuals and might not be transferable to multidisciplinary and multi-agency teams.

Team-building refers to a whole host of activities focusing on anything from joint planning of work activities to assisting team members in examining their roles and relationships within the team. There are numerous instruction manuals aimed at improving team-working (Health Education Authority 1994, Woodcock 1989). Many of these adopt ideas from the organizational development and management literature focusing on issues such as role clarification, interpersonal relationships or approaches to problem solving (Tannenbaum et al 1992).

There is mixed evidence as to the effectiveness of team-building interventions. Porras and Berg (1978) found that 45% of team-building studies showed significant positive changes on 'process' variables, such as trust, communications, support, involvement and problem solving. Boss and McConkie (1981) describe a team-building intervention, which so improved group cohesiveness that the employees' loyalty to the team far exceeded their loyalty to the organization, thus decreasing organizational effectiveness. The design and conduct of this intervention was highly effective, certainly in improving the scores of the intervention team on the Likert (1967) Profile of Organisational Performance Characteristics and the Friedlander (1968) Group Behaviour inventory in comparison with the control group. However, the researchers highlight five major issues emanating from the experience:

♦ It is possible to build a group of people into a team that is so strong in terms of interpersonal support and trust that loyalty to the group exceeds loyalty to the organization.

♦ Methods should be developed to facilitate team member's re-entry to the organization and this may involve informing the wider organization of the goals and objectives developed during team-building sessions.

♦ Problems that surface during team-building sessions should afford opportunities for skill development among individual participants.

♦ Building a strong team does not ensure that the intervention will have a positive impact on the organization. It is important to make sure that any new norms developed support rather than hinder the organization's goals and objectives.

♦ The interventions illustrate (Boss & McConkie 1981) the central role of the consultant. In this instance although the consultant was highly successful in facilitating team-building he failed to help participants to understand the consequences of their decision-making and action plans.

There is little recent valid evidence exploring the effectiveness of team development techniques. DeMeuse and Liebowitz (1981) give a critical analysis of team-building research between 1965 and 1980. They point out that the effectiveness of the team-building experience is often judged on the basis of anecdotal evidence from participants and/or subjective evaluations relating to the value of the experience made shortly afterwards. Although there appears to be some evidence of the effectiveness of team-building interventions it must be pointed out that favourable results should be tempered by the realization that efforts that fail are seldom published. DeMeuse and Liebowitz conclude that although 88% of the evaluations of the team-building interventions demonstrate positive results, the majority of these evaluations were not rigorous enough to determine valid outcomes of the team-building programmes. This is due to weakness in research methods and measurements, which preclude any firm conclusions concerning the efficacy of team-building.

In a more recent review Sundstrom et al (1990) examined empirical research on team development between 1980 and 1988. They found that most research designs had control groups thus yielding more interpretable results than earlier reviews. However, this review still highlights the mixed success of team-building interventions. Team performance improved in four out of nine studies and aspects of team processes improved in eight out of ten studies. The authors conclude that work group effectiveness may have improved in some circumstances but failure of some interventions may be due to focusing only on internal team processes and ignoring the external context in which the group operates.

Guzzo & Shea (1992) summarizing the evidence for the value of team-building interventions suggest that whilst team-building initiatives have a reliably positive effect on member attitudes and perceptions there is no evidence that they improve the performance of the team.

APPLICATION OF TEAM-BUILDING IN PRIMARY CARE

Team-building initiatives in primary care developed in response to the shift in focus from disease orientation to health promotion. In 1987 the Health Education Authority (HEA) initiated a team workshop strategy aimed at assisting primary care teams to develop health promotional activities in relation to coronary heart disease. Up to the end of March 1991, 452 teams from regions throughout England had participated in these workshops. The format varied but the focus was on facilitating the teams to develop action plans for health promotion and disease prevention within their practice population (Spratley 1989).

These workshops have been evaluated locally and nationally. A quantitative study using a pre- and post-intervention design, but without equivalent control groups involved 39 primary care teams (Poulton 1995). All members of these teams (n = 329) completed the Team Climate Inventory (Anderson & West 1998), a validated measure of team functioning which examines the following aspects:

- clarity of team objectives
- participation in decision-making in the team
- commitment to quality of task performance
- support for innovation
- mutual role understanding.

Comparison of pre- and post-test scores demonstrated significant improvements in team member ratings of communication, participation in decision-making, clarity in the value of shared objectives, role understanding and commitment to quality of task performance. These findings support evidence from organizational psychology literature, which suggests that team-building interventions have an impact on team process variables (Guzzo & Shea 1992, Porras & DeBerg 1978, Sundstrom et al 1990). However, the design of the study had several limitations. For example, by adopting a quasiexperimental design, characterized by a pre- and post-intervention measure, no control groups were used, therefore the 'Hawthorne effect' or effects of history cannot be excluded as confounding factors (DeMeuse & Liebowitz 1981). In other words there are several other factors unrelated to the workshop which may have contributed to improvements in team processes. For instance, the impetus of the GP contract, GP fundholding and the Patients' Charter may have influenced changes from above.

More recently West and Pillinger (1996) reviewed the HEA team-building initiative by surveying the Local Organizing Teams (LOTS) responsible for the planning and delivery of the workshops. Questionnaires were sent to 70 LOT representatives and 32 responses were received. The questionnaire asked about methods used in team-building workshops, the attendees, the underlying principles and perceived effectiveness of the workshops. West and Pillinger concluded that the HEA workshop programme was helpful in developing primary care practitioners' awareness of team-working. However, the main focus of the workshops appeared to be on building team cohesion, which has been shown to have only limited impact on team effectiveness. Respondents often reported feeling inadequately prepared to facilitate the workshops and although enthusiastic themselves there was a feeling that wider organizational support for the initiative was lacking.

The HEA team development programme has been used as a template for several smaller-scale initiatives (Poulton and Lynch 2000, West et al 1995). Similar results have emerged in that the most enthusiastic teams invest time and commitment to developing new ways of working only to find that there are insufficient resources and wider organizational support to carry through the ideas generated. It is interesting to note that Hackman, 'the guru of team research', has now turned his attention to these issues, summarized in the following statement:

To ask whether organisational performance improves when teams are used to accomplish work is to ask a question with no real answer. A more tractable question is what differentiates those teams that go into orbit and achieve real synergy from those that crash and burn. The answer to the second question has more to do with how teams are structured and supported than with any inherent virtues or liabilities of teams as performing units. (Hackman 1998, p. 245)

EVALUATING THE EFFECTIVENESS OF TEAM-WORK IN HEALTH AND SOCIAL CARE

The preceding section explored the role of team development in improving team-working in health and social care. It emerged that improving team processes (e.g. communication, participation in decision-making, trust and support) does not necessarily lead to improved effectiveness for the team concerned. Before this issue can be addressed it is necessary to clarify what constitutes effective health and social care.

Over the past decade, the need to control expenditure on health care has created the stimulus to search for measurable criteria of effectiveness in all areas of health care, not least measurable outcomes of community health and social care services. Although there is a growing body of evidence of specific outcomes, disease-focused research, the nature of community health and social care services is so diverse it is difficult to identify clear measurable outcomes of activity (Wilkin et al 1992).

In its broadest sense outcome refers to a visible effect for a specific intervention. Wilkin et al suggest that: 'in the context of health and illness, outcome is usually defined in terms of the achievement of, or failure to achieve desired goals' (Wilkin et al 1992, p. 5).

The authors argue that in this context, outcome is closely aligned to need, suggesting that the two can be considered as different sides of the same coin. In assessing patient/carer (consumer) outcomes, therefore, many of the criteria identified will relate to consumer needs. Such needs tend to focus practitioner attention on the way in which the service is provided, rather than on specific outcomes of clinical interventions. Measurement of the outcomes of clinical interventions from the consumer perspective will involve examining specific disease processes; the impact that health-care interventions have on the progression of these conditions, and the subsequent effect on quality of life for the patient.

Acknowledging the complexities of defining the concept of effectiveness in organizations, several organizational psychologists (e.g. Cameron & Whetton 1983, Goodman et al 1986) argue that research in this area should be abandoned given the lack of a single model or theory which can be applied across organizations. The literature on organizational effectiveness distinguishes between efficiency (doing things right) and effectiveness (doing the right things) (Sundstrom et al 1990).

Efficiency can be defined as the output for a given input and how a team compares with similar teams on set criteria. For example, community nursing is currently measured in terms of the number and duration of patient/client contacts. Effectiveness is much more difficult to quantify in the short term, but would involve a more innovative approach to achieving the desired goals as negotiated with the consumers of the service. Teams can therefore be seen as more or less effective depending on the criteria used. Consequently, the assessment of team effectiveness has come to be seen as a political as much as an empirical process.

In response to this, some psychologists have proposed a 'constituency approach' (Connally et al 1980) which aims to incorporate all significant views in the judgement of team effectiveness. Each of the major constituents, or stakeholders in the process, is identified and the effectiveness criteria they would use are adopted as an indicator. Effectiveness can then be measured using multiple indicators rather than an aggregate, since effectiveness in one area may imply ineffectiveness in another.

As with other models the constituency approach also has its disadvantages as constituencies may use effectiveness criteria, which are unrelated or strongly negatively related. Health and social care teams exist to maintain and improve the health of the population through health promotion, treatment and rehabilitation. Patients and their carers are therefore major stakeholders in this process but, as much of their care is provided free at point of delivery, the allocation and management of resources rests with other stakeholders, notably the Health Authorities/ Boards and Trusts acting as commissioners and providers of health care, respectively. These major groups of stakeholders will have conflicting criteria of effectiveness: that patients and carers be given high-quality care which may be costly; that service commissioners and providers provide this care within allocated resources.

The multiple constituency approach was tested out using key stakeholders in primary care (Poulton & West 1994). A group of 40 stakeholders was brought together to generate measures of primary care effectiveness from their own perspective. These included representatives of consumer groups (patients and carers); practitioners (medical, nursing, practice administration); providers (community unit managers); commissioners (fundholding GP; Health Authority/ Board); policy makers (Department of Health); policy analysts and influencers (Royal College of Nursing, Royal College of General Practitioners).

This exercise yielded effectiveness criteria in four major areas: consumer outcomes; quality of care; team viability; and organizational issues. These measures were subsequently used in a study relating primary care team processes to effectiveness (Poulton & West 1999). An adaptation of these criteria of effectiveness has been used to evaluate a range of team initiatives within primary care. For example, the Joint Ventures Initiative (JVI) referred to earlier was evaluated in terms of services to patients; quality of teamworking among members of primary care team members and between primary care teams and outside agencies, particularly social services; effectiveness and efficiency of primary care services in relation to such aspects as appropriateness of referrals and user satisfaction.

Relating improved outcomes for patients to organizational change is fraught with difficulties. Patient satisfaction studies have been seen as a way of evaluating user views of the services they receive. However, as McIver (1993) points out most patient satisfaction questionnaires are based on a review of other questionnaires and there is a lack of qualitative studies which explore patients' views as to what constitutes high-quality care. For this reason it was decided to collect qualitative information via client/patient interviews, for the JVI project. These results are reported elsewhere (Poulton 1999b).

Another way of encouraging a team approach to care in the community is to use a multidisciplinary audit. One such project was carried out with six primary care teams in England (Poulton 1996). Using a health needs assessment of their practice populations teams were encouraged to identify priorities for intervention and audit the extent to which they were delivering user-centred, cost-effective care to their practice population.

For example, one team identified a high number of young disabled people within the practice population and set out to develop more appropriate services to meet the needs of this vulnerable group of patients. The initiative was evaluated overall by using the Team Climate Inventory to measure team-work and interviews with key members of teams to ascertain the extent to which they felt they had achieved the objectives they set for themselves.

THE FUTURE FOR TEAM-WORK WITHIN CHANGING HEALTHCARE ORGANIZATIONS

Over the last decade we have witnessed major changes in the organization and delivery of health care in the UK. There has been a shift from an acute lead service to a primary care-led NHS. In parallel to these organizational changes, the rise of consumer sovereignty and the emphasis on a needs-led rather than a professionally led service has demanded that primary health and social care respond more effectively to the needs of local communities.

Changes in the organizational structure of healthcare and policy initiatives such as the 'New Deal' for junior doctors have resulted in a blurring of roles between doctors and nurses. Consequently there has been a proliferation of new nursing roles facilitated by the introduction of the UKCC Scope of Professional Practice (UKCC 1992) which allowed for extension of nursing practice to cover activities traditionally undertaken by doctors (Humphris & Masterson 2000). Furthermore the introduction of nurse prescribing for qualified district nurses and health visitors, soon to be extended to other groups of appropriately qualified nurses (DoH 2000), increases the ability of community nurses to better meet the needs of the families and communities they serve.

All four governments of the UK have pledged a commitment to public health (DHSSPS 2000). However, it is not always clear what is meant by the term 'public health' and how it might be reconciled with 'primary care' conflict the Public Health Alliar a public health model of primary care ᴵᴵᴵᶜ ing primary care, public health and community (Public Health Alliance 1998).

Both Scotland and Wales have reviewed aspects of their community nursing provision in the context of public health. In Wales the review addressed only health visiting and school nursing services (Clark et al 2000) and concluded that whilst these services had the potential to deliver the Assembly's agenda for health in Wales both were underdeveloped, undermanaged and under-resourced. The Welsh review proposes pilot studies to test out a range of options. Pilot sites would have health visitors and school nurses seconded from relevant trusts to Local Health Groups (LHG) where they would provide health visiting and school nursing services to the LHG population. Additionally, health visitors and school nurses would undertake a health needs assessment and health profile of the LHG area and in conjunction with the local community develop a Health Plan for the area. Health visiting is envisaged as carrying out three roles: generalist health visiting to children and families; generalist health visiting to particular groups identified by the health needs assessment (e.g. elderly, travellers); and public health and community development. Whether these roles are carried out independently or combined will be decided from the results of the pilot studies.

The review of the nursing contribution to improving the public's health in Scotland (Scottish Executive 2001) focuses on the whole range of community nursing disciplines and is far more radical in its recommendations. The review proposes the development of a public health nursing role, which incorporates the roles of health visitors and school nurses. In addition the review proposes implementation of the family health nurse concept currently being piloted in the Highlands, Western Isles and Orkney. The WHO Ministerial Conference on Nursing and Midwifery pledged support for 'family-focused community nursing and midwifery programmes and services, including where appropriate, the Family Health Nurse' (WHO 2000, p. 2). The role of the family health nurse is envisaged as involving four major types of intervention – primary, secondary and tertiary prevention and crisis intervention/direct care (WHO 1999).

Such changes in roles and structures will undoubtedly have an impact on the functioning of primary health and social care teams. The crux of making any team work is that team-working is about sharing skills and not preserving roles to suit entrenched professional groupings. It is arrogant to suggest that specialist skills and knowledge gained through education automatically provide empirical proof of professional expertise and integrity. The Bristol Inquiry (DoH 2001), whilst focusing on secondary care, has implications for communication and team-working in primary care (Baker 2001). Nursing roles within health and social care have proliferated in the last decade. There is pressure on the UKCC (now Nursing and Midwifery Council) to recognize the nurse practitioner role within the post-registration community nursing specialist programme. However, these professional arguments do nothing to help the establishment of team-working. Gardener warns against territoriality when he says, 'health visiting doesn't matter … district nursing doesn't matter … practice nursing doesn't matter … nurse practitioners don't matter … what matters is people!' (Gardener 1998). In the future, skills to meet the needs of communities will be more important than titles.

CONCLUSION

There is no doubt that team-working in health and social care remains high on the health care agenda. However, it is not always clear what makes a team work well as a team and more importantly whether teams that work well are more effective in improving the health and well-being of the populations they serve. Whilst team development has been shown to improve team processes (communication, trust and support) there is little or no evidence to suggest that there is any lasting improvement to team performance. What is clear is that organizational structures and roles within health and social care have evolved

considerably over the last decade and will continue to do so. The encouraging factor is that health service users are being given more power in influencing the type and delivery of the health and social care they receive. The hope is that in future they will work as equal members of health and social care teams alongside health and social care practitioners. As Clinical Governance takes hold in the new world of the NHS, team-work has got to be an integral part of our practice as in the words of Benjamin Franklin: 'We must all hang together or most assuredly we shall all hang separately.' (remark at the signing of the Declaration of Independence, 4th July 1776). (See Chapter 4 for further discussion of quality issues related to clinical governance.)

SUMMARY

Effective teams in organizational settings are characterized by:

◆ a defined group of individuals who perceive themselves as members of the team

◆ defined roles within the team respected and understood by all team members

◆ regular interaction between team members

◆ clear, shared team goals

◆ equal participation in decision-making by all team members.

The positive effects of team development appear to be:

◆ developing practitioners' awareness of the benefits of team-working

◆ improving communication

◆ improving shared decision-making

◆ improving problem solving

◆ improving trust and support.

The negative effects of team development are:

◆ improved cohesion in the team may be developed at the expense of loyalty to the wider organization

◆ there is no evidence of improvement in overall team performance

◆ innovations may be short lived due to lack of ongoing support from the wider organization.

Using a constituency approach to define effectiveness for health and social care teams the following key areas have been identified:

◆ consumer outcomes

◆ quality of care

◆ team viability

◆ organizational issues.

Subsequent evaluations have narrowed these down to the following:

◆ benefits to patients

◆ benefits to the team

◆ benefits to the wider organization.

DISCUSSION POINTS

1. Do you consider you work in a team and if so what are the characteristics of this team?

2. Assess your team using the following criteria:

   ◆ We have regular formal and informal meetings.

   ◆ Everyone is involved in the decision-making process.

   ◆ Team members support each other in times of stress.

   ◆ We regularly seek the views of the client / patient group we serve and review our practice accordingly.

   ◆ The team is always open and responsive to new ideas that will improve the quality of our service.

REFERENCES

Anderson N, West MA 1998 Measuring climate for work group innovation: development and validation of the team climate inventory. Journal of Organizational Behaviour 19: 235–258

Audit Commission 1992 Homeward bound: A new course for community health. HMSO, London

Baker M 2001 The Bristol Report: implication for clinical governance in primary care. Journal of Clinical Governance 9(3): 109–111

Bales RF 1950 Interaction process analysis: a method for the study of small groups. University of Chicago Press, Chicago

Bales RF, Cohen S 1979 SYMLOG: A system for multiple level observation of groups. Free Press, New York

Bond J, Cartilidge AM, Gregson BA, Philips PR, Bolam F, Gill KM 1985 A study of interprofessional collaboration in primary health care organisations, Report No. 27, vol. 2. Health Care Research Unit, University of Newcastle-upon-Tyne, Newcastle-Upon-Tyne

Boss RW, McConkie ML 1981 The destructive impact of a positive team-building intervention. Group and Organization Studies 6(1): 45–56

Brown R 1988 Group processes: Dynamics within and between groups. Blackwell, Oxford

Burke W 1997 A diplomatic service. Nursing Times 93(3): 42–44

Cameron KS, Whetton DA (eds) 1983 Organizational effectiveness: A comparison of multiple models. Academic Press, New York

Campbell DT 1958 Common fate, similarity, and other indices of the status of aggregates of persons as social entities. Behavioural Science 3: 14–25

Carpenter J (ed) 1986 Training for team-work. Paper presented at a study day on Interprofessional Education at Bristol Polytechnic. Centre for the Advancement of Interprofessional Education, University of Bristol, Bristol

Clark J, Buttigieg M, Bodycombe-James M, et al 2000 Recognising the potential: The review of health visiting and school health services in Wales. School of Health Sciences, University of Wales, Swansea

Connally T, Conlan EJ, Deutsch SJ 1980 Organizational effectiveness: A multiple constituency approach. Academy of Management Review 5: 211–217

Cook G, Gerrish K, Clarke C 2001 Decision-making in teams: issues arising from two UK evaluations. Journal of Interprofessional Care 15(2): 141–151

De Meuse KP, Liebowitz SJ 1981 An empirical analysis of team-building research. Group & Organization Studies 6: 357–378

Department of Health 1997 The new NHS: Modern – Dependable. DoH, London

Department of Health 1996 Primary care: Delivering the future. The Stationery Office, London

Department of Health 2000 Consultation on proposals to extend nursing prescribing. DoH (www.doh.gov.uk/nurseprescribing)

Department of Health 2001 Learning from Bristol: the report of the public inquiry into children's heart surgery at the Bristol Royal Infirmary 1984–1995, CM 5207. The Stationery Office, London

Department of Health, Social Services and Public Safety (DHSSPS) 2000 Building the way forward in primary care. DHSSPS, Belfast

Department of Health; Welsh Office; The Scottish Office (Health Depts. Of Great Britain) 1996 Choice and opportunity: Primary care: the future. The Stationery Office, London

Farrell MP, Schmitt MH, Heineman GD, Roghmann K 1996 The Team Anomie Scale. Unpublished Manuscript University of Buffalo, SUNY

Farrell MP, Schmitt MH, Heineman GD 2001 Informal roles and stages of interdisciplinary team development. Journal of Interprofessional Care 15(3): 281–295

Friedlander FA 1968 A comparative study of consulting processes and group development. Journal of Applied Behavioral Science 4: 377–399

Gardner L 1998 Leading primary care: time for action. Health Visitor 71(1): 21–22

Goodman PS 1986 Impact of task and technology on group performance. In: Goodman PS (ed) Designing effective work groups, pp. 120–176. Jossey Bass, San Francisco

Guzzo RA, Shea GP 1992 Group performance and intergroup relations in organizations. In: Dunnette MD, Hough LM (eds) Handbook of industrial and organizational psychology, Vol. 3. Consulting Psychologists Press, Palo Alto

Hackman JR 1992 Group influences on individuals in organizations. In: Dunnette MD, Hough LM (eds) Handbook of industrial and organizational psychology, Vol. 3. Consulting Psychologists Press, Palo Alto

Hackman JR 1998 Why teams don't work. In: Tindale RS, Heath L (eds) Theory and research on small groups: social psychological applications to social issues, Vol. 4, pp. 245–267. Plenum Press, New York

Health Education Authority 1994 Group facilitation skills toolbox: manual for use with primary healthcare teams. Health Education Authority, London

Hodder P 1999 Integrated nursing teams: sprouting up everywhere? In: Elwyn G, Smail J (eds) Integrated teams in primary care. Radcliffe Medical Press Ltd, Abingdon

Homans GC 1950 The human group. Harcourt, Brace and World, New York

Humphris D, Masterson A (ed) 2000 Developing new clinical roles: a guide for health professionals. Churchill Livingstone, Edinburgh

Iles PA, Auluck R 1990 From organizational to interorganizational development in nursing practice: Improving the effectiveness of interdisciplinary team-work and interagency collaboration. Journal of Advanced Nursing 15: 50–58

Janis IL 1989 Crucial decisions. The Free Press, New York

Lewin K 1948 Resolving social conflicts. Harper Row, New York

Likert R 1967 The human organization: Its management and value. McGraw-Hill, New York

McIver S 1993 Obtaining the views of users of primary and community health care services. Kings Fund Centre, London

Owen A 1998 Self managed teams: the West Berkshire approach. Health Visitor 71(1): 23–24

Porras JI, DeBerg PO 1978 The impact of organization development. Academy of Management Review April 1978

Poulton BC 1995 Effective multidisciplinary team-work in primary health care. Unpublished PhD thesis, Institute of Work Psychology, University of Sheffield

Poulton BC 1996 Multidisciplinary audit in primary health care. Daphne Heald Research Unit, Royal College of Nursing, London

Poulton BC 1997a Evaluation of Cardiff Community healthcare practice based teams project. Daphne Heald Research Unit, Royal College of Nursing, London

Poulton BC 1997b Joint ventures initiative for primary care team development in Hillingdon. Daphne Heald Research Unit, Royal College of Nursing, London

Poulton BC 1999a Evaluation of the Shankill Primary Care Project. University of Ulster, Belfast

Poulton BC 1999b User involvement in identifying health needs and shaping and evaluating services: is it being recognised? Journal of Advanced Nursing 30(6): 1289–1296

Poulton BC, Lynch C 2000 Southern Health and Social Services Board primary care team development. Evaluation Report, University of Ulster, Belfast

Poulton BC, West MA 1994 Primary health care team effectiveness: Developing a constituency approach. Health & Social Care in the Community 2: 77–84

Poulton BC, West MA 1999 The determinants of effectiveness in primary health care teams. Journal of Interprofessional Care 13(1): 7–18

Public Health Alliance 1998 A public health model of primary care – from concept to reality. Public Health Alliance, Birmingham

Rogelberg SG, Barnes-Farrell L, Lowe CA 1992 The stepladder technique: An alternative group structure facilitating effective group decision-making. Journal of Applied Psychology 77: 730–737

Russell J, Mitchell R 2000 The assessment of a nurse-led deliberate self-harm service. Health Bulletin 58(3): 221–223

Scottish Executive 2001 Nursing for health: A review of the contribution of nurses, midwives and health visitors to improving the public's health in Scotland. The Scottish Executive, Edinburgh

Sherif M, Sherif CW 1969 The adolescent in his group in its setting. In: Sherif M (ed) Social interaction. Aldine, Chicago

Spratley J 1989 Disease prevention and the health promotion in primary health care: team workshops organised by the Health Education Authority (HEA). HEA, London

Sundstrom E, De Meuse KP, Futrell D 1990 Work teams: Application and effectiveness. American Psychologist 45(2): 120–133

Tannenbaum SI, Beard RL, Salas E 1992 Team-building and its influence on team effectiveness: an examination of conceptual and empirical developments. In: Kelley K (ed) Issues, theory, and research in industrial/organizational psychology. Advances in Psychology 82: 117–153

Tuckman BW 1965 Developmental sequence in small groups. Psychological Bulletin 63: 384–399

United Kingdom Central Council for Nursing, Midwifery and Health Visiting (UKCC) 1992 The scope of professional practice. UKCC, London

Usherwood T, Long S, Joesbury H 1997 The changing composition of primary care health teams. In: Pearson P, Spencer J (eds) Promoting team-work in primary care: A research based approach. Arnold, London

West MA, Pillinger T 1996 Team-building in primary health care: an evaluation. Health Education Authority, London

West MA, Poulton BC, Hardy G 1995 New models of primary health care: The Northern and Yorkshire Region Micropurchasing Project. Northern and Yorkshire Region, Harrogate

Wilkin D, Hallam L, Doggett A 1992 Measures of need and outcome in primary health care. Oxford University Press, Oxford

Woodcock M 1989 Team development manual, 2nd edn. Gower Press, Aldershot

World Health Organization 1999 Family health nurse curriculum. WHO, Copenhagen

World Health Organization 2000 Munich Declaration: nurses and midwives: A force for health. WHO, Copenhagen

FURTHER READING

Elwyn G, Smail J (eds) 1999 Integrated teams in primary care. Radcliffe Medical Press, Abingdon

This book explores the concept of integrated nursing teams in primary care. Not only does it examine innovative models of a nursing team approach but it also explores legal responsibility and devolved budgets, using practical examples.

Pearson P, Spencer J (eds) 1997 Promoting teamwork in primary care: a research based approach. Arnold, London

This text draws together the work of a multiprofessional group of contributors from the field of primary care, community health, management and psychology. It uses research in primary care to examine the ways in which teamwork can be promoted to achieve high-quality care.

Leadership in community nursing

E. Thomas

INTRODUCTION

The issue of leadership in the NHS is at the top of the Government's modernization agenda. Another high-priority agenda is the delivery of transformed primary care. To achieve both of these ends, nursing is regarded as essential. This chapter explores the issues associated with leadership in community nursing, and the pivotal role it must play in delivering the new agenda.

POLICY BACKGROUND

In 1997, the Secretary of State introduced a White Paper that heralded major changes in health service funding and organization (Secretary of State for Health 1997). General practice fundholding, central to the NHS 'internal market', implemented by the previous government, was replaced by a network of new Primary Care Groups in England and Northern Ireland (PCGs), Local Health Groups in Wales (LHGs) and Scottish Primary Care Trusts in Scotland (SPCTs). These reforms were intended to improve efficiency, reduce variation and fragmentation, and achieve more seamless patient care. The new government made a strong commitment to tackling inequalities in health, by improving patients' access to services, particularly for those groups that were disadvantaged. In the following year, proposals for improving the quality of health care were released in a further White Paper (NHSE 1998). (See Chapter 4 for further discussion about quality improvement.)

The creation of Primary Care Groups, Local Health Groups and Scottish Primary Care Trusts was the first stage in a process that brought together a board consisting of representative GPs, community nurses, social services, the local community and the health authority. They were charged with delivering three core functions:

◆ Improving the health of people and addressing health inequalities
◆ Developing primary and community health services
◆ Commissioning community and hospital services.

Primary Care Groups were expected to evolve into independent Primary Care Trusts. In April 2001, there were 164 Primary Care Trusts providing care to 47.7% of the population in England (Wilkin et al 2001). By April 2004, all Primary Care Groups are expected to have achieved Trust status. (See Chapter 2 for further discussion on recent health and policy changes.)

While Primary Care Groups were rapidly becoming Trusts, other changes and additions to healthcare policy had a dramatic impact on what is required of NHS staff. The NHS Cancer Plan and the New National Service Frameworks for Coronary Heart Disease, Mental Health and Older People were launched (NHSE 2000a,b,c, 2001). These provide models of good practice and standards against which the progress of PCTs, LHGs and SPCGs can be measured. However, the most important policy to be introduced to the NHS was the National Health Service Plan (NHS Plan), which sets out a ten-year programme of modernization and reform (NHSE 2000). Included in this document are many references to the importance of leadership in the delivery of a far-reaching agenda.

A MODERNIZED NURSING SERVICE?

The NHS Plan requires a modernized health service with new roles for nurses, strengthened education and training, new career structures, improved quality of nursing practice and building of clinical leadership (NHSE 2000). Much of this document mirrored the earlier government strategy for nursing, *Making a Difference* (DoH 1999), which set out a new direction for nursing, advocating improved clinical leadership through training and a new career structure for nurses. Furthermore it formalized the need for benchmarks against which nurses could compare and develop their practice, as a means of reducing variation and improving quality.

The *Essence of Care* (DoH 2001) is a toolkit of benchmarks which details assessment processes for nursing and other care providers. It was published by the Department of Health, for nurses and organizations to use as part of their quality improvement programmes. Developed by patients, consumer groups, and professionals and in response to complaints, it provides best practice guidance in eight fundamental aspects of clinical care. Areas covered include:

◆ principles of care
◆ personal and oral hygiene
◆ nutrition
◆ continence and bladder care
◆ pressure ulcer prevention and care
◆ safety of clients with mental health needs
◆ record keeping
◆ privacy and dignity.

Assessing whether community nursing is making progress towards a new modernized service, in terms of achieving new roles, falls to a number of processes, including the annual Performance Assessment Framework. The 'ten key skills' for nursing are included in this. These were announced in April 2000 and are basically ten aspects of nursing practice that are being undertaken safely and effectively by nurses in some parts of the country, but not yet in others. The Government wants all Trusts to implement these whenever possible. The ten key skills that the Government wants nurses to undertake are to:

1. Order diagnostic investigations, such as pathology laboratory tests and X-rays.
2. Make and receive referrals, such as directly to a therapist or a pain consultant.
3. Admit and discharge patients for specific conditions and with agreed protocols.

4. Manage a caseload, such as for diabetes or rheumatology.
5. Run their own clinics, for example, ophthalmology and dermatology.
6. Carry out a wide range of resuscitation procedures, such as defibrillation and intubation.
7. Perform minor surgery and outpatient procedures.
8. Use computerized decision support and triage patients to the most appropriate health practitioner.
9. Take a lead in the way local health services are organized and run.
10. Prescribe medicines and treatments.

NURSE MANAGEMENT IN COMMUNITY NURSING

Historically, nurses wishing to advance their careers had to select promotional opportunities either in management or education. Clinical grading resulted in a much flatter career structure with fewer opportunities for senior nursing roles. Analysis of nurse manager roles was difficult because they were heavily influenced by the health system of which they were a part. This resulted in wide variations between roles which meant that comparative evaluation was virtually impossible. In consequence, there were wide-ranging opinions and anecdotal evidence about what the roles should focus on, especially regarding levels of clinical involvement. This approach is quite different from that taken in medicine and most other clinical professions, where clinical practice is maintained even in the most senior management roles.

Prior to the inception of Primary Care Groups, Local Health Groups and Scottish Primary Care Trusts, nursing in the community was usually divided into separately managed groups: learning disability nurses and mental health nurses linked to a different Trust from the other specialist groups (school nurses, health visitors, district nurses and community children's nurses) while practice nurses and occupational health nurses remained outside this management structure. Community Trusts commonly had clear hierarchies and accountability frameworks, so that although titles might have varied in different parts of the country, the actual management frameworks were very similar. In consequence, groups of nurses were usually managed in pyramid speciality groups, with first and second-line management, service management and ultimately a Nurse Executive Director as a full member of the Trust Board. The addition of a Nursing Director in NHS Trusts was made a requirement when NHS Trusts were introduced in the mid 1990s. These posts were also subject to wide variation but usually had a professional leadership function.

The accountability of practice nurses was, and largely remains, directly to their GP employers, in some cases through practice managers. Some support, and in some situations, professional leadership has been provided by nurses based in health authorities. Where this currently exists, this will change as PCTs, LHGs and SPCTs assume greater control.

Different approaches to the management and accountability between community trust employed nurses and general practice employed nurses, resulted in different types of work being undertaken. In addition, different training and development opportunities were available to practice nurses (Hibble 1995, Jewell & Turton 1994). Bringing community employed and general practice employed nurses together to provide more integrated nursing care is now regarded as an extremely high priority (Adams & Thomas 2001, Wilkin et al 2001). (See Chapter 17 for further discussion of practice nursing.)

The role of nurses on the Boards of Primary Care Groups and Trusts is innovative. They must be filled by practising community and primary care nurses. Effectively, this change has produced a potential cadre of new community nurse leaders from practising clinical nurses, rather than the more hierarchical approaches to nurse manager appointments in the past. In many parts of the country traditional management lines continue alongside the nurse board members, while others have progressed to integrated management structures and fully integrated nursing teams (Headland et al 2000).

In addition to differences in management and accountability structures between Trusts and Boards, there are also differences nationally between the most senior roles of nurses. In PCTs for example, some have appointed Nursing Directors, with widely varying portfolios, including professional leadership. Other PCTs have not gone down this route and in some situations clinical accountability arrangements remain unclear. (See Chapter 4 for further discussion on quality improvement and practice.)

NURSING LEADERSHIP

There is much written about the importance of clinical leadership in nursing, and as the largest occupational group in the NHS, this is understandable. Sarah Mullally, the Chief Nursing Officer for England, suggests that while good leadership is central to the delivery of the NHS Plan, strong nursing leadership is crucial (Mullally 2001).

In practical terms, why is nursing leadership so important to the modernization agenda? There are several reasons why effective leaders are crucial; these include the impact of high workload pressures, issues relating to recruitment and retention, new primary care structures, and nursing care quality.

WORKLOAD PRESSURES

Nurses in the community are experiencing increased workload pressures including the impact of an ageing population, quicker hospital discharges, increased palliative care at home, community care and packages of care for vulnerable children and adults, and more demands of training and clinical governance (Ross 1999). In an increasingly hectic work environment, it is easy to fall into the trap of responding to the urgent while giving the important a lower priority. Reacting to day-to-day responsibilities leaves little time to think and plan, and without an overall plan, service development becomes difficult, if not impossible to achieve.

According to Walsh (2000), nurses do not have spare time on duty. If roles and tasks are to be incorporated into nurses' everyday work, something has to go. Some aspects of practice will need to be set aside to make room for new work. Evidence-based decisions regarding which work to select, or diminish, are a critical aspect of the leadership role, and one which has not been particularly well undertaken in the past. Evidence from patients, from epidemiological sources and from priorities included in Health Improvement Plans and National Service Frameworks, should be informing the direction that nursing takes in the future. This in turn will inform the type of training and the kind and number of staff that are required to deliver quality care. No amount of workforce reorganization initiatives will be effective without a vision of what nursing should be achieving in the light of patient and population-based evidence. The development of a vision with a clear strategy and the goals towards achieving this, is a central element of a leader's role.

RECRUITMENT AND RETENTION

Delivering the best possible patient care, while modernizing that care, requires sufficient nurses, in the right numbers, of appropriate skill and calibre. The recruitment and retention of nurses is now an issue of national concern and nursing in the community, once insulated from the worse effects of staff shortages, is in many areas feeling the impact of shortages of registered nurses. Most Trusts in the United Kingdom, as internationally, report shortages in qualified staff (Buchan & Edwards 2000), especially in areas of greatest deprivation and in high housing cost areas. Research has demonstrated that effective nursing leadership diminishes burnout, which is in turn related to retention among nurses. New staff are likely to be more easily recruited to an area where the nursing leadership is dynamic and where the leader has good interpersonal skills. In addition, effective leadership is likely to lead to improved retention (Stordeur et al 2000).

NEW PRIMARY CARE MANAGEMENT/ACCOUNTABILITY STRUCTURES

For many community nurses, previous lines of management will change in the near future and new accountability structures will be introduced as a result of PCTs, LHGs and SPCTs. There is evidence that, whatever the structure, when effective leadership is observed at the top levels of an organization, it is also found at lower levels, because of modelling and a cascading effect (Bass et al 1987). This suggests that an essential role of nurse board members and others in establishing Trusts, is that they create the cultural norms which will enable the development of open and facilitative ways of working, and the modelling of effective leadership styles.

NURSING CARE QUALITY

There are many publications which point to the correlation between the quality of patient care, staff morale and effective nursing leadership (Antrobus & Kitson 1999, Cunningham & Whitby 1997, Kitson et al 1996, Manley 1997, Stordeur et al 2000). Effective nursing leadership provides a clear direction for patient care (Allen 2000). Leaders work with others to ensure standards are maintained and quality of care enhanced, and support staff to achieve that level of care consistently (Alimo-Metcalfe 1996).

LEADERSHIP VS MANAGEMENT

There has been much written about the virtues of leadership over management in the past ten years, particularly from US sources. Kotter (1990) for example, proposed that although there are differences between management and leadership, they are not separate roles, but parts of the same continuum. He suggested that management is concerned with maintaining a degree of predictability and order, while leadership is about producing change and transformation. In consequence because management tends to be based on an exchange or a transaction (you do this for me and I will reward you), management, which focuses on the day-to-day operations, is also closely akin to a form of leadership known as transactional leadership (Manfredi 1994).

Bass (1985) derived his theory of transformational leadership from earlier work (Burns 1978). A central tenet of Bass's (1985) theory is that transformational leaders develop, intellectually stimulate and inspire followers to transcend their own self interests for a higher collective purpose. Bass suggests that transformational leaders have charisma, and an ability to demonstrate concern for individuals. Furthermore, he proposed that transformational leaders concentrate their efforts on long-term goals and vision, and inspire their followers to do likewise.

Transformational leadership is seen to facilitate individuals performing beyond expected levels of performance, as a result of the leader's influence (Bradford & Cohen 1998). Howell and Avolio (1993) investigated the effects of transactional and transformational leadership styles among 78 managers. Results of this study indicated that a more positive contribution to unit performance came from behaviours associated with transformational leaders. Because it is considered to be the approach most liable to result in change and be effective in changing environments, a transformational style is widely regarded as the most appropriate approach for a leader to adopt during modernization processes (Lindholm et al 2000). According to Goleman (1998), for effective organizational change, traditional management is not enough; a charismatic transformational leader is called for (p. 196).

There are many examples in a wide range of publications that describe the characteristics of transformational leaders. Bass suggests that 'Transformational leaders motivate others to do more, more than they thought possible' (Bass 1998).

The transformational leader is described as collaborative, consultative, consensus seeking, and with advanced interpersonal skills (Markham 1998). These advanced interpersonal skills are not tools to manipulate but are a sign of an individual's interest and concern for their colleagues.

Advanced interpersonal or social skills have also been termed 'emotional intelligence', and these are suggested as an essential component of transformational leadership skills.

Emotional intelligence (Goleman 1998), is reported to have five components:

♦ Self-awareness – the ability to recognize and understand your moods, and the effects these have on others. This he suggests is closely related to self-confidence.

♦ Self-regulation – the ability to control your own disruptive moods and impulses, and to think before acting – a hallmark of which is openness to change.

♦ Motivation – a passion for work that is not related to monetary gain and a capacity to pursue goals persistently. Optimism, and a strong organizational commitment, Goleman suggests, demonstrates this.

♦ Empathy – the ability to see things from other people's point of view, which results in building and retaining staff trust and subsequently talent.

♦ Social skill – the ability to build relationships and rapport, of which the hallmarks are expertise in building teams, persuasiveness and effectiveness in leading change.

According to Goleman (1998), these components can be learned, and will therefore be possible to explore in an interview situation. And in order for training opportunities to be effective in achieving the development of these skills, organizations must refocus their training programmes to include an individualized, personal development plan which involves the exploration of perceptions and feelings. Furthermore Goleman (2000) advocates that seminars alone will not help because they usually only involve cognition and not the engagement of perception or emotion.

Emotional intelligence is not only important for leaders but for all community nurses. In fact, the five components of emotional intelligence, are also fundamental aspects of the best clinical nursing practice. Goleman (1998) suggests that emotional intelligence is the new yardstick by which people will not only be judged by their training and expertise but how well people

handle themselves and each other. He furthermore proposed that low emotional intelligence in leaders lowers everyone's performance. He suggests that it causes a waste of time, creates acrimony, corrodes motivation and commitment, and builds hostility and apathy.

WHAT DO EFFECTIVE LEADERS DO?

Leaders must pull their organizations into the future by creating a positive view of what the organization can become, and simultaneously provide emotional support for individuals during the transition process (Tichy & Devana 1990). The mental health report, *Finding and Keeping* (Sainsbury Centre for Mental Health 2001), identifies the following as key aspects of an effective clinical leadership role:

♦ Creating a shared vision among team members and the provision of direction.
♦ Decision-making, accountability and taking responsibility in a rapidly changing environment.
♦ Managing change effectively.
♦ Articulating the achievable goals of the team.
♦ Motivating and mobilizing staff energies towards achieving long-term goals.
♦ Attracting, retaining and developing good-quality staff.
♦ Dealing effectively with external and internal challenges to provide effective team functioning.
♦ Providing incentives to improve performance.

Dunham and Klafehn (1990) undertook a study of those nurse leaders identified by their subordinates as 'excellent'. This study demonstrated that excellent nurse leaders had transformational skills and qualities. These skills include the ability to think 'outside of the box' and find solutions to problems that may not have been considered previously. This applies particularly during periods of change (O'Keeffee 1998).

The ability to work in a transformational way within an organization is matched by the importance of working in effective coalition with external agencies. Effective leadership is regarded as central to this (Mizrahi & Rosenthal 2001).

Leadership is crucial to effective coalitions because it addresses three critical issues simultaneously: sustaining movement towards external and mutual goals, maintaining internal relations with colleagues to keep them on board, and developing trust and accountability from, and between, coalition members (Rosenthal & Mizrahi 1994).

The capacity to handle both internal and external complex issues requires sustained commitment and skill, together with knowledge of, and adept use of, change management strategies (Trofino 1995). Central to this is the ability to plan, and plan towards a clearly defined vision and its goals. Community nursing management has, in the past, tended to be internally focused and concerned with the day-to-day issues associated with running services. In many respects, planned nursing services based on population, or practice health needs, and the reactive model of community nursing provision, remains highly prevalent. Responding to individual patient and client care needs, will continue to remain a priority for nurses, but in addition the provision of new and more patient/carer focused innovative services, is a requirement of the modernization process. This demands information upon which to base and develop strategies and plans for patient care and public health, based on needs assessment and patient/population generated information (Robinson & Elkan 1996). Delivering strategic aims in times of significant change requires effective leadership. (See Chapter 24 for a discussion of innovative ways of working.)

DEVELOPING EFFECTIVE COMMUNITY NURSE LEADERS

As a consequence of its investment in staff resources, the Government has signalled its belief that training in leadership skills can have a positive effect on leadership behaviour. Initially training for 'f' and 'g' grade nurses was offered; this has now been extended to other grades of nursing staff and clinical groups. The government-funded programmes, provided by the Royal College of Nursing Clinical Leadership Programme, and the Leading Empowered Organizations (LEO) initiative led by Leeds University in England, are the subject of on-going national evaluation. However, there are reports of positive impacts upon staff as a result of leadership training programmes (Antrobus & Kitson 1999, Krejci & Malin 1997, Williamson et al 2001). In addition, the newly created NHS Leadership Centre has already commenced work with senior managers and Trust directors. However, these approaches aimed primarily at first-line leadership and senior managers may leave out, at least in the initial stages, the nursing staff that have leadership roles in PCTs, LHGs and SPCTs. While many NHS Trusts have instigated training programmes for the current H and I grades, this is not universal.

As mentioned earlier, transformational skills can be learned (Goleman 1998) and this is also true of other attributes that will increase the effectiveness of leaders. Developing assertiveness and negotiation skills for example, will also assist community nurse leaders during periods of change. However, interpersonal skills alone do not make an effective leader who must also demonstrate diverse intellectual ability. In our complex healthcare environment, competence in budgetary management, a working knowledge of statistics to understand epidemiological concepts, an ability to work strategically and use information sources efficiently are also important. In the future, in order to develop a cohort of new leaders, there is a view that leadership preparation should be introduced during initial nurse registration training (Cook 2001). (See also Chapter 4.)

In addition to training and personal development, the role of mentorship is considered to be crucial to the continued development of leaders (Dunham-Taylor 2000). A mentor is usually a senior individual who assists a junior in knowing proper protocols, often those that are cultural and unwritten. They will coach and model appropriate behaviour and will inform the junior about important people, in terms of decision-making. Furthermore, the mentor gives the protégé more visibility by exposing their work to higher-level influential individuals. In a study of female managers, it was found for example, that those who had mentors advanced more rapidly than those without. It is also suggested that having a mentor may be more important for women than for men (Brooks & Brooks 1997).

The style that mentorship takes is extremely important for its success. Models of clinical supervision are considered essential to the development of an individual nurse's competence and skills, and therefore patient care. It may therefore be appropriate that similar reflective approaches are taken, in the provision of mentorship.

There is an untapped wealth of creativity and knowledge in staff who deliver individual patient care. To release it and help it to flourish requires effective leadership and encouragement to help people provide the best possible patient care. Just as leaders require mentorship, so also do other levels of staff. In this respect, leaders should mentor their own protégés and help them develop in the ways that they themselves have received help to develop in the past.

BARRIERS TO LEADERSHIP IN COMMUNITY NURSING

The NHS will be characterized by the modernization agenda for some time to come. Delivering this agenda requires leaders in nursing with the ability to influence change, provide a sense of direction and empower others (Cook 2000). However, there may be some barriers to the development of leadership in community nursing, such as culture, career structures and accountabilities, recruitment and retention, workloads, and training.

Mullally (2001) advocates the importance of culture when considering innovation and change in the NHS. Antrobus and Kitson (1999) for example, demonstrated the significance of culture as it influences the leadership ability of nurses. However, it is not just the effect that culture has on effective leadership, but also the culture of nursing itself which may act as a barrier to effective leadership. Antrobus and Kitson (1999), in their research report, suggest that the impact of nursing leadership is restricted by its internal focus, which impacts on its ability to be truly effective.

Nurses are on the whole considered to function with relatively little power in health care (Ford & Walsh 1994, Salvage 1989). They may feel that they are particularly unable to influence the forces shaping their work, since they are employed by organizations strongly dominated by medicine (Kavi & Michels 1991). In their research, Wilkin and colleagues (2001) demonstrated that although nurses in primary care were likely to have been consulted about clinical governance, health improvement and primary care development, they were consulted less than GPs and less likely to have an impact on decision makers. It seems that this research suggests that patterns of nursing's relative powerlessness may be perpetuated in the new primary care world, unless the potential risks and their consequences are recognized and appropriate remedial actions taken.

The changes produced by the nurse grading initiative produced a relatively flat management structure, which meant that for many community trust employed nurses, a 'g' or 'h' grade was the highest clinical post available to them. The most senior roles in nursing were usually nonclinical management posts. For most practice nurses, this career ceiling stayed commonly at 'g' grade. The choice of education or management is not one that appeals to all nurses, a large proportion of whom want to maintain patient contact and their clinical expertise.

Nurse members of PCTs, LHGs and SPCTs are required to have a clinical role, the nature of which varies widely around the country. There are also variations regarding the criteria for appointments of Nursing Directors to these boards. In consequence, in some areas, the opportunities for career advancement are far from clear. It may, for example, be very difficult for nurses to obtain sufficient experience at a sufficiently senior level for them to be eligible for Nurse Consultant posts, the vast majority of which remain in hospital nursing and mental health (Kings Fund 2001). Apart from the impact this may have on the opportunities for development open to nurses, there is also an implication for professional accountability. In clinical governance terms, clear lines of professional accountability are crucial; in many PCTs, LHGs and SPCTs this has yet to be achieved.

WORKLOAD

Limited nursing resources may also constitute a barrier to the development of leadership in community nursing. This could operate on two levels; the first relates to staff that are delivering direct patient care. When staffing resources are low, there may be a tendency for nurses to focus on the 'must dos', which can leave little time for planning, a key element of effective leadership at all levels. Leadership needs to occur whenever a nurse is responsible for a team, a project or for patient care and the NHS modernization agenda provides exciting opportunities for nurses to develop and undertake new and innovative leadership roles. In addition, roles such as those outlined in the 'ten key skills', provide nurses with the potential to expand their practice in a number of different ways. Part of this leadership function lies in helping colleagues to develop and manage their work and resources creatively. The second aspect relates to the limited amount of time allocated for 'board' nursing work, which can be as little as three sessions a month. This may curtail leadership potential and limit opportunities for development.

Although the Government is investing substantially in nurse training, recruitment and retention, shortages, particularly in difficult-to-recruit areas such as inner cities, may persist for some time. It may appear that innovation amidst nursing staff shortages will be difficult but the key to developing new ways of working does not lie in simply continuing to do more of what nurses currently do now. Developments must be founded on what is required to provide a modern nursing service. This must be based on a systematic approach to evaluating the benefits of current clinical practice, matched with what should be done to meet patient and population health needs, within the context of modernization. This process also provides the framework for developing a workforce plan, not a plan based around predetermined establishments, but one which more accurately reflects actual requirements for the nursing resource, and one that can be further used to indicate the training and development needs of nursing staff.

In England, Primary Care Trust board nurse members spend a limited amount of time on board work, although this generally exceeds the time allocated for it. There are a number and range of new agendas in which these nurses are required to play an increasingly important and demanding role. New skills are required in a range of topics and the potential for time commitment is formidable. While the specific responsibilities of PCT, LHG and SPCT board nurses vary, most carry a portfolio for the integration of nurses within the organization. Integrating the community and practice workforce is a key task for Primary Care Trusts. In England, Wilkins et al (2001) found that 77% of PCGs planning to become Trusts, mentioned integration of primary and community nurses as one of the most important reasons for wanting to become a Trust. They also found in their survey, that in most areas the nursing workforces are still managed and work separately. Leading integration initiatives is essential in bringing groups of nurses together. Each group with its own history, culture and approaches to clinical practice is a challenge but one which must be met to reduce the continuing issues of overlap and duplication.

Processes for developing a vision and strategy, and managing its delivery, can be learned from conventional training programmes. However, while the processes are relatively straightforward they do require able and creative leaders to be able to see what the future might look like, based clearly around patient care needs. It also demands a capacity to inspire and motivate others to work towards the vision, and the interpersonal skills with which to support them.

Transformational leadership skills will equip most nurses with the potential to overcome the barriers to community nurse leadership. In terms of organizational and professional cultures, transformational leaders will need to work with people to change cultures from within. This is unlikely to occur overnight but in building alliances and positive relationships inside the organization, a solid basis for the future can be formed. In maintaining external coalitions, the political position and influence of nursing can be extended. Because transformational leaders thrive in climates of change, in part because they are not threatened by change, they will be at the forefront of innovation and development. They will want to examine, with their colleagues, whether there are better ways of providing direct patient care, and will enthusiastically support the implementation of new ways of working, that benefit patients and that are logical for the development of nursing.

CONCLUSION

Modernizing the NHS – and community nursing in particular – requires innovative and resourceful leaders who are fully committed to transformational processes. The traditional, hierarchical approaches to management will need to be replaced by a much more facilitative style of leadership, and by nurses who are trained to lead and who will flourish in the new world.

SUMMARY

◆ Leadership in community nursing plays a key role in delivering the modernization and transformed primary objectives of the current Labour Government for the NHS.

◆ Leadership is about producing change and transformation, whereas management is about maintaining order.

◆ Effective leaders in nursing are needed in particular because of the workload pressures, recruitment and retention issues, new primary care structures and nursing care quality.

DISCUSSION POINTS

1. Consider the differences between management and leadership.

2. In what ways might your community nursing service be developed by using leadership skills?

3. What options are open to community nurses in your area for leadership development?

REFERENCES

Adams C, Thomas E 2001 The benefits of integrated nursing teams in primary care. British Journal of Community Nursing 6(6): 271–274

Allen D 2000 The NHS is in need of strong leadership. Nursing Standard 14(25): 25

Alimo-Metcalfe B 1996 Leaders or managers? Nursing Management 3(1): 22–24

Antrobus S 1999 Nursing leadership: influencing and shaping. Journal of Advanced Nursing 29(3): 746–753

Antrobus S, Kitson A 1999 Nursing leadership: influencing and shaping health policy and nursing practice. Journal of Advanced Nursing 29(3): 746–753

Bass BM 1985 Leadership and performance beyond expectations. Free Press, New York

Bass BM 1998 Transformational leadership: Industry, military and educational impact. Lawrence Erlbaum, Mahwah, New Jersey

Bass BM, Waldman DA, Avolio BJ et al 1987 Transformational leadership and the falling dominoes effect. Group and Organisational Studies 12: 73–87

Bradford DL, Cohen AR 1998 Power up: Transforming organisations through shared leadership. John Wiley & Sons, New York

Brooks D, Brooks L 1997 Seven secrets of successful women. McGraw-Hill, New York

Buchan J, Edwards N 2000 Nursing numbers in Britain: the argument for workforce planning. British Medical Journal 320: 1667–1670

Burns JM 1978 Leadership. Harper and Row, New York

Cook MJ 2000 The renaissance of clinical leadership. International Nursing Review 48(13): 38–46

Cook MJ 2001 The attributes of effective clinical nurse leaders. Nursing Standard 15(35): 33–36

Cunningham G, Whitby E 1997 Power redistribution. Health Management September: 14–16

Department of Health 1999 Making a difference – Strengthening the nursing, midwifery and health visiting contribution to health and health care. Department of Health, London

Department of Health 2000 The NHS plan: A plan for investment a plan for reform. The Stationary Office, Norwich

Department of Health 2001 Essence of care: Benchmarking in clinical practice. HMSO, London

Dunham J, Klafehn K 1990 Transformational leadership and the nurse executive. Journal of Nursing Administration 20: 28–33

Dunham-Taylor J 2000 Nurse executive transformational leadership found in participative organisations. Journal of Nursing Adminsitration 30(5): 241–250

Ford P, Walsh M 1994 New rituals for old. Butterworth, Oxford

Goleman D 1998 Working with emotional intelligence. Bloomsbury, London

Goleman D 1998 What makes a leader? Harvard Business Review November–December: 93–102

Goleman D 2000 Leadership that gets results. Harvard Business Review March–April: 78–90

Headland C, Crown N, Pringle M 2000 Integrated nursing in primary care and analysis of nurses' caseloads. British Journal of Nursing 9(11): 708–712

Hibble A 1995 Practice nurse workload before and after the introduction of the 1990 contract for general practitioners. British Journal of General Practice 45: 35–37

Howell JM, Avolio BJ 1993 Transformational leadership, transactional leadership, locus of control, and support for innovation: Key predictors of consolidated business-unit performance. Journal of Applied Psychology 78(6): 891–902

Jewell D, Turton P 1994 What's happening to practice nurses? British Medical Journal 308: 735–736

Kings Fund 2001 An evaluation of nurse consultant roles. Kings Fund, London

Kitson A, Ahmed L, Harvey G et al 1996 From research to practice: an organisational model for prioritising research based practice. Journal of Advanced Nursing 23: 430–440

Kotter J 1990 A force for change: How leadership differs from management. Free Press, Oxford

Krejci JW, Malin S 1997 Impact of leadership development on competencies. Nursing Economics 15(5): 235–241

Lindholm M, Sivberg B, Uden G 2000 Leadership style among nurse managers in changing organisations. Journal of Nursing Management 8: 327–335

Manfredi CM 1994 Leadership preparation: an examination of master's degree programmes in nursing. Holistic Nursing Practice 9: 48–57

Manley K 1997 A conceptual framework for advanced practice: an action research project operationalising an advanced practitioner consultant nurse role. Journal of Clinical Nursing 6: 179–190

Markham G 1998 Gender in leadership. Nursing Management 3(1): 18–19

Mizrahi T, Rosenthal BB 2001 Complexities of coalition building: Leader's successes, strategies, struggles and solutions. Social Work 46(1): 63–78

Mullally S 2001 Leadership and politics. Nursing Management 8(4): 21–27

National Health Service Executive 1998 A first class service: Quality in the NHS. Department of Health, London

National Health Service Executive 2000a A national framework for coronary heart disease. Department of Health, London

National Health Service Executive 2000b A national framework for mental health. Department of Health, London

National Health Service Executive 2000c The cancer plan. Department of Health, London

National Health Service Executive 2001 A national framework for older people. Department of Health, London

O'Keeffee J 1998 Business beyond the box, p. 2. Nicholas Brealey, London

Robinson J, Elkan R 1996 Health needs assessment. Churchill Livingstone, London

Rosenthal B, Mizrahi T 1994 Strategic partnerships: How to create and maintain interorganisational collaborations and coalitions. Hunter, New York

Ross F 1999 Nursing's response to the primary care led NHS. In: Sims I (ed) Primary health care sciences. Whurr, London

Salvage J 1989 Take me to your leader. Nursing Times 85(25): 34–35

Secretary of State for Health 1997 The new NHS: modern, dependable, Cm 3807. The Stationary Office, London

Stordeur S, Vandenberghe C, D'hoore W 2000 Leadership style across hierarchical levels in nursing departments. Nursing Research 49(1): 37–43

Tichy NM, Devana MA 1990 The transformational leader. John Wiley, Chichester

Trofino J 1995 Transformational leadership in health care. Nursing Management 26(8): 42–47

Walsh M 2000 Nursing frontiers: Accountability and the boundaries of care. Butterworth-Heinemann, Oxford

Wilkin D, Gillam S, Coleman 2001 The national tracker survey of primary care groups and trusts 2000/2001: Modernising the NHS? Kings Fund/University of Manchester, London

Williamson T, Taylor S, Petts S 2001 Assessing leadership development and training. Nursing Times 97(36): 42–43

FURTHER READING

Department of Health 2001 Essence of care: benchmarking in clinical practice. HMSO, London

Goleman D 1998 Working with emotional intelligence. Bloomsbury, London

Kotter J 1990 A force for change: how leadership differs from management. Free Press, Oxford

Tichy NM, Devana MA 1990 The transformational leader. John Wiley, Chichester

Shifting the boundaries of community practice

This section explores the boundaries of practice in seven of the eight areas included in the Community Specialist Framework outlined by the UKCC (1996). It is inclusive of:

◆ practice nursing
◆ district nursing
◆ health visiting / public health nursing
◆ community mental health nursing
◆ community learning disability nursing
◆ community children's nursing
◆ school nursing.

There are several additions to this section, over and above that presented in the first edition of the book. New areas include school nursing, community mental health nursing and community learning disability nursing. It was considered essential to include these important dimensions of community nursing, in an attempt to present a total picture of the provision of nursing care in community and primary care settings.

The first chapter provides an overview of the changing role of the practice nurse, following its interesting evolution, through to present day practice. This is followed by Chapter 18, which focuses on district nursing and how it can rise to the challenge of the recommendations made in the Audit Commission Report: First Assessment (1999).

Chapter 19 discusses health visiting/public health nursing and the opportunities that the political agenda provides, for expanding public health nursing practice to include influencing the broader issues that affect health. Chapter 20 concentrates on community mental health nursing and how policy development has shaped current practice. Chapter 21 on community learning disability nursing discusses the needs of clients with a learning disability, the move to community care and the role of the community learning disability nurse in empowering clients.

Chapter 22 focuses on the community children's nurse, outlines various models of service provision across the United Kingdom and discusses the concept of family nursing. The final chapter describes the history of the school nursing service and highlights opportunities for future development, in the context of a child-centred public health role.

This section is by no means inclusive of all issues influencing community nursing practice. It is meant to provide a 'spring board' for discussion and debate and to promote an understanding of the dimensions of nursing currently practised in community and primary care environments.

17

Practice nursing

L. Carey

INTRODUCTION

Practice nursing has reached an important pinnacle in its development; no longer struggling to identify a clear role for itself, it has emerged as a discipline in its own right, acknowledged as making a significant contribution to the provision of care. The realization that practice nurses are accepted members of the primary healthcare team stands as an exceptional achievement to the individual nurses who have shaped a role to meet the changing needs of care provision. Indeed, practice nurses have grown and adapted in response to the shifting boundaries of primary care provision, from a generalist role to one where the nurse has developed a specialist area of practice. The role evolving from one characterized by directly delegated work, to one recognized as a specialist in both health screening and chronic disease management within general practice.

Yet, practice nursing now faces a new set of challenges, perhaps greater than before, that of meeting the demands for health care within the changing structure of the National Health Service. Indeed, the new agenda for healthcare delivery offers practice nurses one of their greatest opportunities to shape and develop practice. Specifically, the direction of modernization in primary care, as set out in the NHS Plan, requires an accessible and flexible workforce; equipped to meet diverse health needs and address relevant inequalities (DoH 2000). This challenge is set against the backdrop of a health service facing a reducing pool of general practitioners to meet growing demand and changing patient expectations.

Arguably, if healthcare provision is going to meet increasing demand, there is a need to examine creative mechanisms to enable individuals to make the most efficient use of the available services (Pencheon 1998). Practice nursing is fundamental to the success of this policy. Indeed, the initiatives will enable practice nurses to identify their contribution to healthcare provision, and redefine its boundaries of practice. Central to this progression is the characteristic flexibility and the responsive nature of practice nursing that has enabled practitioners to respond to different agendas whilst developing a role which meets the needs of the population (Atkin & Lunt 1996).

In examining the shifting boundaries of practice nursing this chapter will specifically explore how the practice nurse's role has been shaped by both central government, and the changing nature of healthcare provision. It will explore how the potential of the practice nurse can be achieved in meeting the new agenda for health and shifting the boundaries of practice.

HEALTH POLICY AND THE PRACTICE NURSE

Given that within the UK healthcare provision is dependent upon central government funding, it is inevitable that the specific nature of care delivery and indeed the roles of the practitioner are shaped by politicians; and consequently dependent upon the prevailing political ideology. The inevitable politicization of healthcare provision is not a new phenomenon, given that the development of a National Health Service in 1948 was an overt political gesture, aimed primarily at satisfying a national desire for change following the deprivation of the preceding depression and interwar years (Jones & Novak 1999). However, for many practitioners the political agenda is far removed from the day-to-day issues surrounding care delivery. This distance is associated with a continuing representation of nurses as fundamentally altruistic in nature, and, therefore situated outside the political domain. Hence, groups

such as nurses are less likely to be identified with an overtly politicized agenda. This does not imply, simplistically, that nurses are apolitical. Indeed, at times they have demonstrated a strong vein of radicalism (Hart 1985).

However, if practitioners are to effect and shape practice, relevant to the needs of the population, it is necessary to acknowledge that the structure and organization of health is moulded by the political economy of health and the prevailing policy agenda. This is particularly important when considering the development of the practice nurse role, for this group of practitioners owe more to their development to specific healthcare policy, in the form of the 1990 General Practitioner Contract (DoH 1990), than any other group. Indeed, the development of the role undertaken by the nurse in general practice has fundamentally been shaped, not as one would suspect by either the needs of the population or through the impact of nursing as a wider profession, but as a response to the healthcare political agenda. (See Chapter 1 for more detailed discussion of health and social policy development.)

Specifically, the new general practitioner contract (DoH 1990), in offering a clear indication of the political shift away from curative to preventative healthcare delivery was crucial in the development of new nursing roles. Faced with a requirement to increase the services provided within general practice, general practitioners sought the solution in the employment of practice nurses. As such, this piece of legislation offered nursing an important opportunity to develop a new role outside the constraints of traditional nursing management hierarchy. Even though the number of practice nurses grew exponentially at this time a degree of confusion existed, with the range of duties, and the actual role undertaken varying greatly (Atkin et al 1993). Atkin and colleagues (1993), in a national census of practice nursing identified their role as ranging from chronic disease management and health promotion through to practical tasks, such as venepuncture. Similarly, a survey of practice nurses in South West Thames region concluded that the role of the practice nurse remained ill defined, with at times inadequate preparation for the role undertaken

(Ross et al 1994). Subsequent studies, such as Mackereth's (1995) national survey of nurses working in general practice observed an emphasis on practical tasks rather than expanding practice. It can be argued that this variability of practice is in part due to the domination of individual general practitioners in practice nurse development (Deenhan et al 1998).

Undoubtedly, throughout the early 1990s, the activities undertaken by the practice nurse continued to be shaped by government policy. During this period a culture of individualism prevailed (Jones & Novak 1999). For medicine this led to an emerging challenge to a number of traditional myths, including the notion that the doctor 'knows best', and associated deferential attitudes towards practitioners. This in conjunction with both the advancement in technology, and a widening of the public's access to knowledge changed the nature of the consultation in primary care. In tandem, the increasing demand for health care, and transformation in health policy, has resulted in an increase in the perceived workload of the general practitioner (Kumar & Gantley 1999). For example, Gill et al (1998) in an evaluation of one practice in Oxford suggest demand is increasing exponentially with respect to both the number attending and the number of frequent attendees. In contrast, however, Pedersen and Leese's (1997) literature review fails to identify any substantial evidence of increased workload; though acknowledging that this does not necessarily mean there is no problem. In particular, they argue that increased administrative burden and expectations of patients may be contributory factors to general practitioners' workload perceptions.

Yet the changing demand and expectations of healthcare provision have necessitated a refocusing of government health policy. The ideology of New Labour's health policy is clearly represented in the NHS Plan (DoH 2000). In particular, this legislation offers an opportunity to both redefine roles in practice, and reconfigure healthcare delivery based upon multidisciplinary working, though at a cost to the traditional roles undertaken within general practice. In recognizing the increasing demands upon primary care, delegation is perceived as a potential solution.

The move towards delegation is, however, not a new proposal. As early as 1994 Handysides argued that general practitioners would benefit from greater delegation, thereby enabling the practitioner to move towards the role of the general physician within the community. This alteration is a key factor in changing the nature of healthcare delivery, and impacting upon the role of the practice nurse leading to a situation where the remit of the nurse has expanded to incorporate roles previously undertaken by the doctor.

Delegation and relinquishment of traditional roles is crucial to the provision of primary care. Though such developments are as yet to be fully realized, Jeffreys and colleagues (1995) identify the potential for complementary additions to and devolution from nurses' roles. Within their analysis of two general practices, they highlight the potential for practice nurses to take on roles previously undertaken by the general practitioner, with the delegation of some of their existing duties delegated to support staff. The delegation of a limited number of duties currently undertaken by practice nurses to support staff is also described within Brown's (1995) descriptive study of the impact of such support workers. Though not methodologically robust this evaluation recognized the benefit to practice nurses of delegation of duties such as administration, venepuncture and specific health promotion activities. This reinforces the view that practice nurses are still undertaking roles that primarily support the general practitioner rather than achieving nursing's own potential. Indeed, the delegation of nursing tasks may enable nurses to undertake more appropriate roles, though it is questionable whether practice nurses are currently in a position to determine what these new roles are. (See Chapter 24 for further discussion on emerging roles and new ways of working in nursing practice.)

SHIFTING THE BALANCE OF POWER

If practice nurses are to shift the boundaries of practice then there is a clear need to grasp the opportunities placed before them. Specifically, the drive towards a multidisciplinary approach to healthcare delivery provides a key moment in time for practice nurses to move away from a model of care dominated by the general practitioner. The support for a responsive healthcare workforce, including the practice nurse, is laid out within the government document *Shifting the Balance of Power* (STBP) (DoH 2001). In calling for a shift in the balance of power towards both front-line staff and the local communities, away from the traditional centralized approach to management, this document recognizes a significant change in the culture of the NHS; one based upon meeting the needs of the local population. Within the primary care context this necessitates both an increase in the power and responsibilities of the Primary Care Trusts, and the staff working with these organisations. Even though general practitioners currently still directly employ many practice nurses, the changes set out within this document have the potential to impact upon their ability to deliver care.

A central theme here is the concept of empowerment, this both in terms of changing a culture that enables the patient to influence and take control over their own health needs, and in placing power with practitioners who are responsible for care delivery (DoH 2001). Yet, for this policy to be realized in practice, practitioners must be empowered to change the culture and work within a new framework. STBP characterizes empowerment as ensuring that practitioners are able to develop and fully utilize their skills (DoH 2001). This statement is particularly pertinent for practice nurses given that the potential to shape and deliver practice at present, is ultimately controlled by the general practitioner. This is not to undermine the innovations of individual practitioners in developing practice, but recognizes both the positive and negative influences upon the role by the employing general practitioner. Yet if practice nurses, as a group, are to shift the boundaries of their practice then they must consider the concept of empowerment and its relationship to their practice. It is the realization of practice nurses' potential that will enable them as a group to articulate their specific contribution to

improving the population's health, within a nursing context. (See Chapter 7 for further discussion on the community as a framework for health promotion.)

Empowerment itself is a complex concept, that Kuokkanen and Leino-Kilpi (2000) argue is directly related to the broader issues of power, and knowledge base. Kuokkanen follows Kanter (1979) in suggesting that power should not be examined in terms of coercion and domination, but as a means to goal orientation. In relation to practice nursing this offers a new and wider perspective of the organization within which care is delivered. In particular, Kanter (1979) considers that power is generated by the individual, through the creation of opportunities, effective information and support from the organization. Practice nursing has clearly demonstrated the ability to create opportunities in the care provided to the population; with a number of nurses delivering innovative population-centred care. Though it remains doubtful whether opportunities have been created within the wider organizations impacting upon care provision, most notably the Primary Care Trusts. Equally true are the questions raised in relation to how practice nurses have effectively communicated their role.

The lack of clearly defined boundaries for practice has resulted in a position where both the population as a whole, and other practitioners are uncertain of the role. This uncertainty has resulted in other health and social professionals appearing willing to delegate part of their role to the practice nurse without any real consideration of practice nursing as a coherent discipline. Similarly, with regard to organizational support practice nurses are in a confusing position. Some gain extensive support from general practitioners, though may not be as well supported at Primary Care Trust level. Such differences can be traced to the historical development of practice nursing. Initially separated from other community nurses, they developed within a model similar to that of the general practitioner (Carey & Jones 2000). If practice nurses, therefore, are to claim power in order to shape practice, their effectiveness in promoting their role and gaining support from other professionals in the delivery of primary care needs to be considered. (See Chapter 15 for an analysis of team working in health and social care.)

In an alternative analysis to Kanter, Foulcault (1978) identifies the importance of knowledge in relation to power, and its dissemination in human interaction. The Foucauldian analysis highlights the role of powerful discourses, medicine for example, in form of social control. Importantly, the exercise of this power always has a corollary of resistance to the dominant knowledge. However, reflection upon the historical development of practice nursing has resulted in a situation where there is no specified knowledge base of nurses who work within this clinical environment. This has in part been addressed through the inclusion of practice nursing within the specialist community practitioner education programmes. However, the continuing reality of nurses being employed and utilizing the title 'practice nurse' without a distinct knowledge base arguably raises doubts regarding the power base through which they practice. Effectively their domain is subject to the continuing domination of individual general practitioners in shaping and dictating the boundaries of practice. If practice nurses are to develop and utilize their skills to their full potential there is a need to clearly articulate their role, both in its present form and in recognizing its potential. This potential must be sought both in relation to the needs of the organization, and importantly the needs of the local population. The remainder of this chapter will explore the potential of the practice nurse to meet the newly emerging agenda.

ACHIEVING THE POTENTIAL

EXPANDING THE PRACTICE NURSE'S ROLE

Any exploration of a health service committed to the delivery of cost-effective care, necessitates an exploration of the impact of skill mix. This needs examination in relation to the practice nurses' role, and specifically whether the extension and expansion of the nurses' role is appropriate to delivery of care in the primary care setting.

Focusing on the concept of skill mix in primary healthcare teams, Jenkins-Clarke et al (1998) assert that the best-qualified practitioner possible should deliver care. Through working together, the team will be able to deliver optimally effective care. In examining the potential for skill mix changes within primary care Jenkins-Clarke and colleagues (1998) concluded that at least 17% of general practitioners' current work could be wholly delegated to other members of the primary healthcare team. Within this study of ten general practices, participant observation techniques identified that other members of the team, the nurse in particular, could appropriately manage advice giving, screening, management of skin conditions and prescriptions. They conclude that delegation of a number of the duties presently undertaken by the general practitioner were both acceptable and possible. Though quantifying the minimum proportion of work eligible for delegation Jenkins-Clarke et al (1998) question whether it is possible to compose a 'reality' for all primary healthcare teams; highlighting the different ways within which teams worked together, with smaller practices more likely to have shared objectives. (See Chapter 15 for a more detailed account of team-working in primary care.)

In reflecting on skill mix issues, practice nurses need to be active participants in any discussions of how general practice will effectively meet the challenge of 24-hour access to health care, and 48-hour access to a general practitioner. Indeed, Jenkins-Clarke et al (1998) highlight the specific need for further exploration of how the change in role boundaries is negotiated. Associated concerns include the issue of training for nurses and the question of who should manage the organization of care through triage. This is intriguing given that other studies have assumed that the nurse is the most appropriate practitioner to triage those patients suitable for general practitioner consultations. Indeed, Reveley's (1998) comparative examination of the role of the nurse practitioner and second on-call doctor, in triaging same-day patients within one general practice, reports on the acceptability of the nurse with patients and practitioners. Though a small-scale study, the paper suggests that when the role of the nurse in relation to triage is clearly defined then it is less likely than other nurse roles to threaten cultural boundaries between the doctor and nurse.

Similarly, Yerrell (1998) explored the drivers and requisite development for nurses in undertaking an expanded role in the general practice setting. This case study describes the potential for nurse practitioners to extend their role, enabling them to filter patients to the doctor and other nurses. Though the single-site nature of the evaluation determines that the findings are not generalizable, it does highlight how role development impacts upon the surrounding nursing team. Yerrell (1998) suggests that the development of the role be undertaken as part of a wider strategy aimed at effectively managing clinical time. This he argues will contribute to inclusion, partnership, co-operation and shared values as central components to delivery of person-centred services. Though both Yerrell's and Reveley's studies identify the role of triage as belonging to the nurse practitioner, the current demand for this strategy suggests that it is likely to fall within the boundaries of practice nursing. (See Chapter 24 for new ways of working in primary care.)

One area where the role of the nurse in general practice has expanded is the management of minor illness. Though there are a number of studies exploring this issue, there is little consistency in relation to the preparation of the nurse to undertake this role. Training varies from recognized degree programmes through to an informal period of observing the general practitioner. This suggests that if practice nurses are to formally undertake this role, then concerns surrounding competency and appropriateness to practice will need to be explored in greater depth. Nevertheless, there is clear evidence to suggest that the practice nurse may appropriately expand her sphere of practice to include minor illness management. In particular, Shum et al's (2000) randomized controlled trial conducted in five general practices in south-east London and Kent, examined the impact of a nurse-led minor illness session as an alternative to general practitioner service. This study concluded that even though the majority of patients attending did not indicate a preference for whom they consulted with, there were no identified adverse clinical outcomes as a result of the nurse consultation. The higher satisfaction levels reported by those patients attending the nurse reinforce the acceptability of the nurse as an alternative to the general practitioner consultation. However, on a cautionary note, the authors suggest that this may be due to a different style of consultation utilized by the nurse.

The suggestion that the nurse is as effective as the doctor in the management of minor illness is supported by Venning and colleagues (2000). This multicentre randomized control trial confirms that nurse practitioners were as effective as general practitioners both in terms of cost, prescribing and impact on health status. Even though the nurse had longer consultation times and was more likely to carry out tests, and call patients back, the cost of care delivered by the nurse practitioner was comparable with the general practitioner. Similar to the findings of Shum et al (2000) higher satisfaction levels were recorded for those patients attending the nurse practitioner. Venning et al (2000) suggest that if the consultant time of nurses or the returns reduced, without a loss of satisfaction, then they will become a realistic alternative to general practitioners for patients requesting a same-day consultation. In Kinnersley and colleagues' (2000) randomized controlled trial of nurse practitioners versus GPs for patients requesting same-day consultations the length of the consultation period was identified as a potential contributor to patient satisfaction. Though reporting similar findings to the Shum (2000) and Venning (2000) studies, this small-scale randomized control trail of ten general practices in south Wales and south-west England concluded that variation in patient satisfaction was due to the variation between practitioners' individual approach rather than a professional grouping. Marsh and Dawes' (1995) descriptive single-site study similarly reaffirms the appropriateness of a nurse in the management of same-day consultations. This paper, however, questions whether the introduction of the nurse actually reduces general practitioner consultation, or whether it leads to an increase in the number of patients attending given that there is no longer a waiting time.

Given the acceptance of the role of the nurse in the management of minor illness and same-day consultations, we must turn to the questions raised over preparation of the nurse to fulfil these roles. The importance of this was recognized within the early implementation of the nurse practitioner within Derbyshire (Chambers 1994). Evaluation of this project, covering three general practice sites identified training issues as a factor, recognizing both the increased burden of in-house training and a degree of scepticism concerning whether the taught programmes result in suitable trained practitioners. The development of the nurse to undertake roles previously identified as within the domain of the medical profession is further explored by Brown and Olshansky (1997). Their paper argues that the nurse requires not only formal education, but also a post-training period where the practitioner legitimizes their skills within the clinical setting.

Though a number of the studies have focused upon the nurse practitioner, the transferability of the skills identified is undoubtedly appropriate to the emerging role of the practice nurse. This is particularly so, given a central feature of the practice nurse's role is their adaptability as a resource in realizing health policy objectives (Atkin & Lunt 1996). Reiterating this point Salisbury and Tettersell (1988) state that flexibility and corresponding accessibility are recognized as significant components of the nurse's role, with participants reporting patients accessing nurses in order to prevent the unnecessary use of services of the general practitioner. Williams et al (1997), in recognizing the move towards nurses being perceived as a substitution for doctors within the primary care sector, argue that the nurse has a culturally different relationship with the patient than the general practitioner. This fact raises the question whether the breakdown of traditional boundaries can lead to a loss of cultural identity, and uncertainty in the perceptions regarding the change in role undertaken, suggesting the need for a clearer legal infrastructure to support role development of nurses. (See Chapter 13 for further discussion on the legal framework for professional practice.)

THE MANAGEMENT OF CHRONIC DISEASE

It would be inappropriate to consider the evolving role of the practice nurse solely in terms of the addition of new responsibilities devolved from other practitioners. Instead it must include the development of areas of practice already identified as significant to the nurse's role. In particular, practice nursing is now in a position to claim the management of the individual with chronic disease as a core component of their work. Within the context of care delivery the role of the nurse in the management of chronic disease enables the nurse to offer a different service to that of the general practitioner. Specifically, the role of the nurse centres upon encouraging the individual to consider the impact of lifestyle and behaviour on the disease process. The role of the nurse being to act both as a support and educator in enabling the individual to manage the disease process for themselves. Central to this process is a philosophy of caring, requiring the practice nurse to challenge the medical model as a foundation for practice, and instead draw upon distinct health promotion models and frameworks to underpin practice. (See Chapter 27 for further discussion on health promotion.)

The recognition of the nurse's role in the management of chronic disease is exemplified in the implementation of the National Service Framework (NSF) for Coronary Heart Disease (DoH 2000). This and other National Service Frameworks will significantly impact upon the boundaries of practice nurses' care provision. Importantly, the targeting of health care is inextricably bound up with the issue of clinical effectiveness. In this regard, the prevailing health policy aims to place clinical effectiveness on a par with securing cost effectiveness. Given that the task of meeting the NSF for coronary heart disease has predominantly fallen to the practice nurse, nurses must rise to the challenge of identifying the effectiveness of the care they deliver. This will require nurses to consider the care delivered in relation to distinct measurable outcomes. This Spilsburgy and Meyer (2001) argue is difficult given that nursing, as a humanistic discipline, cannot in simple terms measure the impact of the human relationship. (See Chapter 4 for further information on quality improvement.)

Nevertheless, central government requires outcomes for healthcare practices. Indeed, in relation to the management of coronary heart disease the specific role of the nurse and subsequent effectiveness has been challenged (Muir et al 1994). Specifically, Langham and colleagues (1996) in analysing the cost effectiveness of the coronary heart disease prevention, question whether the cost of nurse intervention was effective in relation to improved quality of life. In particular, given that the relative cost of the nurse intervention is high they argue that it is important to identify the impact in terms of other health outcomes. (See Chapter 26 for further discussion on achieving 'value for money' in healthcare provision.)

The cost of ensuring the effective use of nursing care is important given the relative expense of the practice nurse to the health service; though it is important to state that the majority of this cost is not borne by the general practitioner. To date much of the research concerning the role of the nurse has focused upon tasks undertaken with little focus on how effective it is. In this context the delivery of proven effective interventions is fundamental to healthcare delivery, yet as Kitson and colleagues (1996) state, the drive towards evidence-based practice is not always apparent in the care delivered. Nevertheless, the subsequent rise of the clinical governance agenda and increasing emphasis on effectiveness related to both the practice nurse role and interventions will be a central influence upon the practice nurse's role as it continues to evolve. (See Chapter 4 for further discussion on clinical governance.)

TAKING ON THE CHALLENGE OF MENTAL HEALTH

The refocusing of care based upon the needs of the local population is pivotal to both central government, and the development of practice nursing. This re-emphasis has brought previously neglected health issues to the forefront of practice. This shift in culture, enabling mental health to be placed upon the agenda of all healthcare

practitioners, including the practice nurse, requires nurses to expand their practice. It is estimated that mental health problems contribute to 20% of all consultations within the general practice setting (Gray et al 1999). This high incidence has led to a number of studies to examine the impact of practitioners in meeting the needs of this client group.

Gray and colleagues' (1999) survey of practice nurses examined the current role of the nurse in this arena. This survey concludes that whilst practice nurses indicated regular contact with patients, they reported having had little mental health training, and as such may be failing to recognize mental illness. Despite the perceived lack of knowledge their role included administration of antipsychotic medication and management and detection of depression (Gray et al 1999). The resultant need for education of practitioners within primary care is supported by Warner and Ford's (1998) examination of mental health facilitators in primary care. Though a small-scale survey of mental health facilitators' perceptions of their role, it highlights the need for education to link primary care and specialist mental health workers. This may be particularly relevant to practice nurses whose experience of mental health issues is likely to be limited, though there are a number of examples of good practice, where nurses have developed collaborative links with mental health workers. (See Chapter 20 for further discussion on mental health nursing.)

Developing an awareness of mental health issues, is however, important for practice nurses on another level. In particular, given that the sphere of practice centres upon supporting the individual with chronic health needs, nurses should also consider the psychological impact of the disease process upon the individual. McKeown (2000) argues that physical health problems will always have an emotional impact upon the individual and as such impact upon how they are able to live their lives. As such the recognition of mental health considerations is central to the nurse in the move towards a holistic philosophy of care delivery and away from the medical model. (See Chapter 9 for a psychological perspective.)

WORKING WITH THE POPULATION

Contemporary healthcare policy recognizes the necessity of addressing health inequality, and, in particular, the contribution of primary care in meeting this agenda (DoH 1997). However, the reduction in health inequalities can only be achieved if the link between socioeconomic factors is truly integrated into healthcare provision (Smeeth & Heath 1999). The awareness of wider social inequality upon health, though acknowledged, is not easily addressed under a medical model of care provision, which emphasizes an individualistic approach to health. Therefore, if practice nurses are to meet government-set health targets, then there is a need to work in a different framework; one that specifically addresses a public health approach to care provision. (See Chapter 6 for a more detailed discussion on poverty and health.)

Central to the move towards a public health focused primary care service are the identification of local health needs for the population, the development of locally accepted plans and strategies related to health and the building of community self-sufficiency (Chalmers & Bramadat 1996). In the UK, this role has traditionally fallen within the remit of the health visitor, and more latterly, all community specialist practitioner nurses. Yet, as Pearson et al (2000) highlight, it is not necessarily evident in routine practice. As practitioners working within the community, practice nurses have a responsibility to deliver health care that is responsive to local population health needs. This requires practice nurses to not only acknowledge, but also recognize, the impact of socioeconomic factors upon individual health. This realization necessitates that practice nurses identify their potential in working with the community to affect change.

This is not to state that practice nurses should be solely responsible for public health, rather that practitioners must utilize their skills appropriately. Indeed, Mason et al (1999) argue that community health development workers rather than existing health professionals are best placed to support the public health agenda in primary care. This ethnographic study of two small rural communities in Northern Ireland suggests health professionals work at present as disparate groups, each with a distinct aim and client group and therefore do not address the whole community's needs. This challenges all practitioners, including practice nurses to consider how care delivery is organized and co-ordinated to meet patient needs.

MANAGING THE POTENTIAL

IMPROVING TEAM-WORKING

Pivotal in the drive towards both a primary care led NHS, and the realization of the potential of the practice nurse is the need for collaborative working. Zwarenstein and Bryant (2000) define this as 'to work jointly'. Effectively this involves the sharing of responsibility for the care of a patient, sharing of information, co-ordination of work, and joint decision-making on aspects of patient care. This definition of collaborative working is particularly relevant to team-working within primary care, where care is never delivered totally by one individual. Indeed, Hall and McHugh (1995) highlight that without effective team-working it is not possible to achieve enhanced patient outcomes. Though, for practice nurses, collaborative working must be considered both in relation to working within a multidisciplinary team and in relation to its impact on increasingly integrated nursing.

A central principle for team-working within the primary care setting is the need for joint decision-making. However, Richards and colleagues' (2000) literature review suggests that there is only limited evidence of this process existing in practice. West and Poulton (1997) explored the extent of team-working within primary healthcare teams within the UK. These teams compared unfavourably to other teams, from both a commercial and health and social background, in relation to team participation, support for innovation and commitment to team objectives, only scoring higher on task orientation. They conclude that the failure to develop clear and shared objectives is a major problem for primary healthcare teams (Poulton & West 1999). A corollary of this was a need for team objectives based upon primary health care and not a general medical practice focus. Poulton and West (1999) also argue that all team members should be employed by and responsible to one primary healthcare organization, thereby enabling the organization to provide the support and resources to permit the team to function effectively.

The findings of West and Poulton's (1997) study are further reiterated within Williams and Laungani's (1999) study of 30 teams within one inner city NHS Trust. The findings suggest that attention should be paid to removing the barriers to team-working in primary health care. Elston and Holloway (2001) explored the impact of primary care reforms, and specifically primary care groups on interprofessional working in primary care centres. They identified the different philosophical and educational background and identities of team members, and an inherent power imbalance as a key challenge. This was particularly important where general practitioners employ other members of staff. The authors stress that the general practitioners did not want to exercise more power, but expressed a fear of losing their existing power to others. Similarly, they highlight the strong professional identity within groups as a continuing barrier to team-working, suggesting that this may only be negated through interprofessional education. Nevertheless, Long (1996) in an evaluation of a team-working initiative within one primary health team, highlights the value of collaboration in raising awareness of practitioners' roles. This very limited, nongeneralizable study offers insight into the difficulties in communication and interpersonal relationships that existed within the team. Long (1996) argues that unless these issues are addressed they will act as significant barriers to effective primary healthcare team working. Similarly, Bennett-Esslie and McIntosh (1995) in a small-scale study of health professionals suggest that the frequency of multidisciplinary meetings is the most important factor in promoting collaboration within the team.

It is questionable, however, whether the traditional structure of general practice allows for creative working relationships. In reality, the direct employment of the practice nurse by the general practitioner has been viewed as both an opportunity for nurses to move away from the hierarchy of

nurse management, or an iniquitous trap, subject to the exercise of medical power (Carey & Jones 2000). In particular, the employment of nurses by different organizations, namely general practitioners and Trusts, creates a potential barrier to the sharing of practice between nurses. Yet, the sharing of ideas is central to the development of integrated nursing teams. Practice nurses must consider the organization of nursing within these new structures, given that they offer a potential means of reducing the overlap between existing community health nurses' roles and enhancing care delivery. However, little robust evidence exists in relation to the effectiveness of such an approach to care delivery. Though most studies have reported a positive outcome in terms of job satisfaction there is little evidence in relation to clinical outcomes (Black & Hagel 1996, Carnwell & MacFarlane 1999, Headland et al 2000). This is particularly relevant where the concept of the integrated nursing teams is imposed upon the nurses rather than developed as a positive choice. This imposition may prohibit the identification of a shared philosophy of practice, and therefore inhibit change (Goodman 2000). Indeed Galvin et al (1999) suggest that without positive choice teams are likely to experience further problems of communication.

In supporting the development of a sharing of ideas, and a common philosophy for care provision, a central feature to emerge from a number of studies relating to the development of the integrated nursing team is the completion of health needs assessment, this forming an important unifying element of the process of team-working (Black & Hagel 1996, Carnwell & MacFarlane 1999, Headland et al 2000). The examination of health needs for the population enables the team to explore who was best placed to deliver care. This wider approach importantly enables the concept of the team to be broadened to incorporate both individuals and the population as a whole. (See Chapter 15 for a more detailed analysis of team working in primary care.)

CONCLUSION

Practice nursing has at last reached a stage in its development were nurses are recognized as valuable members of the primary healthcare team, from both a patient and professional perspective. This recognition has the potential to enable nurses to examine and explore the power bases that underpin their practice, and in doing so enable them to redefine their scope of practice. However, in exploring the future scope of practice nurses' practice we must be mindful to realize that as part of a wider national health service, the role will be at least in part shaped by central government policy. Yet, if practice nurses are to shape their practice in a meaningful way, it is crucial to deliver care that meets the needs of the local population. This will require nurses to be flexible and responsive in the delivery of health care. Indeed, this will necessitate the acquisition of new sets of skills and tasks that in the short term will address the need for wider access to healthcare provision, address the public health needs of the population and expand practice to incorporate the individual's mental as well as physical health needs. Given that the agenda set out by central government demands the shifting of boundaries of practice, practice nurses now have an opportunity to work in partnership with the population to define these boundaries in the best interests of the profession and the patients.

SUMMARY

◆ The role of the practice nurse has been, and continues to be, shaped by central government and the changing nature of healthcare provision.

◆ The role of the practice nurse has been expanded to include many tasks previously of a solely medical nature.

◆ Roles already identified as belonging to nurses are also being developed and enhanced.

DISCUSSION POINTS

1. How can the practice nurse work as a more effective member of the primary healthcare team?

2. Consider how the practice nurse could identify the broader health needs of the population the practice serves and work towards a public health agenda.

3. Access to primary care services is difficult for marginalized and vulnerable groups in society. Consider how the practice nurse could work as part of a team to improve access to these groups.

REFERENCES

Atkin K, Lunt N, Parker G, Hirst M 1993 Nurses count: A national census of practice nurses. Social Policy Research Unit, The University of York, York

Atkin K, Lunt N 1996 Negotiating the role of the practice nurse in general practice. Journal of Advanced Nursing 24(3): 498–505

Bennett-Emslie G, McIntosh J 1995 Promoting collaboration in the primary care team – the role of the practice meeting. Journal of Interprofessional Care 9(3): 251–256

Black S, Hagel D 1996 Developing an integrated nursing team approach. Health Visitor 69(7): 280–283

Brown J 1995 The handmaiden's tale. Practice Nurse 10(4): 257–260

Brown M, Olshansky EF 1997 From limbo to legitimacy: A theoretical model of transition to the primary care nurse practitioner role. Nursing Research 46(1): 46–51

Carey L, Jones M 2000 Autonomy in practice – Is it a reality? In: Carey L (ed) Practice nursing. Baillière Tindall, London

Carnwell R, MacFarlane L 1999 Integrating a primary care nursing team: one approach. Community Practitioner 72(8): 252–255

Chalmers KI, Bramadat IJ 1996 Community development: theoretical and practical issues for community health nursing in Canada. Journal of Advanced Nursing 24(4): 719–726

Chambers N 1994 Evaluation of the nurse practitioner project. FHSA, Derbyshire

Deenhan A, Templeton L, Taylor C, Drummond C, Strang J 1998 Are practice nurses an unexplored resource in the identification and management of alcohol misuse? Results from a study of practice nurses in England and Wales in 1995. Journal of Advanced Nursing 28(3): 592–597

Department of Health 1990 General medical service council – New GP contract. HMSO, London

Department of Health 1997 The new NHS: Modern, dependable. The Stationery Office, London

Department of Health 2000 National service framework for coronary heart disease. HMSO, London

Department of Health 2000 The NHS plan. The Stationary Office, London

Department of Health 2001 Shifting the balance of power. HMSO, London

Elston S, Holloway I 2001 The impact of recent primary care reforms in the UK on interprofessional working in primary care centres, Journal of Interprofessional Care 15(1): 19–27

Foulcault M 1978 The archaeology of knowledge. Tavistock, London

Galvin K, Andrewes C, Jackson D, Cheesman S, Fudge T, Ferris R, Graham I 1999 Investigating and implementing change within the primary health care nursing team. Journal of Advanced Nursing 30(1): 238–247

Gill D, Dawes M, Sharpe M, Mayou R 1998 GP frequent consulters: their prevalence, natural history, and contribution to rising workload. British Journal of General Practice 48: 1856–1857

Goodman C 2000 Integrated nursing teams: in whose interests? Primary Health Care Research and Development 1: 207–215

Gray R, Parr AM, Plummer S, Sandford T, Ritter S, Mundt-Leach R, Goldberg D, Gournay K 1999 A national survey of practice nurse involvement in mental health interventions. Journal of Advanced Nursing 30(4): 901–906

Hall E, McHigh M 1995 Family practice health care making collaborative practice a reality. N&HC: Perspectives on Community 16(5): 270–275

Handysides S 1994 Enriching careers in general practice: New roles for general practitioners. British Medical Journal 308: 513–516

Hart C 1985 Political funds. Fighting for the fund. Nursing Times 81(35): 18–19

Headland C, Crown N, Pringle M 2000 Specialist nursing. Integrated nursing in primary care and analysis of nurses' caseloads. British Journal of Nursing 9(11): 708–712

Jeffereys LA, Clark AL, Koperski M 1995 Practice nurses' workload and consultation patterns. British Journal of General Practice 45: 415–418

Jenkins-Clarke S, Carr-Hill R, Dixon P 1998 Teams and seams: skill mix in primary care. Journal of Advanced Nursing 28(5): 1120–1126

Jones C, Novak T 1999 Poverty, welfare and the disciplinary state. Routledge, London

Kanter RM 1979 Power failure in management circuits. Harvard Business Review 4: 65–75

Kinnersley P, Anderson E, Parry K, et al 2000 Randomised controlled trail of nurse practitioner versus general practitioner care for patients requesting 'same day' consultations in primary care. British Medical Journal 320: 1043–1048

Kitson A, Ahmed LB, Harvey G, Seers K, Thompson DR 1996 From research to practice: one organisational model for promoting research based practice. Journal of Advanced Nursing 23: 430–440

Kumar S, Gantley M 1999 Tensions between policy makers and general practitioners in implementing new genetics: grounded theory interview study. British Medical Journal 319: 1410–1413

Kuokkanen L, Leino-Kilpi H 2000 Power and empowerment in nursing: three theoretical approaches. Journal of Advanced Nursing 31(1): 235–241

Langham S, Thorogood M, Normand C, Muir J, Jones L, Fowler G 1996 Cost and cost effectiveness of health checks conducted by nurses in primary care: the Oxcheck study. British Medical Journal 312(7041): 1265–1268

Long S 1996 Primary health care team workshop: team members' perspectives. Journal of Advanced Nursing 23(5): 935–941

Mackereth CJ 1995 The practice nurse: roles and perceptions. Journal of Advanced Nursing 21(6): 1110–1116

Marsh GN, Dawes ML 1995 Establishing a minor illness nurse in a busy general practice. British Medical Journal 310: 778–780

Mason C, Orr J, Harrison S, Moore R 1999 Health professionals' perspectives on service delivery in two Northern Ireland communities. Journal of Advanced Nursing 30(4): 827–834

McKeown M 2000 Mental health – does the practice nurse have a role? In: Carey L (ed) Practice nursing. Baillière Tindall, London

Muir J, Mant D, Jones L, Yudkin P 1994 Effectiveness of health checks conducted by nurses in primary care: results of the OXCHECK study after one year. British Medical Journal 308: 308–312

Pearson P, Mead P, Graney A, McRae G, Reed J, Johnson K 2000 Evaluation of the developing specialist practitioner role in the context of public health. English National Board

Pederson LL, Leese B 1997 What will a primary care led NHS mean for GP workload? The problem of the lack of an evidence base. British Medical Journal 314: 1337

Pencheon D 1998 Matching demand and supply fairly and effectively. British Medical Journal 316: 1665–1667

Poulton BC, West MA 1999 The determinants of effectiveness in primary health care teams. Journal of Interprofessional Care 13(1): 7–18

Reveley S 1998 The role of the triage nurse practitioner in general practice: an analysis of the role. Journal of Advanced Nursing 28(3): 584–591

Richards A, Carley J, Jenkins-Clarke S, Richards DA 2000 Skill mix between nurses and doctors working in primary care – delegation or allocation: a review of the literature. International Journal of Nursing Studies 37: 185–197

Ross FM, Bower PJ, Sibbald BS 1994 Practice nurses: characteristics, workload and training needs. British Journal of General Practice 44: 15–18

Salisbury CJ, Tettersell MJ 1988 Comparison of the work of a nurse practitioner with that of a general practitioner. Journal of the Royal College of General Practitioners 38: 314–316

Shum C, Humphreys A, Wheeler D, Cochrane M, Skoda S, Clement S 2000 Nurse management of patients with minor illnesses in general practice: multicentre, randomised controlled trail. British Medical Journal 320: 1038–1043

Smeeth L, Heath I 1999 Tackling health inequalities. British Medical Journal 318: 1020–1021

Spilsburgy K, Meyer J 2001 Defining the nursing contribution to patient outcome: lessons from a review of the literature examining nursing outcomes, skill mix and changing roles. Journal of Clinical Nursing 10(1): 3–14

Venning P, Durie A, Roland M, Roberts C, Leese B 2000 Randomised controlled trial comparing cost effectiveness of general practitioners and nurse practitioners in primary care. British Medical Journal 320: 1048–1053

Warner L, Ford R 1998 Mental health facilitators in primary care. Nursing Standard 13(6): 36–40

West MA, Poulton B 1997 A failure of function: teamwork in primary health care. Journal of Interprofessional Care 11(2): 205–216

Williams G, Laungani P 1999 Analysis of teamwork in an NHS community trust: an empirical study. Journal of Interprofessional Care 13(1): 19–28

Williams A, Robins T, Sibbald B 1997 Cultural differences between medicine and nursing – implications for primary care. National Primary Care Research and Development Centre, University of Manchester, Manchester

Yerrell P 1998 The CliniMed Report – OMNIGePP. The organisation and management of nurses in general practice. Centre for Research in Primary Health Care, Buckinghamshire Chilterns University College

Zwarenstein M, Bryant W 2000 Interventions to promote collaboration between nurses and doctors. Cochrane Systematic Review Vol 4

FURTHER READING

Carey L (ed) 2000 Practice Nursing. Baillière Tindall, London

This is a useful text book for practice nurses and covers the main issues relevant to this professional group.

Jenkins-Clarke S, Carr-Hill R, Dixon P 1998 Teams and seams: skill mix in primary care. Journal of Advanced Nursing 28(5): 1120–1126

This article (and others cited in the reference list) provides insight into skill mix in primary care.

Kinnersley P, Anderson E, Parry K, et al 2000 Randomised controlled trial of nurse practitioner versus general practitioner care for patients requesting 'same day' consultations in primary care. British Medical Journal 320: 1043–1048

This research project outlines the benefits of nurse-led services in primary care.

18

District nursing

W. Warren
C. Alstrom

INTRODUCTION

This chapter sets out to explore the key influences on district nursing practice at the start of the 21st century. The role of the district nurse is expanding and changing to care for patients with complex nursing needs in the community setting and in striving to achieve this, it is essential for district nurses to work as proactive members of the integrated primary healthcare team. This chapter provides an insight into the history and the evolving role of the district nurse, outlines some of the knowledge and skills required to provide effective patient care and discusses managing a nursing team in the changing context of modern health care.

THE EVOLVING ROLE OF THE DISTRICT NURSE

The role of the district nurse is constantly changing and a look back at the history over the last century provides an insight into how fast those changes have occurred (Baly et al 1987). District nursing has evolved from its origins that can be traced back to the mid 19th century. Before formal training and registration was developed for nurses working in the community, standards were variable (Baly et al 1987). During the early 19th century the old Poor Law committees often employed nurses to care for the sick in their own home. Even following the Poor Law amendment in 1834 and the advent of the workhouse this practice continued, as it was often cheaper. During the mid 19th century some charities provided a more well-to-do class of women with some training in nursing to provide care, however this arrangement was not successful as there was no systematic approach to training and care provision.

The work of William Rathbone in establishing the first training school in the 19th century did much to promote recognition of the role and to improve the quality of care (Baly et al 1987). This followed his personal experiences of employing a nurse to care for his terminally ill wife, within the home. His work and the support of senior nurses of the time, including Florence Nightingale, established the foundation of the service that can be seen today. The first trained nurses were educated at Liverpool Infirmary and they began working in the homes of Liverpool in 1863 (Baly et al 1987). In 1887 the Queen Victoria Jubilee Institute for Nurses was established and District Nursing Associations were offered the opportunity to affiliate to the organization providing they could meet the high standards required for the training of nurses (Baly et al 1987). Out of this organization came a new breed of district nurses known as Queens Nurses. These nurses were often superintendents of services and some districts could not afford to employ them. By 1902 the Institute had established examinations and created a community nurse who dealt with a whole range of health and social needs (Baly et al 1987).

In 1919 state registration as a nurse become mandatory and was a prerequisite to undertaking training as a district nurse with the Institute. The Queens Nursing Institute, as it became known, continued to be the training organization until 1968 (Baly et al 1987). Various changes continued to affect the training of district nurses until in 1981 a new training was introduced which was mandatory before a nurse could use the title 'district nurse' (Baly et al 1987).

Since that time the training of district nurses has moved into universities and in 1994 the introduction of the Community Specialist Practitioner Qualification meant that the qualification also gained recognition at first-degree level. Traditionally the key role of the district nurse is as the expert in the care of the sick at home (Baly et al 1987).

This remains predominately true, however the remit has extended to incorporate health promotion and a focus on independence, supporting individuals to reach their personal optimum potential within their health status, and avoiding dependence on both nursing and other services where possible. This concept supports a clear ethic, to respect and maintain the dignity and the individuality of patients and manage care collaboratively in a holistic and proactive way.

The core elements of the district nursing role are to hold the continuing responsibility for the assessment and provision of care to a group of patients within a chosen locality. This involves planning, implementation and evaluation of the care provided, ensuring at all times that research and an evidence base underpins practice (Audit Commission 1999). District nurses also require management and leadership skills to promote effective teamwork within a multidisciplinary setting, across the boundaries of health and social care, facilitating the identification of complementary approaches to meet individual need. (See Chapter 15 for more detailed discussion on multidisciplinary team working.)

The remit of the district nurse has changed significantly in recent years and will continue to evolve in response to changes in the provision of health and social care, such as shorter hospital stays, technological developments and increased life expectancy with its associated morbidity (Audit Commission 1999). The variation in healthcare provision is needs driven and as highlighted in the Audit Commission Report 'First Assessment' (Audit Commission 1999), there is also dependence on local development and delivery of services.

This brief review has shown that the education and training of district nurses has in the past been rather ad hoc. This has however, changed in recent years with district nursing becoming part of the community specialist practice framework recommended by the UKCC (1994). This has resulted in specialist practice outcomes at level 3 (first-degree) and any nurse wishing to work as a qualified district nurse is required to undertake a programme of specialist education to the standard set by the United Kingdom Central Council

(UKCC) and approved by a National Board for Nursing, Midwifery and Health Visiting. On completion of an approved course the NMC enters the qualification against the nurse's name on the NMC register. This move was seen as a positive step and welcomed, but the debate as to what constitutes a specialist nursing role continues. Specialist nurses are described by the UKCC as nurses who are experienced clinicians capable of exercising higher levels of judgement, discretion and decision-making in clinical care. They can influence patient care, utilize leadership skills and use their specialist levels of knowledge and expertise within a multidisciplinary team (Bousfield 1997). Utilizing these skills and drawing on the expertise acquired during pre- and postregistration training and by using his/her expanded knowledge base, the district nurse is ideally placed to develop patient-centred care. Having an understanding of the needs of the patient within this wider context allows district nurses to support patients in making effective decisions about their own care. It also facilitates effective working within primary care organizations aiming to meet the needs of local populations. (See Chapters 1, 2 and 3 for developments in primary care.)

Leadership has become a key focus since the launch of the NHS Plan (DoH 2000). Recognizing the need for leadership skills, the National Nursing Leadership Project has been implemented and district nurses have found themselves alongside other nursing team and ward leaders on courses such as Leading Empowered Organizations (LEO) and the Royal College of Nursing Leadership Programme. However, it would appear that in many NHS Trusts in England only senior nurses are attending these programmes. This may make the introduction of new skills difficult as colleagues and others may not have a shared understanding of leadership concepts. However, a few NHS Trusts have been innovative and have brought the LEO programme into the whole organization and have employed a training facilitator to cascade the information. The concept of leadership is now on empowering nurses and ultimately patients to facilitate high-quality care in a partnership relationship. This is ideally undertaken utilizing a transformational leadership style (Davidhizar 1993), in which leaders seek to understand the problems and issues affecting both nurses and patients and then support them through changes and developing new ways of working. This leadership concept supports the role of district nurses and hopefully these programmes will encourage more effective teamwork. (See Chapter 15 for a discussion of teamworking and team development and Chapter 16 for further discussion on professional leadership and the management of change.)

Another dimension that is having an impact on how nurses provide care is the analysis and review of patient views and satisfaction with services provided. The NHS complaints procedure provides a framework enabling patients to raise concerns about the health care they have received, and ensures that mechanisms are put in place to reduce incidents being repeated (DoH 1996). District nursing needs to consider how it can effectively use complaints to inform practice and to develop new ways of working. Satisfaction surveys help to provide an insight into patients' understanding of district nursing and how services are delivered. One survey has found that: patients are unaware of how to access the service until they are referred; have a perception that nurses are too busy; that they spend too much time on nursing administration; and that visits can be interrupted by mobile phones (Cusick 1998). Another survey indicated that patients wanted a nurse they could trust and who would visit them in their own home, they also wanted to be able to establish a good relationship with that nurse. It went on to highlight that the majority of patients wanted to know what time the nurse would visit, to enable them to be ready and so that they could plan other events in their day (Bartholomew et al 1999). District nurses need to give consideration to these findings in an endeavour to ensure that the professionalism of district nursing is promoted at all times and that patients are aware how to access the services they provide. Further concerns relate to a lack of understanding of the role of the district nurse on the part of patients, some of whom have an expectation that care will be provided in the home, even if it is more appropriately provided in another setting. The district nurse can use the development of service definitions, referral criteria and patient information leaflets to help educate patients and other healthcare professionals accordingly. (See Chapter 4 for further information on clinical governance.)

FIRST ASSESSMENT: A REVIEW OF DISTRICT NURSING

In 1999 a key document was published which continues to have a direct impact on district nurses; *First Assessment: a review of district nursing services in England and Wales* (Audit Commission 1999). This report provides an insight into the pressures on the district nursing service and highlights that there is often a discrepancy between resources, skills and demand for service provision. The report has made a series of recommendations for district nursing providers including the need to set clear service objectives, set referral criteria, establish systematic methods of caseload review, improve the management of patient demands and ensure the appropriate targeting of resources.

This report presents a challenge to district nurses, service managers and Trusts in that the ways in which district nursing services are organized, managed and delivered have to be reviewed. The report also spells out key messages about integrated working, self-managed teams and on the way services are developed and provided to all groups that are involved in the commissioning of services. (See Chapters 2 and 3 for a discussion of recent health and social policy developments and development in primary care).

The district nursing services overall, undertake more than 36 million contacts each year and have approximately 2.75 million patients on their caseload, the majority of these patients are older people (Audit Commission 1999). During 1997/98 expenditure on district nursing services was approximately £650 million (Audit Commission 1999), and questions continue to be asked about how these services are provided and whether they offer best value in both monetary and patient care terms. District nurses have raised concerns about

patients who are being discharged earlier from hospital with more complex needs and the appropriateness of some of the referrals they receive.

The Audit Commission also highlighted the following variations that exist in district nursing services across the country:

◆ Some areas provide 24-hour cover.
◆ Some only provide daytime and evening services.
◆ Variation in the numbers of patients per whole time equivalent district nurse.
◆ Inconsistency in the roles undertaken by the district nurse and members of the nursing team.
◆ Variations in the provision of continence and leg ulcer care in clinic settings.

It has looked critically at service provision and following publication of this report every district nursing service in England and Wales was to be evaluated to establish where it stood against the issues highlighted, and to identify how improvements in the services could be made for the benefit of patients. One of the key issues identified was the need to ensure that the patients being cared for by the district nurse were the right patients.

The scope of district nursing practice if not clearly defined can lead to inappropriate referrals, and ultimately inefficient and ineffective management of resources (Seccombe 1999). By developing locally agreed, clearly stated service definitions and objectives district nurses and service managers can move towards ensuring that they are delivering appropriate and high-quality care. Alongside service definitions and objectives comes the need for clear referral criteria. 'First Assessment' identified as many as one in ten referrals as inappropriate and district nurses provided three main reasons why these referrals were deemed so. Firstly, that the referral should have been made to the practice nurse, secondly, that the patient should not have been discharged from hospital as appropriate services were not in place and finally that no nursing care was required. District nurses also reported that as many as one in five referrals were inadequate and almost one in ten provided misleading or incorrect information about the patient's health status. Information that was missing included incorrect personal information for the patient and no information about whether or not the patient was aware of their diagnosis. However it has been identified that district nurses themselves often have no clear definition of what is appropriate or adequate. This finding confirms the lack of a clear service definition (Seccombe 1999). The development of locally agreed definitions, objectives, referral criteria and documentation, which meet the needs of district nurses and their patients could help to resolve this problem. Recent publications would indicate that these developments are now happening in services across the country.

CASELOAD REVIEW

An area of weakness identified by the Audit Commission was the need for a caseload review in order to improve the management of patient demands and the allocation of resources. The review process allows the opportunity for:

- comparing the numbers of patients on a team's active caseload
- profiling the gender, age, frequency of visits, and dependency of patients
- estimating the overall workload
- comparing the caseload at practice level.

By providing district nurses with information about their caseload, service leaders can support district nurses in:

- encouraging patient discharge or transfer to other more appropriate services
- regularly monitoring change in casemix to ensure effective use of resources
- identifying the type of care patients are receiving
- developing care packages leading to the development of core competencies for the assessment and the delivery of these packages of care.

Few areas have undertaken this type of work and there is little published research in this field, yet, the understanding of the types of care packages required can assist service leaders to identify training needs to meet patient care requirements. On a day-to-day basis caseload analysis can support nurses in prioritizing visits, justify need for bank staff and support the process of appropriate placement of patients in residential and nursing homes.

Work in one community healthcare trust resulted in the development of a casework management tool that is able to provide information about the increased demands on district nursing services. Its emphasis is on defining the complexity of patient care and the equal distribution of the workload within a district nursing team. It also aims to identify areas of inequality between the resourced nursing time and the actual time required to undertake care. It also provides indicators of when a team has reached its patient capacity (Frame & Donnell 1996). However, this project did not state the types of nursing care being provided or if other services were involved and it did not identify a core caseload.

Another dependency tool has been developed to identify the needs of patients and accurately indicate the care that they were receiving (Freeman et al 1999). This has been used as an audit tool for the management of certain conditions. One of the key aspects of this tool is that it can be used to identify district nursing teams, which are under pressure and therefore identify the appropriate distribution of staff. It provides an ongoing profile of the demands on the service and allows informed discussion about the development of services (Freeman et al 1999). However, this tool needs to be evaluated, as no evidence of comparison or transfer to another area is demonstrated. Indeed, the effectiveness and validity of these tools needs to be explored, as they may not meet the needs of every district nursing service.

The Audit Commission report and subsequent service reviews have provided district nursing services with an effective plan for the future and with achievable goals to enable the provision of a service that can demonstrate provision of a high-quality service offering effective and equitable care. (See Chapter 4 for further discussion on quality improvement.)

INFLUENCES ON PRACTICE

The changing context of health care finds district nurses and other community nurses in a leading position within primary care. Through the White Paper *The New NHS. Modern, Dependable* (DoH 1997) the Government provided the opportunity for nurses and general practitioners working in the front line of the primary healthcare team to become clinical strategists. The creation of Primary Care Groups and Trusts, Local Health Groups and Scottish Primary Care Trusts has opened the way for the direct involvement of nurses on the executive and board of these organizations. As a result of these changes, community nurses now find themselves working as employees of primary care organizations that are focused on the commissioning and provision of services. This should allow for a better working relationship with other members of the primary healthcare team. (See Chapters 1 and 2 for information on recent health and policy developments and Chapter 15 for a discussion of teamwork).

The National Service Frameworks (NSF), particularly the recently published NSF for the older person (DoH 2001a), call for a single assessment process for the older person that requires integrated working by all members of the primary healthcare team. This process will enable older people to be assessed effectively and allow the sharing of information between professionals (DoH 2001a). Primary care organizations across the country are considering proposals on how they can achieve a single assessment process. District nurses are ideally placed to participate in the development of strategies to implement the requirement of the NSF, as they have frequent contact with older people, with more than 60% of patients on a district nurse's caseload being aged 65 and over (Audit Commission 1999).

The implementation of 'free nursing care in nursing homes' has implications for the role of the district nurse (Dinsdale 2001). Free nursing care provides patients in nursing homes with a contribution to their fees which equates to the nursing care that they require (DoH 2001a). District nurses are well placed to undertake this assessment process however, there has been little consideration given to the implications on workload (Scott 2001). The Government has recently extended the timescales for the introduction of free nursing care as the guidance was published late and it has been established that organizations needed more time to respond (Kenny 2001).

District nurses have many outside influences on the care that they provide, some like the implementation of free nursing care place extra demands on their time and others such as nurse prescribing allow greater freedom and autonomy. District nursing has waited patiently for the introduction of nurse prescribing which was first mentioned in the Cumberlege Report over 15 years ago (DHSS 1986). In 1999 a 2-year roll out of nurse prescribing education began to allow nurses holding a district nursing or health visiting qualification to undertake this new role, which includes the requirement that district nurses diagnose a limited range of conditions. The products available for district nurses are fairly limited but do allow them to prescribe frequently used items such as wound dressings, catheter products, stoma care products and compression hosiery (British Medical Association and Royal Pharmaceutical Society of Great Britain 2000). The ability to prescribe has helped to improve patient care by saving time, promoting continuity of care and enabling a response to service (Berry & Hurst 1999).

CHANGING DEMANDS

District nurses are no strangers to change, the current role being very different to its origins (Baly et al 1987). However, the current demands on the service are constantly changing due to influences in society, political and medical developments and patient expectations.

The increasing number of older people in the population is now well recognized (DoH 2001a), and the publication of the National Service Framework for the older person (DoH 2001a) reflects the recognition that this group have specific needs which need to be addressed across all areas of health and social care. Older people experience more social and healthcare needs (DoH 2001a) and as a consequence there has been an increased demand for district nursing services. The range of skills required for the management of chronic ill health, when working with the older person, has become more diverse as many more people are cared for at home and in other community settings.

A multidisciplinary approach to the care of the older person and the introduction of the single assessment process (DoH 2000, 2001a) may in some areas require the district nurse to develop better understanding of care management skills and financial assessment. This may be compromising for some nurses and lead them to question the fundamental principles of the provision of health service free at the point of delivery. However the single assessment process should ultimately ensure that the patient receives a more effective service which avoids duplication.

With the Government placing high priority on waiting list initiatives (DoH 2000), there is a great deal of pressure on acute services to achieve a higher level of patient throughput. This has led to early discharge of patients from hospital and a wider use of day surgery which has also placed an increasing demand on district nursing services.

Research undertaken by Macdonald et al (1991) reviewed the changes within acute hospital provision and the impact on district nursing demand. The study identified no change in the number of patients referred to the service, despite one hospital closing and another discharging more patients. The study concluded that the district nursing service enabled patients to remain in their own home for longer when access to acute services were reduced. It also found that the needs of patients on the district nursing caseload were increasingly more demanding and diverse. As the caseload becomes increasingly more dependent, this may over time, limit the input the district nurse can provide for individuals who are less needy (Audit Commission 1999).

The change in demand for services is accompanied by the requirement for district nurses to possess and use a broad range of skills in order to meet needs and manage a wide range of chronic illnesses. They also care for patients who may require more technical and specialized nursing than previously. Close working with specialist nurses particularly those with a community function, may enable district nurses to meet the changing needs whilst ensuring that the access to specialist knowledge continues. However, the specialist nurse's role is to support and in part educate other healthcare professionals and patients (Humphris 1994) and not to provide ongoing care except in specific complex cases. Therefore, district nurses need to continually update their knowledge and ensure evidence-based practice is offered in order to meet a wide diversity of patient needs. (See Chapter 24 for a detailed discussion on new nursing roles.)

The public also has a higher level of expectation and understanding of healthcare provision and this is no less true of the district nursing service. The Patients' Charter (DoH 1995) supported patients having a clear say in care provision and invited their involvement in the evaluation of care received. A more informed public demands a service that they perceive will meet their needs and offer a partnership approach to care.

INTERDISCIPLINARY WORKING

In recent years health and social services have been encouraged to work together to meet the needs of local populations and to provide effective patient-centred care (DoH 1997, 2000). The concept of collaborative working to meet patient needs is not new to primary care. The Harding Committee (Standing Medical Advisory Committee 1981) provided a definition of a primary healthcare team and stressed the need to understand the varying roles and responsibilities of healthcare staff in the community setting. District nurses have a long tradition of working together with other healthcare professionals to determine care provision, often in informal ways due to variations of employment and management (Young 1997). However, recent government policy has advocated those community staff move beyond the informal approach and towards a more structured strategy in an endeavour to ensure a cohesive approach to care. This would incorporate a wide range of staff from health and social care sectors. *The New NHS. Modern, Dependable* (DoH 1997) identified that integrated teams were the way forward, citing not only the need for healthcare professionals to work more closely but also to work across boundaries between health and social care. *Making a Difference* (DoH 1999a) stated that interdisciplinary working was important for all professionals but that nurses would have the skills to support the process. Much work had already been undertaken to develop closer working practices in localities with the creation of self-managed and integrated nursing teams (Gerrish 1999). The Audit Commission (1999) acknowledged that district nurses have played a significant part in the development of these teams, defining clarity and understanding of nurses' roles and working in more co-ordinated and complementary ways to meet the needs of the patients. The success of self-managed and integrated teams seems dependent on a willingness to work together and establishing a shared vision that is owned by all members, to ensure a cohesive approach towards the service to be provided. An understanding of roles is vital and communication at all levels is seen as an essential component (Audit Commision 1999). Rowe (1998) recognized that these teams needed to have the power to make change, but argues that, to function effectively it is vital that district nurses have the skills of team co-ordination as well as clinical skills. Many services now devolve aspects such as budgetary management and collective decision-making to the teams. This move away from traditional ways of working can enable district nurses at all levels to influence future developments (Gerrish 1999), and make a difference to the local provision of care.

Young and Antrobus (1998) identified that self-managed and integrated teams foster creativity and innovation. Given the diversity of care provision now required by community nurses, this may support a greater responsiveness to care. (See Chapter 15 for further discussion of teamwork.)

The concept of team working which crosses boundaries may however be challenging for nurses as boundaries become blurred and traditional roles are questioned. The district nurse's role has needed to be responsive to change and as identified earlier it has evolved and transformed progressively, but it is not a generic role and the nature of district nursing could be challenged if the professional boundaries are not clear.

Leadership may also be an area for concern. District nurses traditionally undertake postregistration qualifications and may expect to engage in a team leader role. Studies relating to self-managed and integrated teams have differing views when considering the need for a team leader (Brumpton 1998, Owen 1998). With the need for collaborative working, the role of co-ordinator is often adopted to ensure the team democratically makes decisions. This may challenge the traditional hierarchical approach within district nursing.

The development of integration and future team working in primary care goes beyond nursing, with many integrated teams already involving care managers (DoH 1998). Also the establishment of Primary Care Trusts, Local Health Groups and Scottish Primary Care Trusts supports the move to greater integration and ultimately interdisciplinary working, particularly between general practitioners, community nurses and social services. The boards of these bodies support nurses, doctors, lay people and social service representatives to work together on national initiatives and local health improvement programmes. With the development of Care Trusts, the opportunities for interdisciplinary working across health and social care providers will grow (DoH 2000).

The 1999 NHS Act (DoH 1999b) enables shared financial arrangements between health and social care agencies and has helped to determine new ways of interdisciplinary working. This requires clear parameters to ensure that patients and clients receive the most appropriate care, and that the skills and expertise of all community practitioners are used effectively. The World Health Organization (1998) recognized that the quality of care provision is improved by interprofessional teamwork. There may currently be many boundaries to cross in order to develop a more cohesive approach to working together in new ways. Initiatives have already begun to shape the future with the emergence of Personal Medical Services (PMS) and Beacon sites that display evidence of patient-focused interprofessional working (NHS Beacon Services 2000). The Peach Report (UKCC

1999) also recognized the need for interprofessional training at prequalification level, and this approach is also being developed at postqualification level. This will influence the way that primary care is delivered in the future, and the district nurse will play a key part in this transition.

CHALLENGES FOR THE FUTURE

The NHS is currently going through a period of transition and the Government's agenda would indicate that this is set to continue. District nurses need to be proactive, accept the challenges they are presented with and find new and innovative ways of incorporating these to ensure that they remain fit for practice. *Extended Nurse Prescribing* (DoH 1999c), *The Essence of Care – Patient Focused Benchmarking* (DoH 2001b), *The Chief Nursing Officers Ten* (DoH 2000), *Free Nursing Care* (DoH 2001a), *The Public Health Agenda* (DoH 1999d) and *The National Service Frameworks* (DoH 2001a) will all change the way that district nursing provides care for patients and also how the service presents to other healthcare professionals. District nurses have to be ready to accept the challenges to traditional ways of providing nursing care to patients in the community and demonstrate that they are both partners and leaders in the provision of primary care nursing. (See Chapter 24 for a discussion on alternative ways of working.)

CONCLUSION

District nursing is constantly evolving and is currently going through a time of immense change and must be prepared to meet the challenges it faces. Influences from national and local initiatives are impacting on working practices and the skills required to meet patient need. The district nurse must ensure that the team is able to embrace the challenges faced. Working in new ways in a community setting will offer exciting opportunities for district nurses as they work more collaboratively with other health and social care practitioners. This may also lead to a review of current working methods and to the abandonment of some of the traditional aspects of their role. The Audit Commission report, *First Assessment* (1999) has provided a framework for district nursing and a template for review and a means of determining the way forward. The ever-changing context of healthcare provision will mean district nurses have to ensure that they are key players in future decision-making. Recent health and social policy changes provide the opportunity, district nurses should ensure that their voice and views are heard and heeded.

SUMMARY

◆ This chapter explores the evolving role of the district nurse and the concept of the specialist practitioner. It considers how good leadership skills can enable district nurses to undertake key roles within Primary Care Trusts.

◆ The impact of the National Service Framework for the older person is reviewed and the implications for integrated working through the use of the single assessment process examined.

◆ The need for collaborative working across health and social care agencies is also explored.

◆ The implications of the Audit Commission Report, *First Assessment*, is discussed, as is the importance of caseload management, referral criteria and the need to establish equity in district nursing service provision.

DISCUSSION POINTS

1. District nurses are changing their roles and function, creating a new ideology based on direction from the Department of Health and patient demand. Consider the impact these changes will have on traditional ways of working.

2. How realistic is the concept of caseload management/analysis and how can it support district nurses in practice?

3. How realistic is the aim to provide district nursing services that are equitable countrywide?

REFERENCES

Audit Commission 1999 First assessment: a review of district nursing services in England & Wales. Audit Commission, London

Baly ME, Robottom B, Clark JM 1987 District nursing. Heinemann Nursing, Oxford

Bartholomew J, Britten N, Shaw A 1999 What they really, really want. Nursing Times 95(12): 30–31

Berry L, Hurst R 1999 Nurse prescribing: the reality. In: Humphries JL, Green J (eds) Nurse prescribing. Macmillan, Basinstoke pp 90–106

Bousfield C 1997 A phenomenological investigation into the role of the clinical nurse specialist. Journal of Advanced Nursing 25: 245–256

British Medical Association and The Royal Pharmaceutical Society of Great Britain 2000 British national formulary. The Bath Press, Avon

Brumpton K 1998 We can work it out. Nursing Times 94(29): 62–63

Cusick K 1998 User views of the district nursing service. British Journal of Community Nursing 3(2): 74–81

Davidhizar R 1993 Leading with charisma. Journal of Advanced Nursing 18: 675–679

Department of Health 1995 The patients' charter. HMSO, London

Department of Health 1996 Complaints listening, acting, improving. Guidance on implementing the NHS complaints procedure. DoH, London

Department of Health 1997 The new NHS. Modern, dependable. Department of Health, London

Department of Health 1998 Modernising social services, promoting independence, improving protection, raising standards. DoH, London

Department of Health 1999a Making a difference. Department of Health, London

Department of Health 1999b The NHS Act. Department of Health, London

Department of Health 1999c. Review of prescribing supply and administration of medicines. Department of Health, London

Department of Health 1999d Reducing inequalities: an action report. Department of Health, London

Department of Health 2000 The NHS plan: a plan for investment, a plan for reform. Department of Health, London

Department of Health 2001a National Service framework for older people. Department of Health, London

Department of Health 2001b The essence of care – patient focused benchmarking for health care practitioners. Department of Health, London

Department of Health and Social Security 1986 Neighbourhood nursing: a focus for care, report of the Community Nursing Review (The Cumberlege Report). HMSO, London

Dinsdale P 2001 'Free' nursing care may lead to a massive shortfall. Nursing Standard 15(49): 4

Frame G, O'Donnell P 1996 Weight-lifters. Health Service Journal 19: 30–31

Freeman S, Shelley G, Gay M, Ingram B 1999 'Measuring services: A district nursing tool'. Nursing Standard 13(47): 39–41

Gerrish K 1999 Teamwork in primary care: an evaluation of the contribution of integrated nursing teams. Health and Social Care in the Community 7(5): 367–375

Humphris D 1994 The basis of role specialism in nursing. In: Humphris D The clinical nurse specialist. Issues in Practice. MacMillan Press Ltd, Basingstoke pp 1–15

Kenny C 2001 Changes to care home funding put back a year. Nursing Times 97(39): 4

Macdonald LD, Addington-Hall JM, Hennessy DA, Gould TR 1991 Effects of reduction of acute hospital services on district nursing services: implications for quality. International Journal of Nursing Studies 28(3): 247–255

NHS Beacon Services 2000 NHS Beacons learning handbook. NHS Beacon Services, Petersfield

Owen A 1998 Self managed teams, the West Berkshire approach. Health Visitor 71(1): 23–24

Rowe A 1998 Self-management in primary care. Nursing Times 94(29): 60–62

Scott G 2001 Minster promises extra funding for special needs. Nursing Standard 16(2): 5

Seccombe I 1999 Listening exercise. Nursing Times 95(25): 56–58

Standing Medical Advisory Committee 1981 The primary health care team: report of a joint working group (Harding Report). Department of Health, London

UKCC 1994 The future of professional practice – the council's standards for education and practice following registration. UKCC, London

UKCC 1999 Fitness for practice. UKCC, London

World Health Organization 1998 Nurses and midwives for health: a WHO European strategy for nursing and midwifery education. WHO, Denmark

Young L 1997 Improved primary healthcare through integrated nursing. Primary Health Care 7(6): 8–10

Young L, Antrobus S 1998 Strategic skills in primary care. Primary Health Care 8(5): 6–8

FURTHER READING

Audit Commission 1999 First assessment: a review of district nursing services in England and Wales. Audit Commission, London

This document provides a strategy for the future of district nursing services and practical tips on how to implement the changes required.

Covey SR 1992 The 7 habits of highly effective people. Simon & Schuster, London

The book is a tool kit for life and leadership, but also provides the principles of adapting to change, and the understanding and power to take advantage of the chances that change can generate.

Department of Health 2001 National service framework for older people. Department of Health, London

This document provides a framework for the future provision of health and social care for the older person, promoting working across boundaries to ensure needs are most effectively met.

19

Health visiting/public health nursing

D. Watkins

INTRODUCTION

The 21st century provides opportunities for health visiting to reaffirm its public health role and make an active and visible contribution to meeting the public health agenda in the United Kingdom. Health visiting has always been firmly rooted in promoting the health of the public with a particular emphasis on maternal and child health (CETHV 1977), however the time is ripe to move into focused activity that addresses the gross inequalities in health between social groups in society and to work in a proactive manner. This ideology is clearly directed by government policy in the present day National Health Service (NHS) (DoH 1999a, 1999b, 2001, Home Office 1998, 1999, SNMAC 1995, Welsh Office 1998a, 1998b, 1999) and in the past history of the development of health visiting (Ministry of Health 1948, CETHV 1977).

Health visiting encompasses an individualistic and a structuralist approach to its work, that seeks to empower individuals and communities to achieve their full potential for the achievement of health, through actions directed at biological, socioeconomic, lifestyle, and environmental determinants of health. The focus of practice is the promotion of health and well-being, protection and prevention (UKCC 2001). The contribution of health visiting to the public health agenda has been reaffirmed by the House of Commons Select Committee on Public Health (2001) and is further supported by the Royal College of General Practitioners (RCGP 2001). They are considered 'major contributors to improving health and to the broader social inclusion agenda' (UKCC 2001, p. 2) and a key resource on public health issues in the community (House of Commons 2001).

This chapter will provide a brief overview of the history of the profession and discuss the origin, and current health visitor's role in public health, maternal and child health, and the protection of children under the age of 5 years in the United Kingdom. It will briefly explore the concept of public health, with an emphasis on the health visitors' work in relation to primary, secondary and tertiary prevention. The chapter will conclude with identifying the emerging opportunities for health visitors to expand their public health role, discussed in the context of current health and social policies.

HISTORICAL PERSPECTIVE

THE PUBLIC HEALTH AND MATERNAL/CHILD HEALTH ROLE

The origins of health visiting practice began in 1862 with the formation of the Manchester and Salford Ladies Sanitary Reform Association. Respectable women were appointed to 'teach hygiene and social welfare, give social support and teach mental and moral health' (Robinson 1982). The notion of household hygiene was one echoed by Florence Nightingale; even in those early days of nursing she recognized the link between child mortality and cleanliness:

The same laws of health or of nursing, for they are in reality the same, obtain among the well as among the sick. The causes of the enormous child mortality are perfectly well known, they are chiefly want of cleanliness, want of ventilation, careless dieting and clothing, want of whitewashing; in one word defective household hygiene (Florence Nightingale 1858 cited in CETHV 1977, p. 12).

Although Florence Nightingale felt this was a call to the nursing profession, she was able to make the division between nursing the sick compared with nursing the well. She acknowledged the importance of a 'nonjudgmental' home visiting service, which would prevent the service becoming unpopular or seen as interference in the lives of families (CETHV 1977:12). A year later in 1892 the first health visiting training programme was established, however it was not formally recognized as such until 1919 when the Ministry of Health and the Board of Education jointly validated a 2-year course of study.

During these early years of health visiting, the emphasis was on promoting public health, through teaching and helping the poor, with activities more related to social work, and improving sanitary conditions, than it was to nursing. However, the importance of maternal and child health grew, influenced by many recruits to the Boer War who were unfit for military service. This led to a realization that investing in the health of children was important for the economy and productivity of the country, and consequently the infant welfare movement emerged. Clinics were established to teach mothers how to care for their babies, the Notification of Births Act (1915) came into operation, and in 1925 the Ministry of Health requested that all health visitors must possess a midwifery qualification. This was influential in promoting the health visitors' role in working primarily with mothers and children, and health visiting became a universal home visiting service extended to middle class families.

The health visitors' work continued to retain a child and maternal health perspective, however it also focused on the field of social medicine and the numbers of health visitors were increased in an effort to reduce child mortality and morbidity. There was a fall in maternal and child mortality between 1901 and 1971, which can be attributed in part to improved maternal nutrition, legal abortion, extending the period of breast feeding, and improved living conditions. Although medical advances, such as immunization and antibiotics, made some contribution to improving the health of the nation, this was considered small in comparison with the impact of efforts to improve environmental and social conditions (Ashton & Seymour 1988).

As the health of mothers and children improved, so the need for health visitors appeared to decline, however Beveridge (Ministry of Health 1948) reinstated the role which reinforced the maternal and child health component, and also widened the scope of the health visitor's work. The NHS Act (Ministry of Health 1948) defined health visitors as:

Women employed by local authority for visiting persons in their homes for the purpose of giving advice as to the care of young children, persons suffering from illness, and expectant and nursing mothers, and as to the measures necessary to prevent the spread of infection (Wilkie 1979).

Although the focus was primarily mothers and young children, the scope of health visiting practice expanded during the early years of the NHS in an attempt to meet the above description of the role. This led to some difficulties in health visitors clearly defining their work and disparities were evident throughout the UK. Some health visitors were 'triple duty' nurses engaged in health visiting, district nursing and midwifery duties, others were working directly in the school health service and some were working with the elderly or diabetics (CETHV 1977).

As a result of the inequities in service delivery and poor recruitment to health visiting training, an investigation was commissioned. The Jameson Report (MoH 1956) was published as a result of this investigation, which advocated a number of changes for the profession. It stated that health visitors must retain their focus with families where there were young children, however they should become family visitors with a primary function of social advice and health education.

THE CHILD PROTECTION ROLE

Whilst health visiting was developing as a profession, in the background there was concern over protecting children's interests. The National Society for the Prevention of Cruelty to Children (NSPCC) campaigned for adult legislation to protect children who were the victims of ill treatment by parents or caretakers (Dingwall 1982).

Parental 'duty' and the 'right' to punish children prevails through the history of child rearing, and has been influential in shaping the construction of childhood and child abuse, and consequently the health visitor's work in working with

families to protect children. Advice to parents in the postwar period referred to not picking up youngsters for fear of spoiling them, and the parent's duty to 'discipline' the child is referred to in present-day literature. The fine line between leniency and discipline is difficult to determine for some, with others basing their child rearing practice on transgenerational family cultures, which may date back to the middle years of the 20th century. Some parents believe they have a right to discipline their child in whatever way they wish (Mayall & Foster 1989). However there has been a move away from parents 'owning their children, to do with as they wish', towards state protection of children as an investment for the country. It was felt that parents held their children in trust, and should they betray that trust, then the state had the right to intervene and monitor the parents to ensure they carried out their duties.

The maternal and child welfare service that developed in response to the above philosophy was seen as best delivered by the health visiting service. It was seemingly nonstigmatizing and the health visitor was considered a 'friend' rather than an inspector (Newman 1980). Dingwall (1982) comments on the suitability of the health visiting service delivering a surveillance service into the 'very heart of every family home in the country', because of 'its compromise between enforcement and libertarian values' (Dingwall 1982, p. 340). Although health visitors had no legal right of entry into families, they rarely made this fact known, they were accepted by communities, and the principles they adhered to revolved around respect, waiting for an invitation to enter, and not acting as an inspector (Dingwall 1982). These values remain inherent today in the professional practice of health visiting.

PRESENT DAY HEALTH VISITING PRACTICE

In 1962 the Health Visiting and Social Work Act set up the Council for the Training of Health Visitors (later known as the Council for the Education and

Training of Health Visitors (CETHV). They offer the following definition for health visiting:

The professional practice of health visiting consists of planned activities aimed at the promotion of health and prevention of ill health. It therefore contributes substantially to individual and social well-being, by focussing attention at various times on either an individual, a social group or a community. (CETHV 1977:8)

This definition is one that is still used today and it outlines the complex nature of health visiting, in that the focus for promoting health is not just the individual, i.e. the child, mother or family, but also social groups and communities. Health visitors assess the health needs of community populations, groups, and individuals and establish appropriate programmes of prevention which contribute to social well-being, as well as physical and emotional health (QAA 2001, UKCC 2001, NMC 2002). Health visiting differs from other dimensions of nursing because of its emphasis on working with communities to address issues of health and social inequalities and social exclusion. This dimension of their work clearly fits into the remit of public health, although it is different from other professionals who practice within this field. Health visitors usually hold a caseload made up of individual clients who are either registered with a general practitioner to whom the health visitor is attached, or make up a defined community, allocated to them on a geographical basis. This allows for personal individual contact, as well as opportunities to work on public health issues with specific groups and communities. (See Chapter 7 for further discussion on working with communities.)

THE PUBLIC HEALTH ROLE OF THE HEALTH VISITOR

Public health has been defined as 'the science and art of preventing disease, prolonging life and promoting health through organised efforts of society' (Acheson 1988). The science and art of preventing disease in health visiting practice has been described by Twinn (1991) who discusses how health visitors combine a scientific approach with the art of health visiting. The scientific basis

to their work encapsulates epidemiology, and the evidence base for practice extracted from research. This is combined with the art of professional judgement based on intuition; the complexities of families and communities, past experiences and the unique situations health visitors find themselves in. There is an art in synthesizing this information, reflecting on and in action and understanding and helping clients to achieve health. Health visiting as previously mentioned is also concerned with 'planned activities aimed at the promotion of health and prevention of ill health' (CETHV 1977), which has a positive effect on the health of individuals and society. (See Chapter 3 for further discussion on innovation and change in public health.)

The public health role of the health visitor is reaffirmed by the UKCC in its standards for specialist community health nursing when 'health visiting' was renamed 'public health nursing' (UKCC 1994). This is further supported by the Quality Assurance Agency (QAA), who developed 'benchmarking standards for health visiting education and practice', that clearly articulate the public health dimension of their work (QAA 2001). The latter document uses the following health visiting principles developed in 1977 (CETHV 1977) to underpin professional practice, which provide a sound basis for public health and are now firmly rooted in research (Cowley and Appleton 2000, CETHV 1977, p. 9):

1. The search for health needs.
2. The stimulation of an awareness of health needs.
3. The influence on policies affecting health.
4. The facilitation of health-enhancing activities.

THE SEARCH FOR HEALTH NEEDS

One of the unique functions of health visiting is searching for health needs, some of which may be self-declared by individuals or communities, whilst others may be unrecognized and require skill by the health visitor to identify. This search, or proactive investigation is essential before an assessment of health needs and planning to meet these can take place. It is working at this stage of 'pre-need' when trying to prevent needs arising in relation to social and health issues (SNMAC 1995), that makes health visiting practice different to any other health professional working within primary or community care and also adds to the complexities of measuring the effectiveness of their practice (Campbell et al 1995, McHugh & Luker 2002). The universal nature of the health visiting service places health visitors in an excellent position to identify needs, which may otherwise have remained suppressed or concealed. Some examples of this work include detecting and working effectively with women suffering postnatal depression (MacInnes 2000), working with children and families 'in need' and identification of child neglect or abuse (Appleton & Clemerson 1999), identifying and working with parents on child-feeding issues, nutrition, behavioural or sleep problems, all of which inadvertently affect child and family health (Acheson 1998, Olds et al 1997, Seeley et al 1996).

Health visitors are also concerned with the broader issues that influence health, for example poverty, housing, unemployment and infrastructures supporting communities, such as public transport. The search for health needs involves looking at these external factors that affect health, which individuals ultimately may have little control over and working at a political level to try to positively influence these issues. (See Chapter 6 for further discussion on structural issues related to poverty and health.)

The work of health visitors in searching for health needs in communities primarily revolves around creating a profile of the local community that takes cognisance of epidemiological data, local information, community and individual needs. This information is used to inform the Health Improvement Programme (HIMP) for that area and ultimately to influence resource allocation (UKSC 2001). (See Chapter 7 for more information on health improvement programmes.)

THE STIMULATION OF AN AWARENESS OF HEALTH NEEDS

The stimulation of an awareness of health needs refers to helping people become aware of what may be possible to achieve in an effort to improve their personal health, or the health of the community (CETHV 1977, UKSC 2001). This can also include working with disadvantaged groups in society who may have limited access to health information and resources (QAA 2001, UKSC 2001). Twinn and Cowley (1992) suggest that stimulating an awareness of health needs should be extended to three different levels:

◆ to clients, individuals and families
◆ to those who take responsibility for the commissioning of health services (Health Authorities, Primary Care Trusts, Primary Care Groups, Local Health Groups (Boards))
◆ to politicians and policy-makers.

In working with all of the above groups, the health visitor may stimulate an awareness of health needs through the provision of knowledge, recognizing that the way in which this is delivered is dependent upon the situation. When working with individuals and communities it is essential to take cognisance of social, educational and cultural backgrounds and people's personal experiences, to respect these and consider how they affect individual perceptions of health. Empowering individuals and communities to gain control over factors that influence their health underpins the application of this health visiting principle in practice and demonstrates the approach used by health visitors when engaging in 'health promotion' as seen in its broadest sense. This is encapsulated in the definition given by the World Health Organization (1986), which states that 'health promotion is about enabling people to increase control over and so improve their health'. The QAA (2001, p. 7) emphasize this point when they describe health visiting as using a 'partnership approach to practice, through which clients are empowered to address issues influencing their health'. This is an essential element of promoting health and preventing ill health and places health visitors in a central position to deliver a public health agenda, based on identified health needs. (See Chapter 27 for further discussion on promoting health.)

It is worth exploring 'empowerment' in more detail in an effort to describe the way in which health visitors undertake practice. Empowerment is a two-way process between professional and client, where the client's needs take priority, and goals are negotiated (Naidoo & Wills 2000). The principles revolve around fostering informed choice, supporting change rather than coercing clients, the provision of knowledge and allowing people to make up their own mind (Tones & Tilford 1994, p. 11). Persuasion, instruction or propaganda does not form part of the process, however clarifying values, building self esteem, and assisting clients to make decisions, which in turn builds self confidence, are essential ingredients to this approach (Tones & Tilford 1994). Naidoo and Wills (2000) categorize the term into 'self empowerment' and 'community empowerment', stating that the underlying intention in both is to use a 'bottom-up approach' which is facilitative and nondirective. This approach is one that is commonly used by health visitors in working with individuals and communities, bringing together both a medical and social model of health, combined with an empowerment approach (Daniel 1999).

When working with politicians and policy makers to stimulate an awareness of health needs it is essential to ensure that links, whether overt or covert are made with the political agenda. To inform this process health visitors need to ensure that health profiles are compiled based on epidemiological data and client experiences, that clearly identify the issues for the community. (See Chapter 3 for further information on epidemiology.)

THE INFLUENCE ON POLICIES AFFECTING HEALTH

Health visitors influence policies on a national and local level and this is pivotal to promoting health and preventing ill health (QAA 2001, UKSC 2001). They are ideally placed in the heart of the community to identify health and social needs and feed this information into health commissioners. For example, there are opportunities for health visitors to become actively involved in Primary Care Groups (Local Health Groups/ Boards), and the emerging Primary Care Trusts to

influence healthcare planning based on accurate needs assessments, ensuring that strategies include issues for prevention (SNMAC 1995). This would incorporate partaking in strategy development that may impact on the health of the community. Examples relate to influencing Health Improvement Plans, Health Action Zones (HAZ) or contributing to services in relation to healthy living centres. Working at an international and a national level with organizations such as the Community Practitioner and Health Visitor Association and the Royal College of Nursing is an effective way to influence policy development and the future profession of health visiting.

THE FACILITATION OF HEALTH-ENHANCING ACTIVITIES

Facilitating health-enhancing activities is a major part of health visiting professional practice and includes the broad remit of public health inclusive of environmental changes, personal preventative activities and therapeutic endeavours (Cowley 1996, p. 280). This may take place through encouraging and enabling individuals to take responsibility for their own health, through facilitating health-enhancing activities which could be community or family based, or by influencing policy formation which positively affects health. Campaigning to establish services in deprived or disadvantaged areas such as nursery school provision, or activities for teenagers are examples of facilitating health-enhancing activities. Monitoring health needs and acting as a health agent who mediates between agencies on behalf of families and individuals and teaches about health-enhancing activities is another element of health visiting.

Sure Start is the cornerstone of the Government's drive to tackle child poverty and social exclusion (Home Office 1998, Welsh Office 1999), and provides excellent examples of health-enhancing activities by health visitors (Bidmead 1999, Daniel 1999). There is substantial evidence to support early interventions with children and much of the work in the United States by Olds et al (1986, 1997) and Kitzman et al (1997) demonstrated the benefits of home visiting in the pre- and postnatal period. The results of these studies indicate programmes can reduce child abuse and neglect, improve parenting skills and the quality of child interactions, reduce subsequent pregnancies and in the long term, reduce criminal behaviour of mothers and children (Olds et al 1998). This evidence base has been used as the basis for Sure Start programmes, which are multiagency and set about to improve the health, intellectual, and social development of children (Home Office 1998, 1999).

The principles of health visiting can be traced through professional practice as demonstrated in the above discussion, however it is worth clearly articulating their role in family visiting and child protection. This vital work continues to dominate health visiting practice and although in some areas different models of health visiting are being implemented, the universal service of home visiting continues in one form or another. The NHS Executive (1996) recommended that all families should receive a visit from a health visitor following the birth of a baby and that future visits after this time should be needs led and left to the discretion of the health visitor. This has resulted in NHS Trusts setting their own frameworks and standards for health visiting practice (McHugh & Luker 2002), however experience and research confirms that the focus of their work remains with children under 5 years and their families (Appleby & Sayer 2001, House of Commons 2001, UKCC 2001).

FAMILY HEALTH VISITING

The nature of home visiting health visitors undertake can be categorized into primary, secondary and tertiary prevention, although Downie et al (1996) warn against the difficulties in defining any health promotion work in this way. They comment on the disease focus, the lack of standard definitions for these three areas thus categorizing prevention in the absence of meaning, and the continued debate between what constitutes primary and secondary prevention. Hall (1996) attempts to attach definitions to the three areas and describes primary prevention as reducing

the incidence of a given disease or condition. Examples of the health visitor's work in primary prevention would be the promotion of immunization programmes to reduce the incidence of communicable diseases; promotion, education and advice regarding breast feeding to promote child immunity and protect from infection and atopic conditions (Latham 1999, Lawrence 2000); education related to the prevention of childhood injuries and home accidents and parenting programmes aimed at enhancing parents' confidence and self-esteem (DoH 1998, Home Office 1998, Kitzman et al 1997). The latter improves children's health and educational attainment, reduces juvenile delinquency and mental health problems in later life, which demonstrate excellent examples of primary prevention (Olds et al 1998).

Secondary prevention is aimed at reducing the prevalence of diseases or conditions, that is reducing the impact, shortening the duration, and early detection of abnormalities resulting in prompt intervention (Hall 1996). Health visitors engage in secondary prevention by early referral to speech therapy for speech problems in children; working with parents in relation to child sleep difficulties (Kerr et al 1997); detection and prompt management and treatment of postnatal depression thus avoiding the potential adverse consequences on child health and development (MacInnes 2000, Seeley et al 1996); identification of child feeding problems and children who fail to thrive; early detection and management of child development and behaviour problems (Sutton 1995) and prompt referral to other professionals.

Tertiary prevention is identified as reducing the impact of disease or disabilities, and assisting people to live within the confines of a disease or condition (Hall 1996). Health visitors have a limited role in tertiary prevention, compared to other nurses who work in the community, particularly the district nurse whose role includes working with terminally ill patients and those with chronic diseases. The majority of the health visitors' work in tertiary prevention relates to working with families where there is a child with special needs.

As previously mentioned, the division between primary and secondary prevention remains blurred and is open to criticism no matter how one defines these elements of prevention. Perhaps a useful way to clarify their meaning is to consider primary prevention as activities undertaken with a particular group or population in which there is no identified risk. Once risk has been identified then activities fall into secondary prevention. An example of this is screening for cardiovascular risk factors such as smoking, obesity and raised blood pressure. Identification is primary, however once any one of these risks has been identified and is treated or monitored, then it becomes secondary prevention, e.g. monitoring and treatment of hypertension, smoking cessation programmes. Tertiary prevention would relate to working with clients postmyocardial infarction in relation to cardiac rehabilitation. Heartline, an initiative by health visitors in Lincolnshire has adopted an approach to prevention of coronary heart disease that encompasses primary, secondary and tertiary prevention. It includes working with families with a new baby, work with schools on lifestyle issues and postcoronary care (Ching & Pledge 1996). (See Chapter 5 for further discussion on disease prevention.)

Domiciliary health visiting has been scrutinized over recent years, in relation to its effectiveness and cost efficiency, and a systematic review was completed by Elkin et al (2000). When considering the results of this review, it is important to note that many of the studies included were American and so may be atypical of health visiting in the United Kingdom. Robinson (1999) reviewed the draft report of the systematic review and commented on the paucity of British research in relation to health visiting, particularly the lack of randomized controlled trials included. The outcome must, therefore be viewed with trepidation. Home visiting effectiveness was demonstrated in (Robinson 1999, p. 16):

◆ improved parenting skills and quality of home environment
◆ amelioration of child behaviour problems
◆ improved child intellectual and motor development, especially in low-birthweight children and failure to thrive
◆ increased immunization uptake

◆ reduced use of medical services
◆ reduced unintentional injury and the prevalence of home hazards
◆ improved detection and management of postnatal depression
◆ enhanced quality of social support to mothers
◆ improved breastfeeding rates
◆ initiatives limiting family size.

The review was inconclusive in demonstrating effectiveness in reducing child abuse and neglect, however surveillance bias was a particular problem in determining the effectiveness of home visiting in this area. Home visiting of the older person was proven as effective in relation to reducing carers' coping stress, enhancing carers' quality of life and reducing mortality and hospital admissions in elderly people. Cost effectiveness was based on six studies from the USA, five of which produced favourable results with the costs of home visiting offset by savings in reduced in- and outpatient care and/or reduced welfare provision (Robinson 1999). (See Chapter 26 for further discussion on achieving value for money.)

THE HEALTH VISITOR'S ROLE IN CHILD PROTECTION

The health visitor's role in child protection has now become a major one, and in recent years particular emphasis has been placed on the profession promoting and protecting the health of children under the age of 5 years. This includes the prevention, detection and management of child abuse and neglect (Home Office 1998, WO 1998a, 1998b). Deaths of children caused by child abuse or neglect has heightened public awareness of the problem and there is acceptance that health visitors intervene in the private life of families, on behalf of the state (Dingwall & Robinson 1993).

The main agencies and professionals who work together in the prevention and identification of child abuse include: National Health Service Trusts (particularly health visitors and school nurses), social services, the police and the National Society for the Prevention of Cruelty to Children (NSPCC).

Health visitors and school nurses do not have legal right of access to households, whilst all other professionals mentioned have statutory powers to investigate cases of actual or suspected child abuse (DoH 1989, Home Office 1991).

The Health Visitors Association (1994) describes the work of the health visitor in the prevention of child abuse as one of observation, assessment, recording and referring. They note that it is 'not the responsibility of the health visitor to diagnose, nor to investigate child abuse' and categorize the role into (HVA 1994, p. 17):

1. the prevention of abuse and neglect
2. the identification and assessment of children causing concern
3. the referral for investigation of children who are at risk of or subject to abuse or neglect.

A variety of interventions are undertaken by health visitors, that aim to prevent the abuse and neglect of children, and these may take place through the universal home visiting service, or community based work. (See Chapter 11 for further discussion on the prevention of child abuse.) Mayall and Foster (1989, p. 64) define intervention as: 'any unsolicited action taken by health visitors to concern themselves with the way parents bring up their children'. It is recognized that home-based interventions by health visitors may stretch across a continuum, depending on the needs of the family. It may extend from 'compulsory supervision of households to ensure children are not being ill treated (initiated by a Court Order), to monitoring health, to promoting development of the child's full potential' (Mayall & Foster 1989, p. 66). The surveillance role of health visitors would also fit into this continuum, although comparable with monitoring it appears to have more of a custodial meaning. This is illustrated by the Collins English Dictionary (1993) definition which refers to surveillance as 'close observation of a person in custody or under suspicion', whilst monitoring is to 'observe or record the condition or performance of a person or thing'.

Many authors comment on the important surveillance role of health visitors (Dingwall 1982, Hall 1996, HVA 1994), which some authors interpret as a 'policing role' (Dingwall 1982), and

others as secondary prevention (Hall 1996). The HVA (1994) remark on the health visitor's prime responsibility revolving around child health surveillance, based on the monitoring of child health, identifying families who may be vulnerable to abuse and agreeing a care plan which assists parents in providing 'more adequate care for their child' (HVA 1994, p. 19). Health promotion theorists may dispute whether surveillance, interpreted as 'policing' and 'compulsory supervision of households' performed by health visitors is comparable with the main principle of health promotion, namely empowerment.

Relating this to the prevention of child abuse and neglect raises some interesting dilemmas for health visitors. It may be necessary to have a hidden agenda and to work towards this when trying to oversee the welfare of children, although health visitors may wish to empower mothers. This raises the question of whether prevention using an empowerment approach and protection, using the definition for surveillance can take place in tandem.

Taylor and Tilley (1989) discuss the difficulty health visitors encounter between establishing a trusting confidential relationship with families, and their policing role. They suggest the problem may be resolved by accepting that the child has priority over the carer, whose needs must take precedence over all other factors. This view is supported by De La Cuesta (1994) who remarks that the family is the secondary concern and the child the primary client. She states the health visitor's relationship or friendship with the mother may continue in a confidential manner, until the primary client is threatened, and it then becomes a policing role on behalf of the state.

Work by Appleton and Clemerson (1999) suggests that 'children in need' may stretch across a continuum, with low need at one end and high at the other. Low need would indicate the family are functioning well and require limited intervention by the health visitor. The focus may be on health promotion activities using an empowerment approach. Children on the child protection register would constitute the highest point on the continuum and would require professional intervention based on protection of the child.

Here health visitors may be required to work in a different way with families, which involves adopting a far more directive approach. A truly empowerment approach to protection work is difficult when a child's life may be at stake.

Although there is diversity, and sometimes confusion in approaches used by health visitors, child protection forms a major element of their role. They act as an advocate for the child, and sometimes this conflicts with parental views. (See Chapter 11 for an in-depth discussion on child protection and the prevention of child physical abuse.)

UK POLICY AND THE CHALLENGES FOR HEALTH VISITING

The Independent Inquiry into Equalities in Health (Acheson 1998) coupled with the 'New Labour' Government has placed public health at the top of the NHS agenda. The evidence base to support prevention is strengthened by the research conducted over the last decade into the impact of poverty on maternal and child health and the implications of poor nutrition, housing, unemployment and poverty on health outcomes for all ages in the population (Acheson 1998). (See Chapter 3 for innovation and change in public health practice.)

Health visitors have been identified as a professional group who have close contact with the well population and are in a position to assess need and initiate appropriate programmes of prevention. The House of Commons (2001) indicate they would like to see health visitors in a key role advising community healthcare professionals and acting as a public health resource. Assessing health needs and taking an active part in commissioning health services that are responsive to local need should comprise a major part of their work (DoH 2001).

The Royal College of General Practitioners (RCGP) were asked how they saw the future role of the health visitor and outlined five future roles (RCGP 2001):

◆ protection of the vulnerable in society (not only children)

◆ health needs assessment and commissioning
◆ action to reduce inequalities
◆ health promotion
◆ primary and secondary prevention.

They propose that training for health visitors should encompass a wider public health role, which allows them to develop the knowledge and skills to lead in the above five elements. This is supported by the Government in *Saving Lives: Our Healthier Nation* (DoH 1999a), *Making a Difference* (DoH 1999b) and the *NHS Plan* (DoH 2001), all of which recommend a public health role for health visitors that moves away from an individualistic approach to practice and concentrates on reducing health inequalities in a wider arena.

Although there are moves in some parts of the UK to shift the focus of health visiting from working primarily with the under-5s and their families into community- and population-based practice, barriers in terms of time and resources remain in some areas. Clark et al (2000) conducted a review of health visiting and school nursing in Wales and found that health visiting was 'under-developed, under-managed and under-resourced' (p. 36). Health visitors are faced with competing demands associated with managing caseloads and undertaking community-based interventions, as well as providing a service to vulnerable groups in society, e.g. travellers. Clark et al (2000, p. 37) recommend that health visiting should be reorganized to support the following three roles:

◆ a generalist health visiting service to families with children
◆ a generalist health visiting service to particular groups identified by the assessment of local needs (e.g. older people, travellers, asylum seekers)
◆ a public health and community development role.

The report also recommends that health visitors and school nurses should be seconded to work with Local Health Groups (Boards) (equivalent to Primary Care Groups in England) and work as part of a team to undertake health needs assessment and develop Health Improvement Plans for the area.

The House of Commons (2001) has also raised questions as to whether all health visitors can continue to work with individuals, families, groups, communities and populations. They also question whether health visitors can continue to include in their role, acting on the determinants of health, empowerment, protection of children, and working at a political level as well as influencing policy. Some decisions need to be made as to how health visitors are used effectively to meet the public health agenda. Opportunities to expand their work in public health relate to the access they have to the population through being placed in primary care, and the interdisciplinary nature of the work they undertake, which puts them in frequent contact with other professionals and agencies who serve the community.

CONCLUSION

This chapter set out to examine the history of health visiting and link current practice with social and health policies. It has outlined the health visitors' work with reference to the existing evidence base, recognizing that health visiting is difficult to measure in some instances because of the nature and diversity of practice, searching out and meeting needs at a pre-need level.

It would be true to say that the future looks bright for health visiting under 'New Labour' where the Government's focus is on reducing inequalities and promoting health. Although the rhetoric found in recent government policies supports the health visitor's role in making a contribution to the nation's health, the conflict in paradigms between individual practice and community and population work needs to be addressed. Health visitors are unable to meet the competing demands associated with managing a caseload, child protection work and public health until extra resources are injected to support the profession. Perhaps as Clarke et al (2000) point out in the study of health visiting and school nursing undertaken in Wales, the time has come to develop different models of health visiting that meet all demands. Health visitors would be employed either to visit families and provide one-to-one advice and support, or to provide

a service to vulnerable groups, or to work with communities using a community development approach. All models would encompass a social and medical model of health, working towards promoting health in a number of different ways, all of which work towards meeting the public health agenda in the United Kingdom.

SUMMARY

◆ Health visiting has its roots in public health and continues to address the public health agenda in the United Kingdom.

◆ Health visitors' work is primarily focused on primary and secondary prevention with limited tertiary practice.

◆ Child protection continues to be a major part of the role of the health visitor, although the focus of activity may need to change from prevention to protection, when the health of a child is at risk.

◆ The political agenda supports health visitors refocusing some of their individualistic practice to working with communities and populations.

◆ The time has come to re-evaluate health visiting and encourage employers to clearly articulate the service they require in line with the health needs of local populations.

DISCUSSION POINTS

1. Compile a profile of your local community using both a social and medical model of health. Identify issues you feel could influence the health of the people residing there and discuss how health visiting could contribute to enhancing the health of the community.

2. Discuss the dichotomy between 'empowerment' and 'policing' families and consider how you may deal with the dilemmas this brings when working with children and families at risk of child abuse or neglect.

3. Government policy places 'public health' at the top of its agenda. Consider how you would prioritize issues for prevention.

REFERENCES

Acheson D 1988 Public health in England. HMSO, London

Acheson D 1998 Independent inquiry into inequalities in health report. The Stationary Office, London

Appleby F, Sayer L 2001 Public health nursing – health visiting. In: Sines D, Appleby F, Raymond E Community health nursing. Blackwell Science, Oxford

Appleton J, Clemerson J 1999 Family based interventions with children in need. Community Practitioner 72(5): 134–136

Ashton J, Seymour H 1988 The new public health. Open University Press, Milton Keynes

Beveridge WH 1946 The National Health Service. Department of Health, London

Bidmead C 1999 Bidding for success; making a Sure Start application. Community Practitioner 72(6): 166–167

Campbell F, Cowley S, Buttigieg M 1995 Weights and measures: outcomes and evaluation in health visiting. Health Visitors' Association, London

Chalmers K 1993 Searching for health needs: the work of health visiting. Journal of Advanced Nursing 18: 900–911

Ching A, Pledge F 1996 A lifelong approach to coronary heart disease prevention. Health Visitor 69(7): 278–279

Clark J, Buttigieg M, Bodycombe-James M, et al 2000 A review of health visiting and school nursing in Wales. University of Swansea School of Health Care Science, Swansea

Council for the Education and Training of Health Visitors (CETHV) 1977 An investigation into the principles of health visiting. CETHV, London

Cowley S 1996 Health visiting and public health. In: Gastrell P, Edwards J (eds) Community health nursing: frameworks for practice. Baillière Tindall, London

Cowley S 1999 Early interventions: evidence for implementing Sure Start. Community Practitioner 72(6): 162–165

Cowley S 2001 Public health in policy and practice: a source book for health visitors and community nurses. Baillière Tindall, London

Cowley S, Appleton J (eds) 2000 The search for health needs. Macmillan, Basingstoke

Cowley S, Billings J 1998 Resources revisited: salutogenesis from a lay perspective. Journal of Advanced Nursing 29(4): 994–1004

Daniel K 1999 Working in partnership. Community Practitioner 72(5): 117–118

De La Cuesta C 1994 Relationships in health visiting: enabling and mediating. International Journal of Nursing Studies 31(5): 451–459

Department of Health 1989 The Children Act 1989 – an introductory guide for the NHS. HMSO, London

Department of Health 1999a Saving lives: our healthier nation. HMSO, London

Department of Health 1999b Making a difference: strengthening the nursing, midwifery and health visiting contribution to health and health care. HMSO, London

Department of Health 2001 Investment and reform for NHS staff – Taking forward the NHS plan. HMSO, London

Dingwall R 1982 Community nursing and civil liberty. Journal of Advanced Nursing 7: 337–346

Dingwall R, Robinson K 1993 Policing the family? Health visiting and the public surveillance of private behaviour. In: Beattie A, Gott M, Jones L, Sidall M (eds) Health and wellbeing: a reader. The Open University Press, Basingstoke

Downie R, Fyfe C, Tannahill A 1996 Health promotion models and values, 2nd edn. Oxford Medical Press, Oxford

Elkin R, Kendrick D, Hewitt M, Robinson J, Tolley K, Blair M 2000 The effectiveness of domiciliary health visiting: A systematic review of internal studies and a selective review of British literature. Health Technology Assessment 4(13)

Hall D (ed) 1989 Health for all children. Oxford Medical Publications, Oxford

Hall D (ed) 1996 Health for all children. Report of the 3rd Joint Working Party on Child Health Surveillance. Oxford University Press, Oxford

Health Visitors Association 1994 The Health Visitors Role in Child Protection. HVA, London

Home Office, Department of Health, Department of Education and Science 1991 Working together under the Children Act 1989. HMSO, London

Home Office 1998 Supporting families: a consultation document. The Stationary Office, London

Home Office 1999 Supporting families: Summary of responses to the consultation document. The Stationary Office, London

House of Commons Health Committee 2000 Memorandum by the Department of Health (Public Health). House of Commons, London

House of Commons Health Committee 2001 Inquiry into public health. House of Commons, London

Kerr S, Jowett S, Smith L 1997 Education to help prevent sleep problems in children. Health Visitor 70(6): 224–225

Kitzman H, Olds D, Henderson C, et al 1997 Effect of prenatal and infancy home visitation by nurses on pregnancy outcomes, childhood injuries, and repeated childbearing. Journal of the American Medical Association 278(8): 644–652

Latham M 1999 Breast feeding reduces mortality. British Medical Journal 318: 1303–1304

Lawrence R 2000 Breastfeeding: Benefits, risks and alternatives. Obstetrics and Gynaecology 12: 519–524

MacInnes A 2000 Findings of a community based group for women with PND. Community Practitioner 73(9): 754–756

Mayall B, Foster M 1989 Child health care. Heinemann Nursing, Oxford

Ministry of Health 1948 National Health Service Act. Ministry of Health, London

Ministry of Health 1956 An inquiry into health visiting. HMSO, London

Naidoo J, Wills J 2000 Health promotion foundations for practice, 2nd edn. Baillière Tindall, Edinburgh

National Assembly for Wales (NAfW) 1999 Realising the potential: A strategic framework for nursing, midwifery and health visiting in Wales into the 21st century. NafW, Cardiff

Newman B 1980 The Betty Newman health care systems model. In: Riehl J, Ray C (eds) Conceptual models for nursing practice. Appleton Century Crofts, New York

NHS Executive 1996 Child health in the community: a guide to good practice. Department of Health, London

Nursing and Midwifery Council 2002 Requirements for pre-registration health visitor programmes. Nursing and Midwifery Council, London

McHugh G, Luker K 2002 Users' perceptions of the health visiting service. Community Practitioner 75(2): 57–61

Olds D, Henderson C, Chamberlin R, Tatenbaum R 1986 Preventing child abuse and neglect: A randomised trial of nurse home visitation. Paediatrics 78(1): 65–78

Olds D, Eckenrode D, Henderson C, et al 1997 Long-term effects of home visitation on maternal life course and child abuse and neglect. Journal of the American Medical Association 278(8): 637–643

Olds D, Henderson C, Cole R, et al 1998 Long-term effects of nurse home visitation on children's criminal and antisocial behaviour. Journal of the American Medical Association 280(14): 1238–1244

Quality Assurance Agency for Higher Education (QAA) 2001 Benchmark statement: Healthcare programmes; health visiting. QAA, Gloucester

Robinson J 1982 An art and a science. Nursing Mirror 3rd November: 24–27

Robinson J 1999 Domiciliary health visiting: a systematic review. Community Practitioner 72(2): 15–18

Royal College of General Practitioners 2001 The future roles of health visitors: a position statement. RCGP, London

Seeley S, Murray L, Cooper P 1996 The outcome for mothers and babies of health visitor intervention. Health Visitor 69(4): 135–138

Standing Nursing and Midwifery Advisory Committee (SNMAC) 1995 Making it Happen. Public health – the contribution, role and development of nurses, midwives and health visitors. Department of Health, HMSO, London

Sutton C 1995 Educating parents to cope with difficult children. Health Visitor 68(7): 284–285

Taylor S, Tilley N 1989 Health visitors and child protection: contradictions and ethical dilemmas. Health Visitor 62(9): 273–275

Tones K, Tilford S 1994 Health education: effectiveness, efficiency, equity, 2nd edn. Chapman and Hall, London

Twinn S 1991 Conflicting paradigms of health visiting: a continuing debate for professional practice. Journal of Advanced Nursing 16: 966–973

Twinn S, Cowley S 1992 The principles of health visiting: A re-examination. Health Visitor Association and UK Standing Conference on Health Visiting Education, London

United Kingdom Central Council (UKCC) 1994 The future of professional practice – the councils standards for education and practice following registration. UKCC, London

United Kingdom Central Council (UKCC) 2001 Developing standards and competencies for health visiting. UKCC Prime Research and Development Ltd, London

United Kingdom Standing Conference for Health Visiting Education (UKSC) 2001 Position statement: Health visiting in the 21st century. UKSC, London

Welsh Office 1998a Better health, better Wales. Welsh Office, Cardiff

Welsh Office 1998b Strategic framework: Better health, better Wales. Welsh Office, Cardiff

Welsh Office 1999 Sure Start: A programme to increase opportunity for very young children and their families in Wales. Welsh Office Circular 21/99. Welsh Office, Cardiff

Wilkie E 1979 The history of the Council for the Education and Training of Health Visitors. George Allen and Unwin, London

World Health Organization (WHO) 1986 Ottawa Charter for Health Promotion. WHO, Geneva

FURTHER READING

Acheson D 1998 Independent inquiry into inequalities in health report: The Stationary Office, London

This report provides an excellent insight into the inequalities in health that exist in the United Kingdom and outlines opportunities for preventative work.

Cowley S, Appleton J (eds) 2000 The search for health needs. Macmillan, Basingstoke

This book is based on sound research into health visiting practice and provides evidence to outline the work health visitors undertake in searching out health needs.

Dingwall R, Robinson K 1993 Policing the family? Health visiting and the public surveillance of private behaviour. In: Beattie A, Gott M, Jones L, Sidall M (eds) Health and wellbeing: a reader. The Open University Press, Basingstoke

This chapter provides an insight into the health visitors' role in protecting children and discusses the difficulties they encounter in undertaking this work.

Olds D, Eckenrode D, Henderson C, et al 1997 Long-term effects of home visitation on maternal life course and child abuse and neglect. Journal of the American Medical Association 278(8): 637–643

Olds D, Henderson C, Cole R, et al 1998 Long-term effects of nurse home visitation on children's criminal and antisocial behaviour. Journal of the American Medical Association 280(14): 1238–1244

The above papers provide evidence of the effectiveness of home visitation and outline issues in relation to primary and secondary prevention.

20

Community mental health nursing

B. Hannigan

INTRODUCTION

The largest of the professional groups charged with the responsibility of providing specialist mental health care is nursing (Sainsbury Centre for Mental Health 1997). Since the 1950s, successive governments have sought to shift the focus of mental health care away from hospitals and into the community. Reflecting this policy, community mental health nurses (CMHNs) have come to play an increasingly important part in the overall provision of mental health care.

Issues addressed in this chapter include: the emergence of 'community care' policies in the UK, and the impact of these on the initial development of community mental health nursing; the appearance of the CMHN as a key professional in the provision of care to people with severe mental health problems; the emergence of the multidisciplinary and multiagency community mental health team (CMHT) as the model for the local provision of care; recent critiques of community mental health care, and the impact of these and of subsequent policy developments; and, finally, some current issues and debates.

THE ORIGINS OF COMMUNITY CARE AND COMMUNITY MENTAL HEALTH NURSING

THE ORIGINS OF COMMUNITY MENTAL HEALTH CARE IN THE UK

The gradual move away from asylum care in favour of care in the community is a trend that has been observed throughout all of Western Europe and North America (Goodwin 1997). Rogers and Pilgrim (2001) observe that a complex set of factors were at play in the UK in the early post-Second World War years, all of which combined together to bring forward the modern era of community care. First were ideological factors, including a generalized post-War distrust of institutions. Other important drivers for community care, Rogers and Pilgrim argue, included concern on the part of UK central government to reduce the cost of asylum care.

The late 1950s and early 1960s were also notable for the emergence, from both inside and outside of the mental health professions, of challenging critiques of inpatient psychiatric care. At the end of the 1950s, Barton (1976) coined the term 'institutional neurosis', to describe the deleterious impact that living in asylums had on patients. Shortly after Barton's book first appeared, Goffman published his celebrated *Asylums*, in which he described the 'total institution' of the mental hospital (Goffman 1961). Critical accounts of mainstream psychiatry were also produced throughout the 1960s by writers such as Laing (see for example, Laing & Esterson 1964). Finally, Means and Smith (1998), amongst other commentators, point to the impact of hospital exposés in driving forward community care. In a number of influential publications, such as Robb's *Sans everything* (Robb 1967), the worst excesses of institutional abuse were revealed.

COMMUNITY MENTAL HEALTH NURSING: THE EARLY YEARS

Modern community mental health nursing emerged in the mid-1950s at Warlingham Park Hospital in Surrey, and at Moorhaven Hospital in Devon (Hunter 1974). Although a relatively young profession, the development of community mental health nursing has been described in an unusually detailed fashion (see, for example, Burke 1996). Information about the growth and characteristics of community mental health nursing has also been enhanced by the completion of a series of 5-yearly national surveys.

THE 1990 QUINQUENNIAL SURVEY OF COMMUNITY MENTAL HEALTH NURSES

The 1990 survey produced a detailed picture of the 5000-strong CMHN workforce at the level of the individual practitioner. One in seven of the CMHNs responding described themselves as specializing in a particular therapeutic approach. Family therapy, behaviour therapy and counselling were the most commonly cited therapeutic specialities. Additionally, just over 40% reported specializing with a particular client group. Of these, almost 60% reported specializing in work with older people. Smaller numbers of CMHNs described themselves as specialists in working with people with long-term mental illnesses; with people with substance misuse problems; with children and young people; in forensic services; or in working with people with HIV-related diseases (White 1993).

White's 1990 survey also generated controversial evidence of a closer identification between CMHNs and primary health care. In the 5 years to 1990 referrals to CMHNs from GPs were seen to have increased as a proportion of total referrals, so that, by the time of White's survey, over a third of CMHN referrals were reported to have originated from GPs. Moreover, clients referred by GPs tended to be less likely to have had previous admissions to hospital, to be less likely to be experiencing 'chronic mental illness', and to be less likely to have a diagnosis of schizophrenia than clients referred by psychiatrists. Finally, White also found that, amongst CMHNs working in England, around one-quarter had no clients on their caseloads with the diagnosis of schizophrenia (White 1993).

POLICY AND PRACTICE: 1990 TO 1997

White's third quinquennial survey came at a critical time. Summing up his findings, White (1993) suggested that many CMHNs might, through focusing on work in primary care with people with 'milder' mental health problems, have lost the skills to work with people experiencing more disabling and longer-term mental illnesses. White also drew attention to the mental health policy framework which was beginning to emerge at the time that his 1990 survey took place. This, as is discussed in detail below, was beginning to point towards a much clearer focus for specialist mental health practitioners – nurses included – in the care of people with 'severe mental health problems'.

White's finding that a quarter of English CMHNs responding in the 1990 survey did not have any clients on their caseloads with the diagnosis of schizophrenia was quickly picked up by other commentators. Gournay (1994), for example, described this situation as 'scandalous'. Gournay also questioned the value of community mental health nursing interventions in primary care, suggesting that the benefits to clients from seeing CMHNs were no greater than the benefits to those who only received treatment from their GPs (Gournay & Brooking 1994). For the sternest critics of community mental health nursing at the start of the 1990s, therefore, CMHNs were not only seeing too many of the 'wrong' sort of clients – the 'worried well' – but were also using clinical interventions with this client group which did not seem to generate any positive health outcome.

CHANGES IN THE ORGANIZATION OF COMMUNITY CARE

From the end of the 1980s onwards, there was a growing concern at the national policy-making level that community care had not 'worked' in the way which had been intended. The White Paper *Caring for People* (DoH 1989a) put the case for a 'mixed economy' of welfare. This, along with *Working for Patients* (DoH 1989b), was incorporated into the NHS and Community Care Act (1990). (See Chapter 1 for a more detailed account of social and health policy development in the UK.)

The NHS and Community Care Act had a significant effect on the work of CMHNs. It became usual for CMHNs to find their services purchased by two distinct agencies: health authorities, on the one hand, and general practitioner fundholders on the other (Muijen & Ford 1996). Unfortunately, these two groups did not always share the same priorities. Health authorities typically required CMHNs to concentrate their efforts on people with severe mental health problems – a continuing policy priority which is discussed at length below – whilst GPs often wanted greater CMHN involvement in primary care with people experiencing a wide range of psychological difficulties (Hannigan 1998).

The impact of the 1990 Act was also felt in other ways. Through the introduction of 'care management', social services departments assumed 'lead agency' responsibility for assessing and reviewing the community care needs of individuals. Significantly for community mental health services, however, 'care management' was not the only mechanism through which care was to be organized and provided. *Caring for People* (DoH 1989a), in addition to setting out details for the organization of community care for all groups of service users, contained an additional section relating specifically to community mental health care. Health authorities, in conjunction with social services departments, were to work together to ensure that all people with mental health needs were to be subject to a 'care programme approach'. This would require the assessment of the continuing health and social care needs of people with mental health problems, the appropriate provision of services, and the appointment of named individuals to co-ordinate overall packages of care (DoH 1989a). However, what *Caring for People* did not make clear was how these two proposed systems of assessing and providing care – care management and the care programme approach – were to integrate together.

THE CARE PROGRAMME APPROACH

The 'care programme approach' (CPA) was formally launched through the medium of a joint health and social services circular at the start of the last decade (DoH 1990). The four main elements of the CPA, as they were summarized in the 1995 document *Building Bridges* (DoH 1995), and again in the more recent *Effective care co-ordination*

Box 20.1 Key elements of the Care Programme Approach

Systematic arrangements for assessing the health and social needs of people accepted into specialist mental health services

The formation of a care plan which identifies the health and social care required from a variety of providers

The appointment of a key worker to keep in close touch with service users and to monitor and co-ordinate care

Regular review and, where necessary, agreed changes to the care plan

---

Department of Health (1995, 1999a).

in mental health services: modernising the care programme approach (DoH 1999a), are described in Box 20.1.

It is only in recent years that the relationship between the CPA and the social services-led care management has been clarified (DoH 1999a). Even in Wales, where the CPA was not formally introduced until 2002 (Welsh Assembly Government 2002) the principles of assessing health and social care needs and appointing keyworkers to oversee care plans were adopted in Welsh Office guidance in the mid 1990s (Welsh Office 1996).

The CPA was firmly aimed at the organization of services for people with severe mental health problems. The 1990 CPA circular, for example, was explicit in its call for the more systematic organization of care for people with 'continuing health and social care needs'. As was foreseen in the early 1990s (White & Brooker 1990), it has been CMHNs who have most frequently assumed the role of CPA community key worker (Community Psychiatric Nurses' Association 1996). More and more, therefore, CMHNs have taken on the role of co-ordinator of care for people with severe mental health problems.

WORKING WITH PEOPLE WITH SEVERE MENTAL HEALTH PROBLEMS

A number of factors came together in the early and mid 1990s, which together urged a refocusing of the work of community mental health nurses

towards meeting the needs of people identified as experiencing severe mental health problems. White's observation, in the 1990 quinquennial survey, that many nurses had drifted away from work with people with more disabling mental illnesses, in favour of a closer association with primary care was one factor. Emerging mental health policy was a further factor. The introduction of the care programme approach, which emphasized the requirement to more systematically organize the care of people with ongoing health and social care needs, was one major policy driver. Another factor was the apparent lack of an evidence base for community mental health nursing interventions with people with 'less severe' mental health problems, as was most notably suggested by Gournay and Brooking's study of CMHNs in primary care (Gournay & Brooking 1994).

The requirement for CMHNs to work exclusively with people identified as experiencing 'severe' mental health problems was also emphasized in the report produced by the Mental Health Nursing Review Team. *Working in Partnership* (DoH 1994) contained 42 recommendations. Recommendation 6 stated that '... the essential focus for the work of mental health nurses lies in working with people with serious or enduring mental illness in secondary and tertiary care, regardless of setting' (DoH 1994, p. 16). The Review Team set this recommendation against the evidence, arising from White's third quinquennial survey, that by aligning themselves with primary care many 'service managers and individual mental health nurses have not always targeted the people in greatest need' (DoH 1994, p. 16).

Government and professional policy initiatives, therefore, were beginning to force a realignment of CMHN practice from the early 1990s onwards. Other factors also urged this refocusing. Whilst doubts were being cast on the value of CMHN interventions with people with 'less severe' mental health problems in primary care settings, the 1990s were also notable for the increasing interest being shown in evidence-based interventions for people with severe mental illnesses.

It became customary from the early to mid 1990s onwards to pool together a range of clinical and social approaches to working with people

> **Box 20.2**   Key components of psychosocial interventions for people with severe mental health problems
>
> Outcome-orientated assessment
> Behavioural family work
> Psychological management strategies
> Case management
> Early intervention
> Psychopharmacology

Brooker 2001.

with severe and disabling mental health problems under the broad title of 'psychosocial interventions' (PSI). The term 'psychosocial interventions', whilst having considerable currency in contemporary community mental health nursing practice, is also one that has defied straightforward definition (Brooker 2001). Brooker notes that, in addition, whilst initially PSI was used to refer solely to family interventions in schizophrenia, the term has latterly appeared to take on a much wider meaning. Box 20.2 draws on Brooker's work, and summarizes what are often now thought of as the main components of PSI.

Often, the theory and research base underpinning the individual components of psychosocial interventions has not been new. The concept of 'expressed emotion', for example, which underpins a range of family interventions aimed at people with schizophrenia and their carers, was first developed in the late 1950s and early 1960s (see Brooker 1990 for a review). Similarly, the psychological management strategies emphasized in psychosocial interventions invariably include the use of cognitive behavioural techniques, an approach which has been developing over a number of decades (Kingdon 1998).

EDUCATION AND TRAINING

Whilst there is evidence supporting the value of the specific components of psychosocial interventions, there has continued to be concern at the lack of implementation of PSI approaches in routine clinical mental health practice. In response to this and other observations, considerable attention came to be paid from the start of the

1990s onwards to education and training, and particularly to the education and training of CMHNs. In an influential study, Brooker and colleagues set out to show that CMHNs could, first, be trained to provide family interventions to people with schizophrenia, and, second, that these interventions could generate measurable health gain (Brooker et al 1994).

At around the same time that Brooker was carrying out his study, the first two post-qualifying 'Thorn' training courses for CMHNs (and other mental health practitioners) also appeared, in London and Manchester respectively. Set up with monies from the Sir Jules Thorn Charitable Trust, these new courses aimed explicitly to prepare practitioners to deliver a range of psychosocial interventions in routine practice (Gamble 1995). There have been modifications to the content of Thorn courses over the years, with modules now including training in psychological interventions, case management and assertive outreach, and family interventions (Gournay 2000). In addition, courses now include an 'integration module', which is intended to equip students with the skills needed to overcome the barriers to the implementation of psychosocial interventions in everyday practice. Courses of this sort have become increasingly popular and sought-after over the last decade. Since the appearance of the first two Thorn programmes in 1992, the number of Thorn and other psychosocial interventions courses in the UK has risen to more than 30 (Brooker & Evans 1999).

WORKING IN MULTIDISCIPLINARY COMMUNITY MENTAL HEALTH TEAMS

Multidisciplinary teams based in community mental health centres started to appear in the UK throughout the 1980s (Sayce et al 1991). In the 1990s, multiagency and multidisciplinary community mental health teams (CMHTs) came to be the accepted method of organizing specialist community mental health services at the local level, and were described as such in contemporary policy guidance (for example, DoH 1995). Research completed in recent years has revealed the widespread growth of CMHTs throughout various parts of the UK (Carter et al 1997, Onyett et al 1994). As a consequence, most CMHNs, having once worked in unidisciplinary teams, now work in teams alongside mental health social workers, psychiatrists, occupational therapists, clinical psychologists and others (Brooker & White 1997). (See Chapter 15 for a more detailed discussion on multidisciplinary team working.)

CMHTs were set up in the belief that they are the best way to deliver flexible and accessible mental health services. Their appearance has not met with universal support, however. Galvin and McCarthy (1994), for example, have argued that CMHTs are prone to both inadequate planning and poor management. Onyett et al (1997) make reference to a number of challenges facing CMHTs and those who manage them, including the tensions for practitioners between being members of both the team and of their profession. Professionals, including those who have traditionally enjoyed considerable autonomy, may also struggle to adjust to the more 'managed' environment encountered in the typical CMHT. Similarly, working in multidisciplinary health and social care teams may also erode the professional identities of individual practitioners, with the result that staff may come to feel both isolated and lacking in support (Brown et al 2000).

POLICY AND PRACTICE: 1997 TO THE PRESENT

THE 1996 QUINQUENNIAL SURVEY OF COMMUNITY MENTAL HEALTH NURSES

A fourth quinquennial survey was carried out in 1996. Brooker and White (1997) found, in this most recent study, that the number of CMHNs working in England and Wales had continued to rise, to almost 7000 in total. Reflecting recent policy requirements, Brooker and White reported that the majority of CMHNs had become members of multidisciplinary CMHTs. Fewer nurses in 1996, as a proportion of the total workforce, reported having a primary care setting as their operational base than was the case in 1990.

The 1996 survey also demonstrated the continuing trend towards increasing specialization within the CMHN workforce. Significantly, in comparison to findings from White's 1990 survey (White 1993), more CMHNs in 1996 described themselves as specializing in the care of people with severe mental illnesses, whilst fewer described themselves as specializing in the care of either older people, or of children and adolescents. Other client group specialities reported in the 1996 survey included work with people with substance misuse problems, forensic work, work with people with eating disorders and work with homeless people. An increased proportion of nurses also described themselves as specializing in particular therapeutic approaches. Counselling, psychosocial interventions and case management were the most commonly cited specialist areas. Finally, in the 1996 survey Brooker and White also drew attention to the difficulties that many CMHNs faced in responding to the different agendas and priorities expressed by those who purchased their services, and the services of the CMHTs in which they worked.

NEW POLICY INITIATIVES

Findings from the fourth quinquennial survey of CMHNs in England and Wales were reported shortly after the election of the new Labour government in 1997. Elected on a platform of 'modernizing' the public services, the provision of mental health care became one of the new administration's key health and social care priorities. Notification of the Government's intentions came with the publication of *Modernising Mental Health Services: Safe, Sound and Supportive* (DoH 1998a). This drew attention to the stigma and misunderstanding which many people with mental health difficulties experience. The document noted, too, that poverty and social exclusion play a powerful part in precipitating and worsening mental ill health. However, the Government also referred in this document to its plans for a review of the Mental Health Act (1983) in England and Wales, and restated its intention to 'address the responsibility on individual patients to comply with their programmes of care' (DoH 1998a, p. 40).

Modernising Mental Health Services also reiterated the administration's controversial position that community mental health care in the UK had 'failed'. Senior members of the Government had first stated this view early in 1998 (see for example, DoH 1998b). These early statements had provoked critical responses from both mental health professionals and campaigning organizations. Margaret Pedler, Head of Legal and Policy Development at the mental health charity MIND, argued that the Government's assertion 'ignores the fact that for many thousands of people the switch to community services has brought, and continues to bring, enormous benefits' (Pedler 1998, p. 4). Thornicroft and Goldberg (1998), writing in a Maudsley Hospital Discussion Paper, weighed the evidence for and against the 'failure' of community care and concluded that, whilst care had not 'failed', it had only been 'half-tried'. A greater invest-ment in community services was needed, they argued, before any definitive judgement could be made.

The Government's solutions to the problems of community mental health care have not, however, been to call for a return to care in institutions. Rather, as Rogers and Pilgrim (2001) have observed, current UK mental health policy is promoting *more* community care, but in a recast form. Both *Modernising Mental Health Services* and the subsequent *National Service Framework for Mental Health* in England (DoH 1999b) include reference to developing and extending the provision of 'assertive community treatment' (ACT) for people with severe mental health problems.

Assertive community treatment has its origins in the United States, where it was developed under the title 'Training in Community Living' (Stein & Test 1980). ACT has been described in a Cochrane systematic review as 'a team-based approach aiming at keeping ill people in contact with services, reducing hospital admissions and improving outcome, especially social functioning and quality of life' (Marshall & Lockwood 2000). Typically, ACT teams are multidisciplinary, with team members pooling their expertise in order to provide a comprehensive and co-ordinated range of services. ACT teams provide highly targeted care, meaning that the ratio of service users to professionals is

low. Interventions include those aimed at improving mental and physical health, plus interventions in other areas such as housing, education and employment (Stein & Santos 1998).

Adherents to the ACT model argue that it represents a highly specified, evidence-based approach to the provision of community mental health care to people with severe mental health problems, and, as such, is quite distinct from 'standard' case management and community mental health team approaches (Marshall & Creed 2000). Interestingly, however, ACT also has its critics in the UK. Tyrer (2000), for example, has argued that the benefits which ACT has brought over 'standard care' in the USA have not been replicated here because 'standard care' in a UK community mental health context already includes many of the features of the ACT approach. It is notable, too, that policy-makers in Wales have not embraced ACT with the same enthusiasm as have their counterparts in England. The National Assembly's strategy for adult mental health services (National Assembly for Wales 2001), for example, notes that controversies surround this way of working, and points out that some service users may be alienated by teams using an 'assertive approach'. The Welsh strategy also casts doubt on the benefits of small caseloads, citing the work of Burns et al (1999) to support this claim.

The appearance of more 'assertive' approaches to community care is one example of how new national strategies for the provision of mental health care – such as the English and Welsh strategies noted above – are reshaping the context of community mental health nursing. England's *National Service Framework for Mental Health* (DoH 1999b) is a detailed and comprehensive document, which contains seven standards associated with five areas. These relate to the promotion of mental health and action to tackle the discrimination experienced by people with mental health problems; mental health in primary care settings and access to specialist services; the provision of care to people with severe mental illnesses; services for informal carers; and the reduction of suicide. The framework also sets out a series of 'fundamental values' which should underpin the provision of mental health services, and establishes a set of guiding principles. These include a commitment to service user involvement; the provision of high-quality and effective care; nondiscriminatory practice; accessible services; services that are safe; offering choice and independence; well co-ordinated care; staff support; continuity of care; and accountability. (See Chapter 4 for a more detailed analysis of quality issues.)

Major changes ahead include the appearance of a new mental health legislative framework for England and Wales. The Draft Mental Health Bill (DoH 2002) proposed the introduction of compulsory treatment in the community. Many nurses had strong misgivings about this, and expressed concerns over the effect that compulsory treatment would have on the relationship between service users and practitioners. The Bill also proposed that the responsibility for undertaking a 'preliminary examination' under the terms of a new Mental Health Act would fall to two doctors, and – unlike at present – not necessarily a social worker with particular training in the workings of mental health law, but *any* other approved mental health professional. For the first time, therefore, it seems likely that community mental health nurses will be expected to play a part in initiating compulsory treatment.

Further changes to the role and function of CMHNs are likely to occur with the anticipated expansion of nurse prescribing. There has already been debate within mental health nursing over the appropriateness of this extension to the mental health nurse's role (see for example, Gournay & Gray 2001). Recent government announcements, however, make clear that nurse prescribing will be extended to cover more 'complex' health difficulties, mental health problems included (DoH 2001).

CURRENT DEBATES

Mental health nursing is a profession characterized by vigorous and healthy debate. These continue to be aired in a variety of places and in a variety of formats, and the reader is referred to the 'Further Reading' section at the end of this chapter for more information. Here, a selection of some of the 'live' issues occupying community mental health nursing is rehearsed.

There has, first, been a sustained debate over what the role and function of mental health nurses should be. This chapter has included an outline of the increase in interest over the last ten or so years in psychosocial interventions for people with severe mental health problems. For some, this concern with the pursuit of 'psychotechnologies' – such as behavioural family interventions and cognitive behavioural approaches – is largely at odds with what the 'proper focus' of mental health nursing should be (see for example, Barker 1995, Barker et al 1997). Rather than concentrating solely on the acquisition of 'evidence-based' skills, Barker has argued eloquently for a very different basis for mental health nursing practice. This approach is one that is primarily concerned with the relationship between nurse and service user, and is characterized by an attention to the 'lived experience' of mental ill health, rather than to 'mental illness' per se.

There has also been debate over the appropriateness of the limiting of mental health nursing activity towards people with 'severe' mental health problems. Barker et al (1998) have expressed strong reservations over the usefulness of the term 'serious', or 'severe', mental illness, and have cautioned against the view that nurses should limit their work to people who are identified in this way. By focusing only on the narrowly defined 'seriously mentally ill', Barker and colleagues argue, mental health nurses may already be failing to contribute to the care of other important groups, including older people with mental health problems, children and young people, and people experiencing depression.

CONCLUSION

Community mental health nurses play a major part in the provision of care to people with mental health problems living in the community. Over the years, the work of CMHNs has changed dramatically. Most now find themselves working alongside social workers, psychiatrists, psychologists, occupational therapists and others as members of multidisciplinary community mental health teams. Many CMHNs, too, now concentrate on caring for people identified as having 'severe mental health problems', and are increasingly expected to offer evidence-based psychosocial interventions to this group of people. Changes in the future practice of CMHNs are likely with the appearance of a new mental health legislative framework, and of a more 'assertive' approach to the delivery of services.

SUMMARY

◆ Over recent decades in the UK, care for people with mental health problems has increasingly been provided in community settings.

◆ It is usual to date the origins of community mental health nursing in the UK to developments which took place from the mid-1950s onwards.

◆ The community mental health nursing workforce has grown considerably over the last 50 years, with the result that CMHNs now play a major part in the provision of care to people experiencing a wide range of mental health problems.

◆ Recent policy has urged CMHNs to concentrate on meeting the needs of people identified as experiencing severe and long-term mental health problems. Reflecting this refocusing, increasing interest has been shown in recent years in new ways of educating practitioners to work with this group of people.

◆ Other recent policy initiatives have grouped together CMHNs and other mental health professional groups in multiagency and multidisciplinary community mental health teams.

◆ Emerging mental health policy since 1997 continues to emphasize the requirement of prioritizing care for people with severe mental health problems. New initiatives include the extension of assertive outreach services, and plans for the introduction of a new – and controversial – legislative framework.

DISCUSSION POINTS

1. Is there a unique role for the community mental health nurse in the context of the multidisciplinary community mental health team?

2. How far do you agree with this statement, taken from the *Working in Partnership* report: 'the essential focus for the work of mental health nurses lies in working with people with serious or enduring mental illness in secondary and tertiary care, regardless of setting'?

3. What should be the role of the community mental health nurse in the primary health care setting?

4. The Government has declared that 'care in the community' has failed. Do you agree? What should be done to improve the care of people with mental health problems living in the community?

5. Think about your own practice as a community nurse. If you are a non-mental health nurse, would you know how to obtain help from your community mental health nursing colleagues in your local area? If you are a community mental health nurse, what can you do to make your skills and knowledge more widely available to your non-mental health nursing colleagues?

REFERENCES

Barker P 1995 Promoting growth through community mental health nursing. Mental Health Nursing 15(3): 12–15
Barker PJ, Keady J, Croom S, Stevenson C, Adams T, Reynolds B 1998 The concept of serious mental illness: modern myths and grim realities. Journal of Psychiatric and Mental Health Nursing 5(4): 247–254
Barker PJ, Reynolds W, Stevenson C 1997 The human science basis of psychiatric nursing: theory and practice. Journal of Advanced Nursing 25: 660–667
Barton R 1976 Institutional neurosis, 3rd edn. John Wright and Sons, Bristol
Brooker C 1990 Expressed emotion and psychosocial intervention: a review. International Journal of Nursing Studies 27(3): 267–276
Brooker C 2001 A decade of evidence-based training for work with people with serious mental health problems: progress in the development of psychosocial interventions. Journal of Mental Health 10(1): 17–31
Brooker C, Evans J 1999 Charting the growth of psycho-social interventions training for mental health professionals in the United Kingdom. School of Nursing, Midwifery and Health Visiting, University of Manchester, Manchester

Brooker C, Falloon I, Butterworth A, Goldberg D, Graham-Hole V, Hillier V 1994 The outcome of training community psychiatric nurses to deliver psychosocial intervention. British Journal of Psychiatry 165: 222–230

Brooker C, White E 1997 The fourth quinquennial national community mental health nursing census of England and Wales. The Universities of Manchester and Keele, Manchester and Keele

Brown B, Crawford P, Darongkamas J 2000 Blurred roles and permeable boundaries: the experience of multidisciplinary working in community mental health. Health and Social Care in the Community 8(6): 425–435

Burke J 1996 Community psychiatric nursing: the development of the service. Nursing Times Research 1(3): 229–237

Burns T, Creed F, Fahy T, Thompson S, Tyrer P, White I (for the UK700 Group) 1999 Intensive versus standard case management for severe psychotic illness: a randomised trial. The Lancet 353: 2185–2189

Carter MF, Evans KE, Crosby C, Prendergast LA, De Sousa Butterworth KA 1997 The all-Wales community mental health team survey. Health Services Research Unit, University of Wales, Bangor

Community Psychiatric Nurses' Association 1996 Untitled report of CPNA survey. CPNA Today, December 2

Department of Health 1989a Caring for people: community care in the next decade and beyond. HMSO, London

Department of Health 1989b Working for patients. HMSO, London

Department of Health 1990 The care programme approach for people with a mental illness referred to the specialist psychiatric services. HC(90)23/LASSL(90)11. Department of Health, London

Department of Health 1994 Working in partnership: a collaborative approach to care. HMSO, London

Department of Health 1995 Building bridges: a guide to arrangements for interagency working for the care and protection of severely mentally ill people. Department of Health, London

Department of Health 1998a Modernising mental health services: safe, sound and supportive. Department of Health, London

Department of Health 1998b Frank Dobson outlines third way for mental health. Press release 98/311. Department of Health, London

Department of Health 1999a Effective care co-ordination in mental health services: modernising the care programme approach. Department of Health, London

Department of Health 1999b National service framework for mental health: modern standards and service models. Department of Health, London

Department of Health 2001 Patients to get quicker access to medicines. Press release 2001/0223. Department of Health, London

Department of Health 2002 Draft Mental Health Bill. The Stationery Office, London

Galvin SW, McCarthy S 1994 Multidisciplinary community teams: clinging to the wreckage. Journal of Mental Health 3: 167–174

Gamble C 1995 The Thorn nurse training initiative. Nursing Standard 9(15): 31–34

Goffman E 1961 Asylums. Penguin, Harmondsworth

Goodwin S 1997 Comparative mental health policy: from institutional to community care. Sage, London

Gournay K 1994 Redirecting the emphasis to serious mental illness. Nursing Times 90(25): 40–41

Gournay K 2000 Role of the community psychiatric nurse in the management of schizophrenia. Advances in Psychiatric Treatment 6: 243–251

Gournay K, Brooking J 1994 Community psychiatric nurses in primary health care. British Journal of Psychiatry 165: 231–238

Gournay K, Gray R 2001 Should mental health nurses prescribe? Maudsley Discussion Paper No. 11. Institute of Psychiatry, London

Hannigan B 1998 Fragmentation or integration? Mental Health Nursing 18(1): 4–6

Hunter P 1974 Community psychiatric nursing in Britain: an historical review. International Journal of Nursing Studies 11: 223–233

Kingdon DG 1998 Cognitive behaviour therapy for severe mental illness: strategies and techniques. In: Brooker C, Repper J (eds) Serious mental health problems in the community: policy, practice and research, pp. 184–203. Baillière Tindall, London

Laing RD, Esterson A 1964 Sanity, madness and the family. Penguin, Harmondsworth

Marshall M, Creed F 2000 Assertive community treatment: is it the future of community care in the UK? International Review of Psychiatry 12: 191–196

Marshall M, Lockwood A 2000 Assertive community treatment for people with severe mental disorders. Cochrane Database of Systematic Reviews, Issue 1

Means R, Smith R 1998 Community care: policy and practice, 2nd edn. Macmillan, Basingstoke

Muijen M, Ford R 1996 The market and mental health: intentional and unintentional incentives. Journal of Interprofessional Care 10(1): 13–22

National Assembly for Wales 2001 Adult mental health services for Wales: equity, empowerment, effectiveness, efficiency. Strategy document. NAfW, Cardiff

Onyett S, Heppleston T, Bushnell D 1994 The organisation and operation of community mental health teams in England. The Sainsbury Centre for Mental Health, London

Onyett S, Standen R, Peck E 1997 The challenge of managing community mental health teams. Health and Social Care in the Community 5(1): 40–47

Pedler M 1998 Mind responds to Dobson's announcement. OpenMind 95: 4

Robb B 1967 Sans everything: a case to answer. Nelson, London

Rogers A, Pilgrim D 2001 Mental health policy in Britain, 2nd edn. Palgrave, Basingstoke

Sainsbury Centre for Mental Health 1997 Pulling together: the future roles and training of mental health staff. The Sainsbury Centre for Mental Health, London

Sayce L, Craig TKJ, Boardman AP 1991 The development of community mental health centres in the UK. Social Psychiatry and Psychiatric Epidemiology 26: 14–20

Stein LI, Santos AB 1998 Assertive community treatment of persons with severe mental illness. Norton, London

Stein LI, Test MA 1980 Alternative to mental hospital treatment. I: conceptual model, treatment programme and clinical evaluation. Archives of General Psychiatry 37: 392–397

Thornicroft G, Goldberg D 1998 Has community care failed? Maudsley Discussion Paper No. 5. Institute of Psychiatry, London

Tyrer P 2000 The future of the community mental health team. International Review of Psychiatry 12: 219–225

Welsh Assembly Government 2002 Adult mental health services. A national service framework for Wales. Welsh Assembly Government, Cardiff

Welsh Office 1996 Guidance on the care of people in the community with a mental illness. Welsh Office, Cardiff

White E 1993 Community psychiatric nursing 1980 to 1990: a review of organisation, education and practice. In: Brooker C, White E (eds) Community psychiatric nursing: a research perspective, vol. 2, pp. 1–26. Chapman and Hall, London

White E, Brooker C 1990 The care programme approach. Nursing Times 87(12): 66–67

FURTHER READING

Books

Barker P 1999 The philosophy and practice of psychiatric nursing. Churchill Livingstone, Edinburgh

This eloquent and accessible book brings together a collection of Phil Barker's papers, together with commentaries from other leading mental health nurses. Barker's perspective on the 'proper focus' of mental health nursing is covered in detail here.

Brooker C, Repper J (eds) 1998 Serious mental health problems in the community: policy, practice and research. Baillière Tindall, London

This edited book includes contributions from a range of authoritative writers, and gives an excellent account of context and practice in the care of people with severe mental health problems.

Hannigan B, Coffey M (eds) 2003 The handbook of community mental health nursing. Routledge, London

This book brings together authoritative contributions from leading mental health researchers, educators and practitioners to provide a comprehensive text for community mental health nurses in training and practice.

Journals

Journal of Psychiatric and Mental Health Nursing. This is probably the UK's leading research-led mental health nursing journal.

Journal of Mental Health, volume 9, number 6. The final edition of this journal in 2000 included a Special Section on mental health nursing, which comprised four separate papers and two commentaries. This is a useful place to start in terms of current debates and perspectives in the field.

Internet

The on-line psychiatric nursing discussion list, owned by Len Bowers of City University, London, can be accessed at www.jiscmail.ac.uk/lists/psychiatric-nursing.html. This is a lively forum for the exchange of news and views, and includes contributions from nurses all around the world.

21

Community learning disability nursing

R. Wyn Williams
L. Rhead

KEY ISSUES

- The values and principles that underpin community learning disability nursing.

- Role of the community learning disability nurse.

- Implementation of clinical governance.

- Influences and opportunities for community learning disability nursing.

INTRODUCTION

The aim of this chapter is to give an overview of the development of community learning disability nursing (CLDN) identifying some of the key issues facing learning disability nurses today. The value base and principles underpinning CLDN are reviewed in light of current legislation and policy. The role of the community nurse is discussed considering current professional guidelines (such as UKCC 1998a), UK policies and national strategies (such as DoH 2001, NHS and Community Care Act 1990, Health Act 1999, NAW 1999, NHS Plan 2000, Scottish Executive 2000). The requirements of clinical governance are discussed with examples given from practice focusing on audit, clinical supervision and reflection. The chapter concludes with future aspirations and challenges for the role such as nurse consultant, prescribing, generic role and health facilitator.

THE VALUES AND PRINCIPLES THAT UNDERPIN COMMUNITY LEARNING DISABILITY NURSING

In the 1970s following the publication of the White Paper *Better Services for the Mentally Handicapped* (DoH 1971), the newly established National Development Team laid out the blueprint for what has come to be the role of the community nurse for people with learning disabilities. The role has evolved as an outreach worker supporting carers (mostly parents) as a way of preventing admission into the largely inappropriate hospital settings. The reprovisioning process gathered momentum throughout the late 1970s and people with learning disabilities began to resettle from hospital.

By the early 1980s community learning disability teams emerged as a way of co-ordinating and supporting new services as well as maintaining their direct involvement with families and people with learning disabilities. In 1982 there were 70 teams in England and by 1987 there were five times that number, totalling 348 (NHS Executive 2000). This huge area of development reflects the view that services for people with learning disabilities should provide support and assistance that is noninstitutionalized.

Services for people with learning disabilities are, and arguably have been, in a constant state of change since the late 1960s, with the resettlement of learning disabled people from institutional facility-based environments to individualized community provision, being the central shift. Latterly, the disabled people movement, value-based and disability theories, primary legislation, contemporary social policy, and nursing have been a part of the enormous changes that have occurred. In response, the role of the nurse for people with learning disabilities has undergone considerable change and several reports have contributed to this transformation; the Briggs Report (DHSS 1972), Jay Report (DHSS 1979), Cullen Report (DoH 1989), DoH (1995a), have initiated and shaped the debate.

The rest of this chapter will focus on three international trends that have shaped the values and principles of learning disability services and discuss the role of the nurse in meeting the needs of people with a learning disability though the three tenets set out below:

1. The ideology of normalization, or social role valorization (SRV) (Wolfensberger 1972, 1983, 1998).
2. The increased legislative basis of rights in society from the United Nations Declaration of Rights (1946), The Human Rights Act (1998), Disability Discrimination Act (1996), Community Care (Direct Payments) Act (1996), and the increased role and empowerment of user groups

and other organizations that represent their needs.
3. The principles of ordinary life as embodied in legislation such as the All Wales Strategy for the Mentally Handicapped (Welsh Office 1983), NHS and Community Care Act 1990, and through influential papers such as An Ordinary Life (Kings Fund 1980) and the seminal five service accomplishments (O'Brien 1987).

It is important to remember in discussing these central themes that they are inherently connected to one another. Therefore no one theme can be seen as being more important than the other and reference should be made to each in any discussion of learning disability service provision.

NORMALIZATION

The history of normalization is long; Bank-Mikkelson (1969) defined the goal of normalization as 'an existence as close to the normal as possible'. Nirje (1969) further refined normalization as 'patterns and conditions of everyday life that are as close as possible to the norms and patterns of the mainstream of society'. Britain and North America have been more influenced by the later redefinitions of the principle by Wolf Wolfensberger (1972, 1983, 1992, 1998). The ideology of normalization in the 1970s was seen partly as an answer to the hospital scandals and fuelled the debate against institutional care. It was seen by some as a blueprint for noninstitutional services.

The goal of normalization is to integrate the devalued individual into society, through the acquisition of enhanced image and competence. As a direct result, it is anticipated that valued social roles will emerge.

Although the influence of normalization can still be seen today in service development and policy, the principles of normalization and SRV are not official policy in the UK. Academics and service planners have accepted the concept of normalization, although Chappell (1992) suggests that these concepts have not filtered down to the practitioners.

However critics of normalization/social role valorization suggest that the ideas inherent within it only further disable and disempower those it purports to serve. Chappell (1992) argues that the notion of cultural valued roles for people with learning disabilities fails to support the valuable characteristics of people with a learning disability. Hence the community nurse for people with learning disabilities has a role in promoting the positive facets of the client group, which will be discussed in relation to empowerment.

RIGHTS

The acceptance that individuals have unalienable rights, and freedom for themselves and protection of these rights from others became a central idea in the international community following the Second World War. The United Nations Declaration on Human Rights (1948) made clear that no one life was in any way less than another and that where infringements to this occurred, action in international law might be pursued.

Rights such as race relations, sexual equality, labour law all served to make a fairer and more equal society. The picture however for people with disabilities in law was quite different, in spite of the constant lobbying of People First, Values into Action, Citizen Advocacy and others, who campaigned tirelessly for equality in law. Legislation such as the 1986 Disabled Person's Act sought to give some measure of rights to disabled people, yet it fell far short of being an effective means to ensure and protect rights for disabled people.

It was not until 1996 that legislation against disability discrimination was enacted. However, even the Disability Discrimination Act (HMSO 1995) fails as an effective means of protecting the rights of people with learning disability within our society. The feelings around the rights of disabled people within the UK at this time, are articulated by Redworth and Redworth (1997, p. 182), who stated that: 'Disabled people are not perceived as nor function as citizens nor do they have full citizenship rights and responsibilities within Western society'.

Although The Human Rights Act (1998) makes it possible for a person to pursue the rights and freedoms guaranteed by the European Convention on Human Rights in the UK courts. However the Act's full significance has yet to be seen and the emerging case law to date suggests the implications for public bodies will be immense. The Act will enable those who feel their rights have been infringed to claim. (See Chapter 13 for further discussion of legal implications.)

Public bodies are having to consider the services they provide and the manner in which they do so, in light of the act. This may facilitate open debate and ensure that basic rights are respected (HMSO 2000). This legislation will impact on CLDNs, who will need to consider their practice within the context of enhanced rights for service users.

ORDINARY LIFE

It has been over 30 years since the last White Paper (1971) and the new White Paper, *Valuing the People. A New Strategy for Learning Disability for the 21st Century* (DoH 2001), sets out how government will provide new opportunities for individuals with learning disability, to live full and independent lives as part of their local communities. In the period following devolution, Wales and Scotland have launched similar strategies to achieve inclusive and participatory lives for people with learning disabilities.

John O'Brien's service accomplishments (1987) have been used to measure the level of participation of people with learning disabilities in community settings (see Box 21.1). Central to this is the premise of choice and autonomy, allowing the individual to govern their own lives. To achieve an ordinary life within the context of learning disability services is paradoxically an extraordinary achievement.

The aim of services today is the development of valued lifestyles in which the people themselves

---

Box 21.1 John O'Brien's (1987) five accomplishments essential to quality of life

1. Community presence
2. Choice
3. Competence
4. Respect
5. Community participation

have greater choice over their lives and are integrated into their local communities (NHS and Community Care Act 1990, O'Brien 1987, Welsh Office 1983). The notion of an ordinary life can be clearly seen in the All Wales Strategy (AWS) (Welsh Office 1983). That is, people with learning disabilities have:

◆ the right to an ordinary pattern of life within the community
◆ the right to be treated as an individual
◆ the right to additional help and support in developing their maximum potential.

These principles underpin the services in Wales and have influenced UK service development for the past 18 years.

The principles of SRV, rights and ordinary living patterns are at the heart of care practice today. However, they do not describe the clinical practice of the community learning disability nurse who works in complex and dynamic settings. Increasingly the competing tensions of addressing health needs within a multiagency and multidisciplinary setting means that the community learning disability nurse requires many skills and attributes in order to deliver best practice. (See Chapter 15 for a more detailed discussion on team working.)

The following section outlines the contexts in which the community learning disability nurse practices, the challenges they face and some approaches that may assist in supporting people with a learning disability.

THE ROLE OF THE COMMUNITY LEARNING DISABILITY NURSE

Using the following headings as a framework for discussion, the role of the community learning disability nurse will be explored:

◆ the appropriate identification and assessment of need
◆ promoting and maintaining health
◆ empowerment and enabling environments
◆ partnerships of care.

THE APPROPRIATE IDENTIFICATION AND ASSESSMENT OF NEED

Assessment is an essential aspect of the CLDN role. It enables the practitioner to obtain information about a client's health needs and wishes, prior to intervention. The client and carer are involved in the assessment process, which often begins with an exploration of health need from a broad perspective. The OK Health Check (Matthews 1996), although basic, provides a reasonable foundation from which to begin such an assessment.

The assessment tools utilized by the CLDN appear to vary from team to team, however they usually address similar areas such as epilepsy, communication, relationships, behavioural difficulties and daily living skills. The client's blood pressure, pulse, body mass index and urinalysis, etc. may also be monitored. This initial assessment often leads to more in-depth exploration of specific areas. The Case study 21.1 provides an example of assessments used.

Case Study 21.1

Sue is a 43-year-old woman who has Down syndrome and lives in a group home with minimal staff support. This lady was referred to the CLD team with symptoms of increased lethargy, urinary incontinence and occasional wandering from home.

Assessment one

The initial assessment revealed that Sue's cognitive and functional ability had gradually declined over a period of months. This had caused relationships within the home to become strained, as Sue was unable to complete her usual domestic tasks. Urinalysis showed no abnormality and an infection was therefore ruled out as a possible cause for the incontinence.

Assessment two

An assessment specifically looking at the health needs of people with Down syndrome was utilized. This highlighted that Sue needed blood tests for thyroid function and vitamin B12 deficiency. The possibility that Sue was suffering from dementia was also identified. This indicated the need for further monitoring and referral to other agencies.

Assessment three

A multidisciplinary risk assessment was carried out due to Sue's vulnerability when in the group home alone. This was reviewed regularly and management strategies amended in line with Sue's changing needs.

PROMOTING AND MAINTAINING HEALTH

When promoting the health of people with a learning disability several different approaches can be used. These are: medical; behavioural; educational; empowerment; and social change. Barr (1998) reports that any of these approaches could be utilized by the CLDN, depending on the needs of the individual and the other people involved. Ideally the approach should reflect the underlying principles and philosophy of care for learning disabled people such as empowerment, autonomy, choice and respect. (See Chapters 19 and 27 for more detailed work on empowerment.)

There are a number of key reasons for health promotion activity in learning disability nursing. Firstly, policy dictates that together with the primary healthcare team, the CLDN has a central role to play in the surveillance and promotion of health (DoH 1995b). Secondly, people with a learning disability experience both intrinsic and extrinsic difficulties when attempting to achieve and maintain optimal health. These difficulties are now explored.

Intrinsic difficulties

Intrinsic difficulties are those that the individual experiences because of the impact of their learning disability. These include the additional difficulties that learning disabled people experience in recognizing the signs and symptoms of illness. For example, people with a learning disability often have limited literacy skills and are therefore unable to access health promotion literature. In addition, they may not have the ability to communicate their health concerns due to intelligibility of speech, limited understanding, and memory and concentration problems (Van der Gaag 1998).

Further intrinsic difficulties may include the physical problems and ill health often associated with specific syndromes such as Down syndrome. These include congenital heart defects, increased incidence of dementia and thyroid dysfunction.

Extrinsic difficulties

Extrinsic or environmental problems include the inequity of access to healthcare services that learning disabled people often face. This can be due to problems with physical access, staff attitudes and transport difficulties (DoH 1998a). People with a learning disability are also known to experience difficulties in obtaining work, which can lead to low income, inadequate housing conditions and poverty. Such poverty is a large part of the everyday lives of learning disabled individuals (Davies et al 1995), and is associated with powerlessness, exclusion and an inability to participate in society (Naidoo & Wills 1998). (See Chapter 6 for a more detailed account of poverty). Circumstances such as these can have a detrimental effect on both the mental and physical health of people with a learning disability. The CLDN should therefore use health promotion activities to address these issues. (See Chapters 6, 7 and 27 for more information relating to health promotion.)

Health promotion is an enabling process which ultimately aims to enable people to improve their own health. (Barr 1998, p. 313).

This process encompasses activities such as health education and primary, secondary and tertiary prevention of health loss.

Health education

A fundamental aspect of health education is to shape the client's beliefs by providing health knowledge. This might include giving the client information on how to look after their body, how to access appropriate health services, or on factors in the wider environment that are detrimental to health (Downie et al 1996). The CLDN can simplify this information to make it interesting and easily understood. Many videos and uncomplicated leaflets now exist which can help with providing health knowledge. Prostheses can also be obtained from health promotion units and used to illustrate screening techniques, e.g. breast prostheses to demonstrate self breast examination. These can aid learning for clients with a learning disability by visually representing health-promoting activity.

The client's attitude and eventually their behaviour may also need to change, in order for health improvement to take place. Increasing the client's self-esteem and enabling them to make choices and be more assertive (Downie et al 1996) can facilitate changes in these areas. These measures should empower clients to resist pressures to conform, and allow them to take greater control of their lives.

In addition to the interventions carried out on an individual level, the CLDN should educate those in positions of power, about the specific health needs of people with a learning disability. This activity may be targeted at local health groups, community health councils and primary healthcare colleagues. The knowledge, beliefs, attitudes and behaviour of carers should also be targeted, as they are the main people who support the encouragement and maintenance of health-related behaviour in learning disabled clients (Sperlinger 1997). (See Chapter 7 for further work on community-based health promotion.)

Preventive measures can be divided into primary, secondary and tertiary prevention of health loss. Vernon (1997) states that action by the CLDN on these three levels will prevent health loss before it occurs, promote early detection of abnormalities and avoid needless progression of health deterioration. The Department of Health (1995b) highlights several areas of health need which the nurse can address through preventive measures. These include coronary heart disease, accidents, mental illness, cancers and sexual health.

Primary prevention

Using coronary heart disease as an example, the CLDN works in partnership with the client, to discourage smoking, reduce their intake of saturated fat and maintain adequately low blood pressure and cholesterol levels. This is important for learning disabled clients who often have reduced levels of fitness and increased obesity (Perry 1996). (See Chapter 5 for a more detailed discussion on coronary heart disease prevention.)

Secondary prevention

The early detection of health loss can be facilitated by routine health checks for learning disabled individuals (DoH 1998a). CLDNs should collaborate with their primary healthcare colleagues in order to facilitate such routine checks, which should include screening for particular conditions such as breast and testicular cancer.

Tertiary prevention

There are a number of ways in which the CLDN can prevent the needless progression of health deterioration. These include the management of physical conditions such as epilepsy or diabetes, teaching the individual to self-administer medication and the management of challenging behaviour and mental illness (Vernon 1997).

EMPOWERMENT AND ENABLING ENVIRONMENTS

Empowerment is the giving to individuals of power to take decisions in matters relating to themselves (Chambers Dictionary 1994). This is particularly important for learning disabled people, many of whom were marginalized, segregated and incarcerated in large hospitals or institutions. This type of institutional care had a devastating effect on learning disabled individuals and undermined their autonomy and self-determination. Factors such as loss of contact with the outside world, enforced idleness, bossiness of staff and loss of possessions, led to varying degrees of institutional neurosis (Barton 1960). This author describes institutional neurosis as a disease characterized by apathy, lack of initiative and submissiveness.

The closure of the large institutions and the increase in community care has had a significant effect on the lives of learning disabled individuals. Services now seek to bring about more valued lifestyles for people with a learning disability, in which they have greater control, representation and autonomy (DoH 1995b, 1998a). Despite these changes, many learning disabled clients continue to be affected by excessive parental control and other social and environmental barriers, which may limit access to work, leisure and education. Empowerment for the learning disabled client is therefore a central aspect of the CLDN role. Empowerment has been seen by Rodwell (1996) as essentially enabling others to recognize their strengths, abilities and their personal power. On an individual level, the CLDN can facilitate empowerment by providing clients with knowledge, skills and opportunities in autonomy, making choices, developing meaningful relationships, risk taking, rights awareness and independence.

The dictionary definition of empowerment appears to place an emphasis on the development of personal skills. However, the literature suggests that empowerment is also about creating empowering environments. Shepheard (1998) for example, states that CLDNs should promote the kind of environment where clients can explore matters of importance to themselves and make choices. (See Chapter 7 for further work on empowerment of communities.)

Family members or paid carers will form an important part of this process, which might be achieved through risk management. It is important to note that families often experience difficulties with empowering their learning disabled children because society does not understand or receive their child (Barnes 1997). Enabling the client to participate in community living from the earliest age should lead to integration and empowerment for these individuals.

PARTNERSHIPS OF CARE

Partnership and collaboration are used in a wide range of contexts and are enthusiastically encouraged as a way forward for services (DoH 1999, Health Act 1999, NAW 2000, 2001, NHS and Community Care Act 1990, NHS Plan 2000, WO 1998). Throughout the UK, CLDNs work in a variety of interprofessional settings.

There is an expectation that community nurses work in collaboration with other professionals to provide a seamless service for service users. Atkins and Walsh (1997) consider collaboration to be a significant factor in improving the quality of services. However, Leathard (1994) suggests that collaborative working is thriving because of the pressure to utilize scarce resources effectively. Lacey (1998) remarks that collaboration has gained a 'common sense' acceptance with 'little research to demonstrate the effectiveness' (p. 43). Conversely, public enquiry has led too often to identifying a lack of collaboration (Waterhouse 2000). As Fowler et al (2000) suggest the advantages of collaboration are sometimes measured by its absence.

Guidance documents such as the *Flexibilities for Joint Working in Health and Social Care* (NAW 2000) and the Health Act (HMSO 1999) encourage practitioners to focus on individual needs and create partnerships with the client and other agencies in providing a seamless service for the client (Mathias & Thompson 2001). Within some parts of the UK the setting up of integrated care trusts with social care and health care working within a single organization has begun. The strength of such organizations will be measured in the future by their collaborative and flexible working practices.

The work of community learning disability nurses depends on their competence in undertaking full and appropriate assessments. In identifying health need and developing effective individualized packages of care, the CLDN forges and facilitates working partnerships that empower the service user or client. However, as health professionals, they are subject to the requirements that clinical governance demands of all practitioners within the NHS today. The following section explores how CLDNs can fulfil their unique role with people who have a learning disability and meet the clinical governance agenda.

IMPLEMENTING CLINICAL GOVERNANCE IN COMMUNITY LEARNING DISABILITY NURSING

Methods which are used by the learning disability nurse, to facilitate clinical governance include the following separate but inter-related measures.

AUDIT

Audit is a continuing cycle of activity, which is aimed at improving services for learning disabled clients (Pougher 1997). Historically, it appears that audit has relied heavily on the scrutiny of nursing records, care plans, etc. This activity continues to be necessary in order to assess the quality of the record and identify areas for improvement (UKCC 1998b). However, in the current climate of client participation, it is essential that the views and opinions of learning disabled individuals are sought, and used as an indicator of service quality.

There are, of course, some inherent difficulties associated with obtaining feedback from learning disabled clients. These include acquiescence, communication difficulties, limited literacy skills and lack of autonomy exacerbated by the sometimes paternalistic attitudes of carers and care agencies. Such difficulties can be addressed or at least minimized, by employing imaginative strategies. For example Simon and Roy (1996) found that using facial expression cards increased the responsiveness of learning disabled clients and enabled them to express their level of satisfaction with services. Acquiescence can be minimized by rephrasing questions and asking clients to give an explanation to support their opinions (Murray et al 1998). The latter approach may only be appropriate for use with clients who have a mild learning disability.

It is essential that such methods are used to facilitate consumer audit for learning disabled individuals. This will lead to positive changes in service delivery and make services more client centred.

RISK MANAGEMENT

The move towards community care, from the segregated environment of the institutions has led to more independent and autonomous lifestyles for learning disabled clients, hence it can be argued that learning disabled individuals are becoming increasingly exposed to risk.

Most people take risks on a regular basis, simply by undertaking their normal daily routine. It is reasonable to assume however, that people with a learning disability may be less adept at calculating risk than members of the general population. For example, some individuals may have led a sheltered lifestyle, which prevented them from taking risks and learning from them. Others may not have the cognitive ability to make carefully considered judgements about certain hazardous situations. The risk management process is one way in which people with a learning disability can be empowered to take reasonable risks and lead more fulfilling lives as a result. Risk taking can provide learning disabled individuals with opportunities for emotional growth and is consistent with theories of social role valorization (Shirtliffe 1995).

The CLDN is therefore presented with conflict between professional accountability and the desire to promote the client's independence and autonomy. For example, it is arguable that O'Brien's (1987) five service accomplishments of community presence, relationships, competence, choice and respect, provide learning disabled clients with both opportunities and risks. It is therefore essential that the risk management process is employed by CLDNs in their daily practice.

Risk management is a systematic and considered process for making professional judgements about risk (UKCC 1998a). An important aspect of risk management is the assessment of potential benefits versus potential harm. This process should involve the client and carer and employ a multiagency, multiprofessional approach (Saunders 1998). These measures, along with accurate record keeping, should enable the CLDN to exercise their accountability, while fostering client independence and empowerment.

Case study examples of risk management in practice

Case Study 21.2

Joan is a 50-year-old lady who has a moderate learning disability. She has recently moved into a small community group home from a large institutional establishment. This lady experienced very limited independence and autonomy prior to moving, and wished to spend short periods of time alone in her new home. Staff however, felt unable to leave Joan alone in the house, even for short periods. This situation was particularly difficult when only one staff member was on duty and brief trips to the local shop, etc. were necessary. Joan would then be expected to leave the activity she was engaged in and go with the staff member, which she very much resented. A systematic, multidisciplinary approach was taken to weighing up the possible risks and benefits of enabling Joan to spend short periods of time alone in the house. Possible risks were then minimized and Joan now enjoys the type of independence and privacy that most of us take for granted. Other benefits to Joan included empowerment, choice, increased self-esteem and respect. The shared sense of responsibility and accountability facilitated by a multidisciplinary, multi-agency risk management process also appeared to allay staff anxieties and enhance decision-making.

Case Study 21.3

Jo is a 15-year-old young man with a mild learning disability. His parents are divorced and Jo was spending much of his time with his father, who actively encouraged him to drink large quantities of alcohol. Jo's alcohol abuse led to incidents of violent behaviour and was of great concern to his mother.

Numerous attempts were made to obtain a social worker for Jo, but to no avail. A multidisciplinary risk assessment was therefore carried out and a copy sent to social services. A social worker was allocated immediately. It appears that a risk assessment can be a powerfully persuasive tool.

CLINICAL SUPERVISION AND REFLECTION

Both reflection and clinical supervision can be used to facilitate clinical governance, through promotion of quality care. Clinical supervision is an exchange between two practising professionals, which aims to improve practice through reflection, problem solving and an increased understanding of professional issues (UKCC 2001). The purpose of reflection is to enable the practitioner to learn from lived experiences and thereby increase clinical effectiveness (Johns 1995). Numerous models can be used to facilitate reflection, such as Gibbs (1988) and Schön (1983).

The shift towards community care for learning disabled clients, has significantly increased the importance of supervision for the CLDN. Working in the community setting, means that the CLDN is more autonomous and therefore more accountable than ever before. Supervision can be viewed as an activity that reduces vulnerability through validation and support, an opportunity to explore and express personal distress, and a regular space for reflection (Rea 1998). Benefits to clients from clinical supervision may include better quality care and more effective risk management by having 'blind spots' in the clinician's practice identified (Cutcliffe & Epling 1997).

EVIDENCE-BASED PRACTICE

Clinical governance is facilitated by practice based on evidence of effectiveness. This is supported by lifelong learning and continuing professional development (UKCC 2001), which will in turn inspire public confidence and meet individual learning need (DoH 1998a). Specialist practitioner status will enable the CLDN to meet these objectives by demonstrating a higher level of decision-making, developing and leading practice and contributing to research (UKCC 1999a). The latter is particularly significant, due to the dearth of research in learning disability nursing.

INFLUENCES AND OPPORTUNITIES FOR COMMUNITY LEARNING DISABILITY NURSING

The extension and expansion of the CLDN role will now be explored and some of the current debates affecting nursing considered in this discussion:

♦ The full impact of the Human Rights Act (1998) is yet to be fully realized and the result may be claims lodged against the NHS under the schedules of the Act. The CLDN is in a prime position to inform clients of the Act so they acquire a greater awareness of what it may mean for them. The effect on service provision may include changes in places of residence, mediation and care planning strategies for people with difficult and challenging behaviour.

♦ The question as to whether CLDNs should prescribe is open to debate. Prescribing has the potential to increase opportunities for nurse-led clinics/units such as Assessment and Treatment Units. However, the ability of the CLDN to prescribe should not replace the right of learning disabled people to access generic primary health care. It is clear that changes in legislation surrounding nurse prescribing will impact on community learning disability nursing. To what extent this would affect their role and practice remains to be seen.

♦ The future 'education' of community learning disability nursing is also a constant subject of debate. Nurses need to take an active part in future decisions relating to education. Issues currently being discussed include generic nursing, learning disability nursing and social work joint training, all graduate status and preparation of unqualified care staff working in learning disability services. Educational providers must work in partnership with learning disabled people and services to ensure that the future provision of education prepares CLDNs that are fit for purpose.

♦ The impact of *Fitness to Practice*' (UKCC 1999b) will need to be evaluated carefully. There is currently discussion as to the number of nursing branches required and the preferred option for the preparation of nurses at a pre-registration level remains a great uncertainty (UKCC 2001).

♦ *Valuing the People* (2001) identifies the role of the 'health facilitator'. Although this document does not identify community learning disability nurses as health facilitators, it could potentially become a nursing role in the future.

♦ The creation of nurse consultants in 1998 heralded a new age for nursing. For some, the role enhances the standing and influence of nurses in an increasingly sophisticated health setting or alternatively it could be viewed as simply dressing up a demoralized workforce. We may see an increase in the number of consultant community learning disability nurses in the future. (See Chapter 24 for more detailed discussion of new nursing roles.)

CONCLUSION

This chapter has provided an overview of some of the issues that have influenced the development of community learning disability nursing, shaped its practice and outlined factors that continue to challenge this area of nursing. Issues relating to professional practice and skilled implementation of care have been discussed in the light of the nurses' role and the importance of collaborative practice has been identified. A brief account such as this cannot be seen as exhaustive; it is simply intended to be a starting point for discussion and reflection. The issues raised within this chapter are pertinent to all disciplines involved with the care and support of people with a learning disability. Through discussion, the developing role of the CLDN can be articulated. It is important that research into this area of nursing is encouraged and national networks established to share good practice and innovation within the field of CLDN.

SUMMARY

♦ The value base of learning disability nursing is strongly influenced by social role valorization, human rights and ordinary life principles.

♦ CLDN practice is framed within a health context. Within this, risk management, evidence-based practice, audit and clinical governance are issues central to their work.

♦ The role of the community learning disability nurse has been viewed through the philosophy of health promotion, empowering relationships, appropriate assessment of need and partnerships in care.

◆ The continuously evolving context of learning disability nursing requires nurses to be flexible and adaptable, utilizing their unique skills to maintain and support the valued lifestyles of people with learning disabilities.

DISCUSSION POINTS

1. Consider ways in which clients could be included in the development of local and national policy.

2. Guidance from government suggests that healthcare professionals should engage in interprofessional work. Examine the ways in which your team engages in interprofessional working practices and list how collaboration might be improved.

3. In relation to clinical governance consider the influence of this framework on your practice and service provision.

4. Identify the possible role of the CLDN in prescribing medication and consider in what contexts the CLDN could utilize the ability to prescribe.

5. In what ways may initiatives such as the consultant nurse and nurse-led clinics develop the role of the CLDN.

REFERENCES

Atkins JM, Walsh RS 1997 Developing shared learning in multiprofessional health care education: for whose benefit? Nurse Education Today 17: 319–324

Bank-Mikkelson N 1969 Denmark. A metropolitan area in Denmark: Copenhagan. In: Kugel R, Wolfensberger W (eds) Changing patterns in residential services for the mentally retarded. Presidents committee on mental retardation, Washington

Barnes M 1997 Families and empowerment. In: Ramcharan P, Robers G, Grant G, Borland J (eds) Empowerment in everyday life: Learning disability. Jessica Kingsley, London

Barr O 1998 Responding to the health needs of people with learning disabilities. In: Thompson T and Matthias P (eds) Standards and learning disability, 2nd edn. Baillière Tindall, London

Barton R 1960 Institutional neurosis. Stonebridge Press, Bristol

Chambers Dictionary 1994 Chambers Harrap Publishers Ltd, Edinburgh

Chappell AL 1992 Towards a sociological critique of normalisation principle. Disability, Handicap and Society 7(1): 35–51

Cutliffe J, Epling M 1997 An exploration of the use of John Heron's confronting interventions in clinical supervision: case studies from practice. Psychiatric Care 4(4): 178–180

Davis A, Eley R, Flynn M, Flynn P, Roberts G 1995 To have and have not: addressing issues of poverty. In: Philpot T, Ward L (eds) Values and visions. Changing ideas in services for people with learning difficulties, pp. 334–345. Butterworth-Heinemann, Oxford

Department of Health 1989 Caring for people: community care in the next decade and beyond (Cullen Report), Cmnd 849. HMSO, London

Department of Health 1995a Continuing the commitment. The report of the Learning Disability Project. HMSO, London

Department of Health 1995b Health of the nation: A strategy for people with learning disabilities. HMSO, London

Department of Health 1998a Signposts for success in commissioning and providing health services for people with learning disabilities. NHS Executive, London

Department of Health 1998b A first class service: Quality in the new NHS. Department of Health, London

Department of Health 1999 Saving lives – Our healthier nation. HMSO, London

Department of Health 2000 NHS plan. A plan for investment. A plan for reform. Department of Health, London

Department of Health 2001 Valuing the people. A new strategy for learning disability for the 21st century. A white paper. CM5086. HMSO, London. Accessed @ http://www.official-documents.co.uk/document/cm50/5086/5086.htm

Department of Health and Social Security 1971 Better services for the mentally handicapped. HMSO, London

Department of Health and Social Security 1972 Report of the Committee on Nursing (Briggs Committee), Cmnd 5115. HMSO, London

Department of Health and Social Security 1979 Report of the Committee of Enquiry into Mental Handicap Nursing and Care (Jay Report), Cmnd 7468. HMSO, London

Downie RS,Tanahill C, Tanahill A 1996 Health promotion models and values, 2nd edn. Oxford University Press, London

Fowler P, Hannigan B, Northway R 2000 Community nurses and social workers learning together: a report of an interprofessional education initiative in South Wales. Health and Social Care in the Community 8(3): 186–191

Gibbs G 1988 Learning by doing: A guide to teaching and learning methods. Further Education Unit, Oxford Polytechnic, Oxford

HMSO 1986 Disabled Person's Act. HMSO, London

HMSO 1990 National Health Service and Community Care Act. Accessed @ http://www.hmso.gov.uk/acts/summary/01990019.htm

HMSO 1995 Disability Discrimination Act. Accessed @ http://www.hmso.gov.uk/acts/acts1995/1995050.htm

HMSO 1996 Community Care (Direct Payments) Act. Accessed @ http://www.hmso.gov.uk/acts/acts1996/1996030.htm

HMSO 1998 Human Rights Act. HMSO, London

HMSO 1999 Health Act. Accessed @ http://www.hmso.gov.uk/acts/acts1999/19990008.htm

HMSO 2000 Human Rights Act. An Introduction. HMSO, London

Johns C 1995 Framing learning through reflection with Carper's ways of knowing in nursing. Journal of Advanced Nursing 22: 226–234

King's Fund 1980 An ordinary life – Comprehensive locally-based services for mentally handicapped people. King's Fund, London

Lacey P 1998 Interdisciplinary training for staff working with people with profound and multiple learning disabilities. Journal of Interprofessional Care 12(1): 43–52

Leathard A (ed) 1994 Going inter-professional. Working together for health and welfare. Routledge, London

Mathias P, Thompson T 2001 Interprofessional and multi-agency working. In: Thompson J, Pickering S (eds) Meeting the health needs of people who have a learning disability. Baillière Tindall, London

Matthews DR 1996 The OK Health Check. Fairfield Publications, Preston

Murray C, McKeenzie K, Kidel G, Lakhani S, Sinclair B 1998 A framework for obtaining customer feedback in a health service community learning disability team. British Journal of Learning Disabilities 26(3): 94–99

National Assembly for Wales 1999 Realising the potential. A strategic framework for nursing, midwifery and health visiting in Wales. NAW, Cardiff

National Assembly for Wales 2000 Flexibilities for joint working in health and social care. NAW, Cardiff

National Assembly for Wales 2001 A plan for the NHS with its partners. Improving health in Wales. NAW, Cardiff

NHS Executive 2000 Community specialist services. Accessed 29/10/01 @ http://www.doh.gov.uk/london/learningdisabilities/css.htm

Naidoo J, Wills J 1998 Practicing health promotion: Dilemmas and challenges. Baillière Tindall, London

Nirje B 1969 The normalisation principle and its human management implications. In: Kugel R, Wolfensberger W (eds) Changing patterns in residential services for the mentally retarded. Presidents committee on mental retardation, Washington

O'Brien J 1987 A guide to lifestyle planning. In: Bellamy GT, Wilcox B (eds) The activities catalog. Paul H Brookes Publishing Co, London

Perry M 1996 Treating obesity in people with learning disabilities. Nursing Times 92(35): 37–38

Pougher J 1997 Providing quality care. In: Gates B (ed.) Learning disabilities. Churchill Livingstone, New York

Rea K 1998 Supervision. In: Thompson T, Mattias P (eds) Standards and learning disability, 2nd edn. Baillière Tindall, London

Redworth M, Redworth F 1997 Learning disability and citizenship: paradigms for inclusion. Journal of Learning Disabilities for Nursing, Health and Social Care 1(4): 181–185

Rodwell CM 1996 An analysis of the concept of empowerment. Journal of Advanced Nursing 23: 305–313

Saunders M 1998 Risk management. In: Thompson T, Mathias P (eds) Standards and learning disability, 2nd edn. Baillière Tindall, London

Schön D 1983 Educating the reflective practitioner. Josey Bass, San Francisco

Scottish Executive 2000 The same as you? A review of services for people with learning disabilities. Tactica Solutions, Scotland

Shepheard J 1998 Learning disability: Empowerment. Nursing Standard 12(17): 49–55

Shirtliffe D 1995 Risk taking for clients with learning disabilities. Nursing Times 91(5): 40–42

Simon F, Roy M 1996 Consumer audit in community learning disability teams. British Journal of Learning Disabilities 24(4): 145–149

Sperlinger A 1997 Introduction. In: O'Hara J, Sperlinger A (eds) Adults with learning disabilities: A practical approach for health professionals. John Wiley and Sons, Chichester

UKCC 1998a Guidelines for mental health and learning disabilities nursing. UKCC, London

UKCC 1998b Guidelines for records and record keeping. UKCC, London

UKCC 1999a A higher level of practice. UKCC, London

UKCC 1999b Fitness for practice. UKCC, London

UKCC 2001 Supporting nurses, midwives and health visitors through lifelong learning. UKCC, London

Universal Declaration of Human Rights 1948 Accessed @ http://www.unhchr.ch/udhr/index.htm

Van der Gaag A 1998 Communication skills and adults with learning disabilities: eliminating professional myopia. British Journal of Learning Disabilities 26: 88–93

Vernon D 1997 Health. In: Gates B (ed.) Learning disabilities, 3rd edn. Churchill Livingstone, New York

Waterhouse R 2000 Report of the tribunal of inquiry into the abuse of children in care in the former county council areas of Gwynedd and Clwyd since 1974 – Lost in care. Accessed @ http://www.doh.gov.uk/lostincare/20102.htm

Welsh Office 1983 The All Wales Strategy for the development of services for the mentally handicapped. Welsh Office, Cardiff

Welsh Office 1998 Better health – Better Wales (Cm 3922). Welsh Office, Cardiff

Wolfensberger W 1972 The principle of normalization in human services. National Institute on Mental Retardation, Toronto

Wolfensberger W 1983 Social role valorization: A proposed new term for the principle of normalisation. Mental Retardation 21: 234–239

Wolfensberger W 1992 A brief introduction to social role valorization as a high-order concept for structuring human services, 2nd edn. Training Institute for Human Service Planning, Leadership & Change Agentry (Syracuse University), Syracuse, NY

Wolfensberger W 1998 A brief introduction to social role valorization: A high-order concept for addressing the plight of societally devalued people, and for structuring human services, 3rd edn. Training Institute for Human Service Planning, Leadership & Change Agentry (Syracuse University), Syracuse, NY

FURTHER READING

This list is not intended to be exhaustive, however it should provide a useful starting point.

Books

O'Hara J, Sperlinger A (eds) 1997 Adults with learning disabilities: a practical approach for health professionals. John Wiley and Sons, Chichester

Thompson J, Pickering S (eds) 2001 Meeting the health needs of people who have a learning disability. Baillière Tindall, London

Two general texts that provide a basis for further reading and discussion of the role of the CLDN.

On-line resources

Many on-line and web-based sites are available. These are useful links to documents and organizations.

Department of Health, accessed at http://www.doh.gov/uk

National Assembly for Wales, accessed at http://www.wales.gov.uk

Northern Ireland, accessed at http://www.dhssni.gov.uk

Scottish Health, accessed at http://www.scotland.gov.uk

Foundation of Nursing Studies accessed at www.fons.org/networks/nnldn. This site follows on the work initiated by Chris Elliot Canon, formally of the ENB. The foundation provides a forum for sharing good practice and also access to the learning disability discussion list.

General learning disability sites with excellent links, regularly updated: http://www.paradigm.org.uk, http://www.bild.org.uk

22

Community children's nursing

J. Muir
A. Sidey

INTRODUCTION

Community children's nursing is a relatively young discipline compared with more established branches of community nursing. As such, the corporate identity of services is still emerging. This lack of a traditional foundation can facilitate more imaginative and flexible approaches to identified care needs, however it can also cause confusion and misunderstanding for stakeholders and affect collaboration with other professional groups. In order to clarify the context of the current situation, this chapter begins with a brief overview of the development of community children's nursing services and then examines four key themes:

◆ roles and responsibilities: the context of community children's nursing
◆ ways of working: family nursing
◆ ways of working: interprofessional and multiagency case management
◆ challenges and opportunities for community children's nursing services.

Case studies will be used to illustrate significant points and to challenge current thinking.

THE DEVELOPMENT OF COMMUNITY CHILDREN'S NURSING

The formal existence of a community children's nursing service was first recorded in 1949 (Gillet 1954). Whilst the development of services has been

271

consistently supported in official reports and government directives since the 1950s, expansion of this provision remained slow until the early 1990s (Whiting 2000). The last decade has witnessed most growth and development in this discipline due to a number of reasons, which include:

◆ Medical advances that have enabled infants and children to survive what were once fatal disorders.

◆ The increased availability of medicines, therapies and technology to support associated care needs.

◆ The government agenda that has pursued a shift from secondary care to primary care alongside a philosophy of increasing consumer expectations.

◆ The recognition of community children's nursing as a discrete community specialist practitioner recordable qualification (United Kingdom Central Council (UKCC) 1994).

However, community children's nursing services are fragmented and anomalies continue to exist that give rise to confusion. For example, in a recent survey Eaton (2001) identified six different models of services in operation in the UK (Box 22.1).

Further to this, little over 50% of the UK have access to a service with only a minimal number able to offer 24-hour access (Royal College of Nursing (RCN) 2001). These variations have occurred essentially because current legislation regarding the care of sick children differs between hospital and community settings. For example, more than a decade ago, the Department of Health (DoH 1991) stated that there should be at least two qualified children's nurses on duty 24 hours a day in all hospital children's departments and wards, a notion that was reinstated following the Beverley Allitt inquiry (DoH 1994). However, such a standard does not apply to the care of sick children in the community, despite being a recommendation following the review of children's services by the House of Commons Health Committee (1997). Consequently, there has been a lack of understanding and commitment by commissioning and purchasing authorities to meet the needs of sick

---

Box 22.1 Models of community children's nursing services

Model 1: Hospital outreach – generalist
Model 2: Hospital outreach – specialist
Model 3: Community-based team
Model 4: Hospital at home
Model 5: District nursing service
Model 6: Ambulatory or assessment unit

---

children and their families in the community in some areas. The National Service Framework (NSF) for children should provide the opportunity to address this issue.

ROLES AND RESPONSIBILITIES: THE CONTEXT OF COMMUNITY CHILDREN'S NURSING

At present, community children's nursing and the role of the community children's nurse (CCN) lacks a clear professional corporate identity, an issue not unique to this discipline. A corporate identity strengthens the culture and values of a service and provides a signpost for all staff. The need to strengthen the corporate identity of the National Health Service (NHS) was a significant factor underpinning the development of the NHS University (DoH 2001a).

A stronger identity within community children's nursing would enhance interdependent working with other care providers. In order to facilitate this, the uniqueness of the CCN's role, alongside other nursing disciplines, needs to be established. A distinction between the titles that are often used synonymously within the literature (community children's nurse, clinical nurse specialist, specialist outreach nurse) follows.

Community children's nurses are registered children's nurses with a community specialist practitioner qualification. This role can be identified with models 1, 3 and 4 (Box 22.1). Based in either an acute or community setting, the CCN facilitates nursing care for a varied, yet defined, caseload of sick children in a range of community settings. The work of the CCN has been described as having seven broad areas (Box 22.2).

Box 22.2 The work of the community children's nurse

Supporting the families of children with long-term nursing needs

Supporting children with a disability

Supporting families who are caring for a child during the terminal phase of his/her life

Neonatal and postnatal care, including the care of children with complex problems arising from prematurity and disorders presenting at birth

Supporting children undergoing planned surgery

Caring for children with acute nursing needs, which can reduce the need for and duration of hospital admission

Follow up and support of children requiring emergency treatment which may assist the promotion of early discharge from hospital

---

Health Committee (1997)

A *clinical nurse specialist* (CNS) may work independent of, or within, a CCN team and concentrate on a disorder-specific subspeciality such as community neonatal nursing. The CNS is a qualified children's nurse, usually with an increased level of expertise and further training in the defined subspeciality but not necessarily in community nursing. This role concurs with model 2 (Box 22.1). Miller (1995) describes the role as clinical expert, resource consultant, educator, change agent, researcher, advocate and mentor. These themes resonate with dimensions of lecturer practitioner and nurse consultant roles and there is a need for clarification of the interface between such roles to minimize further confusion.

Conversely the *specialist outreach nurse* provides care from either a secondary or tertiary health care setting and is often a member of a specialist multiprofessional team. This role links most closely with models 2 and 6 (Box 22.1). The outreach nurse is a registered children's nurse with further training in the speciality but not necessarily in community nursing. The philosophy underpinning practice is often one of 'shared care' either between primary and tertiary settings, between primary and secondary care, or between all three (Hunt 2000). This model is particularly well established in the care of children with malignant disease.

Whilst some differences in these three roles are evident, they each aim to avoid admission to

hospital, reduce the length of hospital stay and provide a high-quality, effective service. This chapter is specifically concerned with the role and responsibilities of the CCN.

In the context of more established community nurses who work with children, such as health visitors (HVs) and school nurses (SNs), there are certain generic aspects that overlap with the CCN role. (See Chapters 19 and 23 for a detailed discussion of the health visitor and school nurse roles.) For example, health promotion and child protection clearly apply to the work of each of these three nurses but with varying degrees of emphasis (see Chapter 11 for a more detailed discussion of child protection issues). However, there are two distinguishing aspects to the CCN role that do not directly apply to other community nurses. Firstly, all CCNs are registered children's nurses and secondly, the main focus of their work is either to provide direct 'hands on' care or to facilitate and co-ordinate this in a range of community settings. This second component requires the CCN to be able to perform complex nursing procedures, such as changing a tracheostomy tube in a fragile baby whilst being observed by parents and untrained carers, and then to teach these same skills to those who may be emotionally vulnerable and lack confidence. This, therefore, demands unyielding confidence and advanced competence in teaching complex tasks to enable parents and other carers to become experts in the child's care.

Case Study 22.1

Roles and responsibilities

John is a young person of 11 years. He has had a complicated 7-year history of intractable constipation and recently had a colostomy performed as a result of this. He is reliant on oral medications. He receives support from a specialist outreach nurse, a CCN, a health visitor and school nurse. The specialist outreach nurse works within the gastroenterology team at the regional hospital. She initially visited John in the children's ward following his operation and now assesses him in a nurse-led clinic in the outpatient setting following his discharge home. Here, she will see him approximately four times per year to oversee the effectiveness of his treatment and provide the link between hospital and community provision. Following his assessment and adjustment to his treatment in the clinic, she liaises with the local team of CCNs to advise his named nurse of his continuing care needs between appointments. The CCN provides regular home visits to John and his family. The aim of these home visits is to teach John and his parents how to manage the colostomy; to assess the effectiveness of his medication and make appropriate changes according to his symptoms, and to act as a resource to the HV and SN. The HV will eventually provide ongoing home visiting support to John and his family once they are independent in his care management and his condition stabilizes, using the CCN as a resource only. She is also organizing a budget to provide regular supplies to the family and in the meantime, these continue to be supplied from the CCN budget. The SN works with the teachers to ensure that John has the necessary equipment, resources and support in school to enable him to attend without fear of being socially isolated. Each member of the team involved in John's care is dependent upon the effective communication of all members to ensure continuity.

Questions

1. How might John's care be configured differently?
2. With the focus on new ways of working, how might services for children in the community be delivered differently in the future?

WAYS OF WORKING: FAMILY NURSING

The ability for parents to negotiate their degree of involvement in their child's home care is limited by a lack of alternatives (Kirk 2001). The dearth of community children's nursing services in the UK means that parents are often required to learn complex skills and assume 24-hour responsibility for their child in order to achieve home care. This involves parents performing highly technical procedures that have previously been considered the domain of professionals, and perhaps extended nursing practice, and therefore adopting a 'neoprofessional' role. For example, this may entail administering intravenous therapy, providing tracheostomy support and administering parenteral feeding.

The terms most often associated with the work of CCN's are 'partnership' working and 'family-centred care'. However, the concept of 'family nursing' is gaining increasing recognition in the UK and may be more appropriate. Friedemann (1989) describes family nursing on three levels:

1. Individual: the nurse treats each individual in the family as an individual client.
2. Interpersonal: the nurse uses communication techniques with two or more individuals to address family processes such as decision-making, limit setting and defining family roles.
3. Family system nursing: the client becomes the whole family system and nursing goals are aimed at changes in the system.

Given the role expected of parents, it is necessary for the CCN to assess how the family works together as a team in meeting the complex demands made on them as a system and to identify their unique needs. This could be reframed into identifying both their personal and 'neoprofessional' needs. Recent evidence from both CCNs and families, as the recipients of services, would seem to support this notion. For example, research commissioned by the English National Board for Nursing, Midwifery and Health Visiting (ENB) identified 17 principles of CCN practice derived from interviews with families (Procter et al 1999) (Box 22.3).

These principles identify the fundamental need for the CCN to work in the context of the family as a whole and to work with the family as a unit of care. Principles such as 'fostering family empowerment' and 'promoting the health of families' relate both to family processes, using skills of 'listening and discovering', and to the client being the whole family system. This is further evidenced in the work of Carter (2000) whose study explored the role and skills used by CCNs caring for children with chronic illness. As a complement to the principles outlined in Box 22.3, CCNs themselves identified the need to have a deeply contextualized understanding of the child's and family's needs and the ability to work within an 'individual family's community'. This requires skilled negotiation and tremendous respect for the way

Box 22.3 Guiding principles of community children's nursing practice

1. Promoting family-centred care rather than child-centred care.
2. Maintaining or improving the quality of life of the family, rather than focusing on medical needs.
3. Minimizing stressful events rather than giving routinized care.
4. Fostering family empowerment rather than learned helplessness / dependency on professionals' solving abilities.
5. Having an approach of partnership rather than the imposition of professional expertise.
6. Appreciating the complexity of a problem rather than oversimplifying it.
7. Solving or reframing problems rather than avoiding them.
8. Recognizing the boundaries of own expertise and knowing where to turn for appropriate help, rather than trying to solve all problems independently.
9. Establishing credibility with paediatric and primary healthcare colleagues through working together openly rather than having an insular approach.
10. Having a flexible, organic, responsive role, rather than a formally directed set of functions.
11. Having knowledge gained through experience rather than procedures.
12. Having the knowledge to anticipate and plan for future directions in the care needs of the child, rather than reacting to crisis.
13. Being available (light touch) for the family when the family wants it, rather than when it is most convenient to services.
14. Promoting the health of families rather than focusing solely on tertiary interventions.
15. Lightening the burden through manner of approach, rather than getting caught up in the anxieties of the situation and reinforcing the burden.
16. Enabling children and families to lead ordinary lives, rather than this being regarded as secondary to biomedical interventions.
17. Listening and discovering rather than imposing ready-made solutions from elsewhere.

families choose to live their lives (Carter 2000). (See Chapter 12 for a more detailed discussion of family nursing.)

Case Study 22.2

Family nursing as a framework for practice

Rashider is 3 years old. She has an undiagnosed degenerative disorder that causes spastic quadriparesis and episodes of severe spasms. She is fully dependent for all activities of daily living. She has feeding problems and requires a gastrostomy tube for overnight feeds and the administration of medication. She is cared for at home by her parents – both aged 26 years – and her grandparents. She has two brothers. Imran is 6 years old and attends the local school. He suffers from severe, uncontrolled eczema. Yusuf is 4 years old and is still at home. She also has a baby sister of 3 months. Her mother is the main carer and is showing signs of stress, appearing withdrawn and tearful. Her father works long hours for a local company. At present the following services are involved in this family's care:

Community children's nurse	Health visitor
School nurse	Geneticist
Pre-school counsellor	Community paediatrician
Consultant neurologist	Asian liaison health worker
General practitioner	Dermatologist
Independent nurse for gastrostomy services	Social worker

Respite care services from a local voluntary agency have been offered but refused by the family

Questions

1. From this list of professionals, who could adopt a more central role in facilitating a family nursing approach, using the three levels as a guide?
2. What might be the goals for this family?

The need for continuity is imperative as the CCN works alongside the family while they develop their confidence and competence in providing highly skilled home care. The blurring of boundaries is an inevitable consequence, as parents become technical and intuitive experts in their child's care, often able to detect symptoms before professionals. This requires both professional maturity and flexibility on the part of the CCN in order to manage and develop appropriate relationship boundaries, which remain fluid as the home situation changes. These combined factors require skills that may be described as 'interpersonal' and 'intrapersonal' intelligence (Goleman 1995).

'Interpersonal intelligence is the ability to understand other people: what motivates them, how they work, how to work co-operatively with them' (Goleman 1995, p. 42). It includes the capacity to respond appropriately to the emotions, motivations and desires of other people. Intrapersonal intelligence, conversely, demands self-knowledge and looking inwards in order to access one's own feelings and to draw on them to guide behaviour. Both attributes are required in order to work with intelligence. This intelligence refers to the ability to 'be with' a situation whilst not needing one's own needs met or needing to have all the answers. Indeed, professionals who acknowledge their limitations have been shown to promote trust in the families they work with (Kirk 2001). It has been otherwise described as the 'emotional side of nursing' and refers to the nontechnical skills or 'soft' skills, including empathy, compassion, facilitation, listening to and being with families (Carter 2000). These skills are fundamental to the creation and maintenance of a supportive relationship with the child and family, an essential part of the CCN's role, and ability to nurse 'with' rather than 'of' the family (Carter 2000). However, there are challenges associated with this humanistic approach to practice, the most demanding of which is about creating the balance between personal and professional involvement. This phenomenon is not unique to CCN's practice. Since there are no guidelines to define the balance between the personal and professional relationship, an individual management strategy is required. For example, such a strategy might include a personal reflective journal coupled with more formal clinical supervision in order to foster an explicit acknowledgement of this area of practice that is often difficult to discuss openly. As part of professional practice, CCNs have a responsibility to work with other practitioners to find ways to uncover and share their experiences and develop flexible approaches to managing relationship boundaries. The notion of interprofessional team supervision could provide a useful framework to take this forward.

WAYS OF WORKING: INTER-PROFESSIONAL AND MULTIAGENCY CASE MANAGEMENT

It is clear that CCNs play a central role in the lives of families where there is a child with health and social needs and that a number of professionals and agencies are likely to be involved. This in itself requires great skill and negotiation on behalf of the CCN to effectively work within, and sometimes co-ordinate, complex packages of care.

Events in health care in recent years have brought the significance of interprofessional practice into sharp focus. Indeed, both the NHS Plan (DoH 2000) and the Kennedy Report (DoH 2001b), following the Bristol Inquiry, provide clear standards and recommendations for practice. No longer can practitioners afford to work in a professional vacuum. Most co-ordinated care requires a multiagency response that demands a collaborative effort of all those concerned with the care of the child and family (DoH 2001b). (See Chapter 15 for a detailed discussion of multiprofessional team working.)

The nature of home care for children with complex health care needs is often constant and long-term, requiring a vast number of professionals and agencies to be involved in supporting the family. It is not surprising that parents feel overwhelmed by a number of factors associated with this experience including:

◆ confusion around the roles and responsibilities of the different professionals
◆ the sheer number of visits from, and to, various professionals
◆ the need to co-ordinate the many services involved
◆ the need to act as advocate on behalf of their child.

These factors often require parents to act as their own keyworker in an attempt to negotiate and meet their needs. Consequently, parents may experience symptoms such as exhaustion, burnout and stress-related illness, directly attributed to the sustained nature of care giving and the lack of co-ordinated available support (Murphy 2001, Whyte et al 1998).

All professionals have a responsibility to act in the best interest of the child and their family and to ensure a co-ordinated programme of care. This requires teamwork and collaboration to break down professional barriers. Essential to this process is effective role negotiation and the clear

---

Box 22.4   Responsibilities of the keyworker

Key aspects of the role:
   Liaise between agencies
   Co-ordinate service provision
   Act as a single point of reference for communication
   Act as an advocate for the child and family
   A source of comprehensive information

To ensure that:
   Services do not overlap
   Gaps in service provision do not exist
   Communication between agencies is accurate and
   speedy
   Equipment is available
   The package of care is appropriate and meets the
   needs of the child and family
   The plan of care is followed

To provide:
   Emotional support
   Access to a range of required resources

To act:
   As a link and an advocate ensuring that total care is
   available

(ACT & RCPCH 1997)

articulation of individual responsibility and accountability for different aspects of care. Collaborative working, which may include selective joint visiting and shared care, assists in role clarification and the prevention of professional rivalry and overlap. Furthermore, the formal identification of a named keyworker is recommended for each family. The keyworker must be acceptable to the family, preferably chosen by them and endorsed by all professionals and agencies involved as the main referral point and channel for discussion and communication (Box 22.4).

Clearly, the provision of an identified keyworker can assist in unravelling the complex variables impacting on the family and enhance interprofessional and multiagency case management. The keyworker should be a separate, statutorily recognized, valued and dedicated person to assist families in the co-ordination of care and services for their children. Where services exist, CCNs are often seen as the most appropriate practitioner to adopt such a role, however, rarely is this role formally acknowledged and identified within the CCN's work or caseload management. The implications of these combined facets are identified in Box 22.5.

Box 22.5   Interprofessional and multiagency case management

Requires:
   Leadership from within the CCN team
   Creative thinking
   Challenging existing ways of working
   Cost analysis and realistic resourcing
   Service commissioning
   Flexibility within commissioning process
   Expanded boundaries from within the CCN role
   Integration of provider organizations including Higher
   Education Institutions
   Strategic planning
   Appropriate service provision
   Collaborative partnerships between agencies
   Innovative and proactive professional expectations
   Planned review processes
   Identification of shared goals and outcomes
   Shared assessment of risks and unmet needs

Can result in:
   New ways of working
   A flexible framework for care provision
   Integrated service delivery
   Greater family autonomy
   Empowered and satisfied families
   Reduction in family burden of care
   Negotiated roles and role release / expansion
   Care delivered by appropriate personnel
   Reduction in parental exploitation
   Clarification of roles and expectations
   Clarification of individual responsibility and
   accountability
   Effective discharge planning
   Increased range of care options
   Pooled budgets
   Reduced funding disputes
   Planned and responsive respite care provision

Home care for sick children that is co-ordinated using an interprofessional and multiagency framework with the support of an identified keyworker can result in an integrated service designed in the best interest of the whole family. If home is to remain the best and first choice as the place for essential care, then this must be negotiated and facilitated within such a framework.

Case Study 22.3

Interprofessional and multiagency case management

Lucy, aged 4 years, suffers from epilepsy. Her convulsions commenced soon after her rapid birth at

26 weeks gestation. During her first year it became evident that other neurological damage had been sustained which resulted in a degree of learning difficulty and profound lack of co-ordination with cough and swallowing reflexes. Subsequently a tracheostomy and gastrostomy were performed to protect her airway and meet her nutritional needs. Her parents became competent in all aspects of her care. The family live in a rural area many miles from the regional children's unit. Initially, supplies were difficult to obtain as the HV was unfamiliar with the care required and no budget was identified to supply the equipment. Whilst Lucy's learning difficulties were recognized the family did not receive support and advice on managing her difficult behaviour. Recently, however, a multidisciplinary community-based service was established in the area for sick children. A CCN ensures the family remains competent in her care. The children's learning disability nurse supports the family in developing effective means of communicating with Lucy and managing her challenging behaviour. The social worker supports the family in addressing their emotional, social and financial needs. The CCN has been identified as the named keyworker at the request of the parents.

Questions

1. Which care provider is the most appropriate to negotiate the level and content of respite care?
2. How can an appropriate budget be negotiated to support Lucy's deteriorating condition and ongoing home care?

CONCLUSION

This chapter has outlined the central role that CCNs play in the delivery and coordination of care for sick children and their families. However, in order to meet the future needs of this group, CCNs will need to review and refine their practice for the emerging new world of integrated health and social care. There has been limited specific reference to community children's nursing services through the radical restructuring of the NHS. Consequently, these reforms (DoH 2000, 2001c) and the interpretation of policy documents for community children's nursing services provide both challenges and opportunities. As a minority service, CCNs have a responsibility to assert the need for appropriate provision for families and to work with other organizations in their development. Above all, this requires strong professional leadership at all levels. (See Chapter 16 for a more detailed account of professional leadership.)

From a local perspective, CCNs must identify the most appropriate communication systems within and across Primary Care Trusts as increasing NHS funds are allocated directly to these organizations (DoH 2001c). These communication channels must be effective and efficient to ensure that services for sick children and their families are at least maintained and/or developed in the context of identified local health needs and health improvement programmes. Furthermore, CCNs must be conversant with national and local policy agenda in order to identify imaginative and creative opportunities and work meaningfully with primary care priorities. The need for new ways of working within the current reforms will require CCNs to challenge their existing perception of how and where they practice and examples may include (see Chapter 24 for a detailed discussion of new roles and ways of working for nurses in primary care):

- flexible proposals for the implementation of the National Service Frameworks for sick children
- the development of expert patient programmes (DoH 2001d) for parents of children with key chronic conditions
- the development of nurse-led clinics for children with acute or chronic health problems within primary care (Muir & Burnett 2000) with investment in independent prescribing practices.

Finally, further opportunities exist to strengthen the national corporate identity of community children's nursing services. For example, the Health Visitor (DoH 2001e) and School Nurse (DoH 2001f) Practice Development Resource Packs, provide a clear focus and identify how these services could be delivered to the entire population. Whilst these resources are based on family-centred and child-centred public health roles respectively, this model could usefully translate to community children's nursing services. However, for any of these initiatives to be grasped, professional leadership is fundamental and requires investment at both local and national levels. (See Chapters 19 and 23 for further information on health visiting and school health nursing public health roles.)

SUMMARY

◆ As parents learn complex skills and assume 24-hour responsibility for their child's care they adopt 'neoprofessional' roles and become experts themselves.

◆ The family as the unit of care remains central to community children's nursing practice.

◆ Managing the parent–professional relationship requires emotional maturity and intelligence on behalf of the CCN in order to develop flexible boundaries in practice.

◆ Care should be planned and delivered from an interprofessional/multiagency perspective with a named keyworker as the main referral point.

◆ A strong corporate identity aids interprofessional and multiagency working.

◆ Professional leadership is the key to the development and enhancement of services.

DISCUSSION POINTS

1. Who provides professional leadership for children with healthcare needs and their families in community settings in your area?

2. Who assesses the parents' confidence and competence to undertake skilled nursing interventions at home?

3. What strategies are in place to meet the anticipated health and social needs of sick children and their families at home in your area of practice?

4. How is the keyworker role identified and evaluated in the delivery of multiagency care packages?

5. Consider what communication systems CCNs can access within primary care organizations.

REFERENCES

Association for Children with Life-threatening or Terminal Conditions and their Families (ACT) & Royal College of Paediatrics and Child Health 1997 A guide to the development of children's palliative care services. ACT, Bristol

Carter B 2000 Ways of working: CCNs and chronic illness. Journal of Child Health Care 4(2): 66–72

Department of Health 1991 The welfare of children and young people in hospital. HMSO, London

Department of Health 1994 The Clothier Report. HMSO, London

Department of Health 2000 The NHS plan. The Stationery Office, London

Department of Health 2001a The NHS University. www.doh.gov.uk/nhsuniversity.htm

Department of Health 2001b The Bristol Royal Infirmary Inquiry: Final Report. The Stationery Office, London

Department of Health 2001c Shifting the balance of power in the NHS: securing delivery. The Stationery Office, London

Department of Health 2001d The expert patient: a new approach to chronic disease management for the 21st century. The Stationery Office, London

Department of Health 2001e The health visitor and school nurse development programme: health visitor development resource pack. The Stationery Office, London

Department of Health 2001f The health visitor and school nurse development programme: school nurse development resource pack. The Stationery Office, London

Eaton N 2001 Models of community children's nursing. Paediatric Nursing 13(1): 32–36

Friedemann M-L 1989 The concept of family nursing. Journal of Advanced Nursing 14: 211–216

Gillet JA 1954 Children's nursing unit. British Medical Journal 684: 1954

Goleman D 1995 Emotional intelligence. Why it can matter more than IQ. Bantam Books, New York

Health Committee 1997 The House of Commons Health Select Committee. Health services for children and young people in the community: home and school. Third Report. The Stationery Office, London

Hunt J 2000 Relationships between outreach nurses and primary healthcare professionals In: Muir J, Sidey A (eds) Textbook of community children's nursing, Chapter 11. Baillière Tindall, London

Kirk S 2001 Negotiating lay and professional roles in the care of children with complex health care needs. Journal of Advanced Nursing 34(5): 593–602

Miller S 1995 The clinical nurse specialist: a way forward? Journal of Advanced Nursing 22: 494–501

Muir J, Burnett C 2000 Opportunities for the development of nurse led clinics in community children's nursing. In: Muir J, Sidey A (eds) Textbook of community children's nursing, Chapter 29. Baillière Tindall, London

Murphy G 2001 The technology-dependent child at home, Part 1: in whose best interest? Paediatric Nursing 13(7): 14–18

Procter S, Biott C, Campbell S, Edward S, Redpath N, Moran M 1999 Preparation for the developing role of the community children's nurse. Researching professional education: Research Report Series, no. 11. English National Board for Nursing, Midwifery and Health Visiting, London

Royal College of Nursing (RCN) 2001 Directory of community children's nursing services, 15th edn. RCN, London

United Kingdom Central Council (UKCC) 1994 The future of professional practice – the Council's standards for education and practice following registration. UKCC, London

Whiting M 2000 1888–1988: 100 years of community children's nursing. In: Muir J, Sidey A (eds) Textbook of community children's nursing, Chapter 2. Baillière Tindall, London

Whyte DA, Barton ME, Lamb A, et al 1998 Clinical effectiveness in community children's nursing. Clinical Effectiveness in Nursing 2: 139–144

FURTHER READING

Muir J, Sidey A (eds) 2000 Textbook of community children's nursing. Ballière Tindall, London

An authoritative textbook, which provides an introduction to the major spheres in community children's nursing including historical perspectives, theory and clinical practice. The four sections of the book cover organizational facets, philosophical issues, dimensions of practice and the advancing picture of community children's nursing.

Association for Children with Life-threatening and Terminal Conditions and their Families (ACT) & Royal College of Paediatrics and Child Health 1997 A guide to the development of children's palliative care services. ACT, Bristol

ACT Bristol. Palliative care for young people 2001 ACT, National Council for Hospice and Specialist Palliative Care Services and Scottish Partnership Agency for Palliative and Cancer Care. ACT, Bristol

These complementary guides provide an overview of the measures that can help families and professionals meet the emotional, therapeutic, spiritual and physical needs of children who experience life-limiting or -threatening disorders.

Health Committee 1997 House of Commons Select Committee. Health services for children and young people in the community; home and school. Third Report. The Stationery Office, London

This is the most comprehensive review of children's services conducted since the Court report in 1976. It reports on a broad examination of nursing services for children at home and in school. In particular it discusses the work of community children's nursing services and makes clear recommendations for the expansion of provision to enable children and their families to have easy and equitable access to appropriately qualified staff. It provides valuable evidence to support the need for community children's nursing services.

Sharing the Care 1999 English National Board for Nursing, Midwifery and Health Visiting. Department of Health, London

A resource pack, which is aimed at supporting community children's nurses to provide care in partnership with other services in the community. Designed to accompany the development of Diana, Princess of Wales Community Children's Nursing Teams it has proved to be a valuable resource for a range of professional and voluntary groups. It contains sections which include shared working, team management and the role of the key worker.

School nursing

D. Watkins
C. Crocker

INTRODUCTION

School nursing as a unique discipline within specialist community nursing practice is faced with challenges and opportunities, in line with recent government policies (DoH 1999a, 1999b, 2001a). Its future role in child-centred public health is one that must be capitalized upon, in an effort to positively influence the health and well-being of school-aged children. Although school nursing has always been based on public health principles, its seems to have lost its way over the last decade, with numbers of school health nurses employed falling (Health Committee 1997), and health visitors performing both a health visiting and school nursing role (Clark et al 2000). The social policy context is set to change this downward trend, with school nursing teams cited as taking responsibility for (adapted from *Saving Lives: our Healthier Nation* (DoH 1999a) and *Making a Difference* (DoH 1999b):

◆ assessing the health and social needs of school communities and children, and developing individual and school health plans

◆ undertaking a key role in immunization and vaccination programmes

◆ contributing to personal health and social education within the school environment

◆ promoting positive parenting through working with parents

◆ working with children, families and the school to support children with medical problems or special educational needs

◆ promoting positive mental health through programmes that offer counselling and support to the school-aged child

◆ providing advice on relationships and sex education

◆ working with the school staff to provide advice and support on health issues

◆ working in a multidisciplinary/multiagency manner, liaising between schools, primary care groups (Trusts) and special services in meeting the health and social needs of the school-aged child

◆ identification of social issues, to include protection from child abuse.

This chapter will explore the historical perspective on school nursing and then describe current practice, comparing this with the roles outlined above. It will conclude with a discussion of the barriers to school health nursing moving forward and present ways of working to address changes in practice.

HISTORICAL PERSPECTIVE

School nursing has existed in the United Kingdom for just over 100 years, supporting the school medical officer and the health visitor (Fletcher & Baldwin 1992). Although there appears to have been a form of school health services since 1893 in some parts of the UK, it did not become universal until 1904. The Government of the day commissioned an investigation into the health of young men recruited to the Boer War, as statements from army personnel indicated they were in poor health, partly attributed to inadequate nutrition in childhood. From this, a report was published by the Interdepartmental Committee on Physical Deterioration (BPA 1995), which recommended that school health nurses and doctors were appointed to meet the health needs of children attending school. The importance of social care, housing and environmental issues were also recognized and the Government sought to improve social conditions. However this was the first time that school health services were considered and

was the beginning of establishing the profession of school nursing.

This milestone was closely followed by the Education Act of 1907, which reaffirmed the recommendations of the above report, by placing in statute the foundations for a universal school health service for all children attending school. A service was developed that aimed to promote and maintain the health of children. This was long before cities and towns had a dedicated service for children attending hospital, the creation of the National Health Service, primary care services and access to general practitioners.

In 1944 a review of the Education Act gave local authorities a legal duty to provide dental and medical services to children in maintained schools and to consider the needs of children who required specialist care. However the service remained variable across the United Kingdom and it was not until the 1970s that we saw a truly universal service provided by school health nurses to school-aged children.

Uniformity in service provision developed when responsibility for school health nursing transferred from local authorities to District Health Authorities in response to the National Health Service Act of 1974. Responsibility for the purchase and delivery of school health nursing became the District Health Authorities' remit, with services such as vaccination and immunization programmes, vision and audiometry screening becoming an essential part of the school nurse's role.

In addition to this the Education Acts of both 1981 and 1993 laid the foundation for the provision of services for children with special educational needs. There is a statutory obligation for education departments to notify health authorities of any child who is likely to require special services to meet their educational requirements. The Act places importance on a multiagency approach to assessing, planning and delivering care to children who have special needs and there is now a greater emphasis on integrating children with such needs into mainstream schools. However this is not always possible for children with severe learning disabilities, who may need to be placed within special needs units in mainstream schools

(Education Act 1981). (See Chapter 21 for a more detailed discussion on learning disability issues.)

The overall aim of an integrated approach between education and health enhances the philosophy of assisting every child to achieve his or her full potential. This echoes the United Nations Convention on the Rights of the Child (1992). As social policy has developed, the emphasis for school health nursing has moved from care of the ill in 1946, to the care and promotion of the well and the prevention of ill health in the 21st century.

CURRENT SCHOOL NURSING PRACTICE

School nursing and the school health service is a fundamental part of child health services and its purpose primarily is to meet the needs of the school-aged child and his or her family, through the provision of primary, secondary and tertiary health care. The service establishes links between the home and school, and aims to promote positive community health and ultimately a healthy and health-conscious school-aged population (Strehlow 1987). 'How' school nurses work towards achieving a 'healthy and health conscious' population is worthy of consideration, particularly as the evidence base to support much of their practice is questionable. There is a distinct lack of empirical-based studies that demonstrate their effectiveness (Fletcher et al 1997, Wainwright et al 1999), however there are studies that outline their work which provide insight into current practice.

The literature appears to divide school nursing into the following categories:

◆ health assessment and surveillance
◆ care and treatment
◆ health promotion.

Each of these areas will now be discussed in detail.

HEALTH ASSESSMENT AND SURVEILLANCE

Health assessment and surveillance appears to form a large component of the school nurse's role and is inclusive of activities such as undertaking universal health interviews when children enter school. Health interviews with parents and children are now part of the child surveillance programme in the majority of NHS Trusts in the United Kingdom and have replaced the traditional school medical. In most areas the health interview is offered as a universal procedure with few using selective interviewing. Selection is based on those children and families where there is a known health or social issue, or where parents request a school interview (Shepherd & Stuart 2001). There is some evidence to support the effectiveness of school health nurses undertaking this role universally and benefits such as detection of problems in children and allowing better use of the school medical officers time to deal with more acute child health needs, have been identified (Bolton 1994). A review of the literature by Barlow et al (1997) commissioned by the Department of Health, examined health interviews in relation to the content of the check and outcomes achieved, which were defined in terms of new disorders identified, referrals for assessment, the outcome of referrals and liaison with teachers and other health professionals.

The studies reviewed included large sample groups, however many were retrospective in nature and relied on past documentation to demonstrate results. Unfortunately the accumulation of information accrued from 47 studies was not sufficient to reach any conclusion. Studies were unsubstantiated in the majority of cases, with limited information available on assessment criteria, referral standards, referral outcomes, health conditions identified and outcomes achieved. The authors comment they are unable to come to any conclusion regarding the effectiveness of health interviews, either universal or selective. More recent research indicates there is little difference in detecting health problems between selective and universal health interviews in detecting health problems in children and that most health issues have been picked up by either the health visitor or the general practitioner before entry to school. Giving parents the choice of a health interview and information on the services the school health nurse provides, presents opportunities for parents to express their concerns and is an effective use of the school nurse's time (Shepard & Stuart 2001).

Screening has always been a fundamental part of the school nurse's role, historically relating back to the foundations of the school medical services, as discussed earlier. However its value in terms of health outcomes is currently being debated (Snowdon & Stewart Brown 1997), although many school health nurses continue to engage in a variety of screening procedures such as vision testing and height and weight measurement. The Hall Report (Hall 1996) advocated a core programme of screening, however this related primarily to pre-school children, resulting in health authorities setting their own core programme, thus leading to inconsistencies in screening school-aged children throughout the United Kingdom (Humphries & Tonge 2000). The differences suggest that many school health nurses are spending unnecessary time and resources delivering screening programmes that are questionable in terms of their effectiveness.

School nurses are also involved in school profiling in some areas, which involves the collection of data pertaining to the school population, and from this information identifying areas for health promotion activity. Profiling is seen as an effective systematic means of assessing health needs, rather than relying on the subjective view of the school health nurse (Naidoo & Wills 2000). Its benefits relate to linking with service planning, however a taxonomy needs to be used that ensures the concept of 'need' is defined in some sort of consistent manner. The problems associated with the assessment of need are well documented (Cowley et al 1996, ENB 1996, Naidoo & Wills 2000) and although the value of detailed health profiles of school-aged children is noted in the literature (Hancock 1994), their value in influencing health strategy has been disputed (Bagnall & Dilloway 1997). This suggests that school health nurses need to be more influential in working with those who commission health services in the future to ensure the needs of school-aged children are met. (See Chapter 2 for more information pertaining to needs analysis and commissioning of health care.)

CARE AND TREATMENT OF CONDITIONS IN THE SCHOOL-AGED CHILD

Preventative strategies to address conditions such as asthma and diabetes have been initiated by school health nurses in many areas. Locally there are examples of school health nurses teaching school staff the basics of asthma prevention, inhaler technique, management of an exacerbation of asthma and developing school-based policies related to the overall management of this condition in the school setting. Pearson and Hart (1996) indicate such work in their studies, however little is included on overall evaluation of such activity. Guidelines on catheterization of children in school is another area that has been developed by school nurses (White 1997) although much of their work appears to be moving away from secondary and tertiary prevention to a primary preventative focus in terms of disease prevention (Wainwright et al 1999). (See Chapters 19 and 27 for further discussion on health promotion.)

Care and support of children with special needs in school is an area of practice school nurses continue to be involved with, and one that is advocated by the Health Committee, House of Commons (1997) and the Welsh Office (1997). Both governments outline the need for children with special health or educational needs to receive a healthcare plan that ensures school staff have the information to understand and support children with long-term health needs. This is drawn up in consultation with the parents and sets out in detail the measures required to support the child in the school setting. The school nurse is considered the first point of contact for school staff, they take responsibility for advising and providing support to the school, the child and the family and liaise with the appropriate professionals and agencies involved in the care of the child. School nurses are not expected to provide 'hands on care' for the child whilst at school; their role is usually purely an advisory, supportive one that acts as a 'liaison between parents, teachers, head teachers, hospitals and consultants, so that the child achieves the maximum from (his or her) education' (Moldauer cited in Health Committee 1997, p. xxiii).

The situation where school nurses work in independent or special schools may be slightly different from that outlined above, with some 'hands on care' taking place. This may include treatment for minor conditions and injuries and care of the child with special health needs (Poulton 1998). (See Chapter 21 for further discussion on learning disability issues.)

IMMUNIZATION PROGRAMMES

There is no doubt that immunization programmes form a large percentage of the work of the school nurse and are delivered according to national policy. Bagnall (1995) reports on the positive outcome achieved by school nurses in the mass immunization programme undertaken to prevent a measles epidemic. Seven million children were immunized by school nurses and this was considered an outstanding success. Many school nurses worked as part of a team and found this beneficial to their working practice (Bagnall 1995). The MMR campaign is another example of the excellent work by school health nurses in preventing epidemics of serious diseases.

HEALTH PROMOTION AND HEALTH EDUCATION

Health promotion and health education are the central components of school nursing practice and are undertaken in a variety of guises by all school nurses in the United Kingdom (Clark et al 2000, Poulton 1998). Their practice has been defined as work with individual children and families, work with groups of children and work in the wider school (Lightfoot & Bines 1996). These areas will now be discussed more fully to facilitate an understanding of the extent of their work in health promotion and health education.

Work with individual children and their families to promote health takes place primarily through screening and health interviews previously mentioned. The degree to which this takes place is variable across the United Kingdom, however a picture of this activity in Wales is available through the latest Review of Health Visiting and School Nursing conducted by Clark et al (2000).

This research found that health interviews were undertaken by school nurses on entry to school, and again during the first year of secondary school in some NHS Trusts, and repeated when the child was aged 15 years in other NHS Trusts. In some instances parents were involved, whilst in others the interview was confidential between the child and the school nurse. The interviews are seen to provide an excellent opportunity for the school nurse to discuss dietary habits, social and health problems and as the child reaches secondary school, issues to do with adolescence, sexual orientation, family planning and lifestyle behaviours such as smoking, alcohol and drug misuse.

Other methods of one-to-one contact involve school nurses running 'drop-in sessions' where pupils are encouraged to attend to discuss anything that may be bothering them. Locally these have proved successful, although concrete evidence of their effectiveness is still to be measured. Other drop-in sessions relate to sexual health inclusive of family planning advice (Clark et al 2000), and a multidisciplinary approach to drop-in sessions has been adopted in some areas (Crowe 2000). The Wick teenage drop-in centre provides advice and support on health-related topics to teenagers who attend the local high school. It is operated by a centre co-ordinator, health visitors, a practice nurse and a school health nurse and the objectives of the service are to (Crowe 2000, p. 796):

- 'improve the general health and well-being of teenagers in the area
- provide a confidential service that is user friendly and one which teenagers have been involved in creating
- provide health information on all relevant teenage issues
- provide a nonjudgemental advisory health service in an endeavour to influence behavioural change
- improve teenage lifestyles allowing them to explore their own values and improve their assertion, decision making and negotiation skills'.

Evaluation of the project outcomes is yet to be completed, however process evaluation suggests that teenagers are attending the centre for advice on emergency contraception, undertake exercise programmes offered and positive comments have been received from the school. It will be interesting to follow this project and ascertain whether it achieves the outcomes set in relation to improving teenage lifestyles and their health and well-being. (See Chapter 4 for further discussion on measuring outcomes and quality improvement.)

School nursing health-promoting practice with groups of children usually revolves around the school curriculum, through teaching input on health-related topics, with the majority of school nurses involved in classroom teaching (Charleston & Denman 1997). The range of topics covered by school nurses includes aspects of sexual health, smoking, alcohol and substance misuse, nutrition and healthy eating, etc. (Wainwright et al 1999). Another method of promoting health with groups of pupils is through specific topic-related group work. Smoking cessation groups is an example where school nurses deliver school-based initiatives (Waley 1995). Fletcher et al (1997) comment on the lack of studies citing school nurses involvement in school-based tobacco control. The one-off sessions in school delivered by school nurses should be viewed with caution, as their effectiveness may be short lived. It is important that all topic-based teaching is delivered as a part of the overall curriculum and that links are made with other relevant subject matter and skills. Areas such as assertiveness, peer pressure and decision-making need to be addressed, thus making the connection between knowledge and the skills required to take personal control over choices available.

The wider school environment and health-promoting activity relates to the 'health-promoting school' philosophy. This is a World Health Organization Initiative that specifies certain criteria for a 'health promoting school' (Box 23.1).

The school presents an excellent setting in which to promote health, as it contains a captive audience who are likely to spend numerous years in attendance. Children spend a considerable proportion of their life in school and the opportunity to positively influence their health and lifestyle choices is significant. Although the author is aware of local activity regarding school nurses working

---

Box 23.1 The 12 WHO criteria for a health-promoting school

1. Active promotion of the self-esteem of all pupils by demonstrating that everyone can make a contribution to the life of the school.
2. Development of good relations between staff and pupils and among pupils in the daily life of the school.
3. Clarification for staff and pupils of the social aims of the school.
4. Provision of stimulating challenges for all pupils through a wide range of activities.
5. Use of every opportunity to improve the physical environment of the school.
6. Development of good links between school, home and community.
7. Development of good links among associated primary and secondary schools to plan a coherent health education curriculum.
8. Active promotion of the health and well-being of school and staff.
9. Consideration of the role of staff as exemplars in health-related issues.
10. Consideration of the complementary role of school meals (if provided) to the health education curriculum.
11. Realization of the potential of specialist services in the community for advice and support in health education.
12. Development of the education potential of school health services beyond routine screening and towards active support for the curriculum.

World Health Organization (WHO) 1993

---

towards the WHO criteria for health-promoting schools, there is little evidence cited in recent reviews (Clark et al 2000, Wainwright et al 1999) to suggest their work has been recognized. Healthy school award schemes have been popular in the United Kingdom, some of which school nurses will have inevitably been involved (Naidoo & Wills 2000).

THE CHALLENGES FACING SCHOOL NURSING IN THE 21ST CENTURY

Comparing current practice with that advocated in recent social policy outlined at the beginning of this chapter indicates that school nurses are already fulfilling the objectives set before them. However the evidence base on the majority of their practice is sparse and requires further research and evaluation to demonstrate effectiveness.

There is a need to strengthen the school nurse's public health role in improving health and addressing inequalities, to build on current innovation and develop a child-centred public health perspective (Mullally 2001). Ways in which this could be addressed is through adopting the following approach to practice (adapted from DoH 2001b):

1. Tackle the causes of ill health.
2. Identify health needs across the school-aged population, rather than focus on individual children.
3. Profile the school population, link this with the community the school serves and plan school nursing practice based on need, an evidence base (wherever possible) and NHS priorities.
4. Influence the local Health Improvement Plan with the evidence collated in the school profile and use this information to plan services.
5. Work collaboratively with other professionals, agencies and sectors to plan and deliver health-promoting services.
6. Prioritize the needs of vulnerable children and groups and target resources to meet these needs.
7. Work as part of a multiprofessional team and ensure actions taken make the healthy choice the easier choice.
8. Influence policies at a national and local level that impact on health.
9. Evaluate both the process and outcome of school nursing practice.

An assumption should not be made that public health work only relates to working with populations and groups, as it can also involve working on a one-to-one level with individual children and families, engaging with children with disabilities, immunization programmes and family/child health interviews. (See Chapter 3 for further discussion on public health issues.)

When working with groups of children or young people it is important to use a 'bottom–up' approach that respects the views of those concerned and provides opportunities for young people to influence services and to 'be heard'. This can help to develop skills of negotiation and

decision-making, which are transferable skills that can assist in other dimensions of life.

The school population and health profiling is an essential element of health promotion activity and used in conjunction with the criteria outlined previously for health-promoting schools, could make a real difference to the school physical and social environment. 'Community development and whole school approaches can be a powerful way to narrow the health gap, increasing social support in deprived communities and getting resources into areas that need them most' (DoH 2001b, p. 15). (See Chapter 7 for further discussion on community development.)

Health profiling may result in identifying that some schools require more services than others. Drug misuse, teenage pregnancy, truancy and bullying are but a few of the health issues that may be identified. School nurses need to recognize the same service will not be delivered to all schools; it is about prioritizing need and ensuring equity in service provision.

ADDRESSING THE CHALLENGES AND FACILITATING CHANGES IN PRACTICE

This section will not focus on management of change theory (see Chapter 16 for a detailed discussion on change management), but simply identify those issues in school nursing that need to be addressed to allow the profession to move forward and engage in innovative proactive practice.

The numbers of school nurses need to be dramatically increased to allow time for them to undertake health-promotion activity. As Wainwright et al (1999) point out, one of the main problems confronting school nurses committed to health promotion, is conflicting priorities and other duties. It is difficult to ascertain up-to-date numbers of school children for whom school nurses are responsible, however recommendations from the School Nurse Review in Wales state that school nurses should serve no more than five schools (Clarke et al 2000).

The image of the school nurse needs to change and the role valued by other professionals. The RCN School Nursing Forum stated in 1997 that school nursing suffered from a poor image and low status (Health Committee 1997). This is portrayed in recent literature, with school nurses themselves commenting on the erroneous perception by parents, children, teachers, doctors and other nurses of what a school nurse does (Humphries & Tonge 2000). To allow for meaningful team working and collaboration on public health issues to occur, the school nurse's role needs to be valued by other members of the multidisciplinary team, however school nurses themselves must be clear of their role and contribution before this can be articulated to others. (See Chapter 15 for further discussion on multidisciplinary team working.)

This chapter has emphasized the lack of an evidence base underpinning much of the school nurse's work. It is essential this is addressed in line with the present culture of quality assurance and clinical governance. School nurses themselves must be proactive in evaluating their work and new innovation must include stringent methods of evaluating effectiveness in the planning stage, thus ensuring the impact of new developments can be measured.

There continues to be diversity in practice across the United Kingdom and whilst it is important that school nurses respond to local need, there are opportunities to develop standards that allow for a uniform approach to school profiling, health interviews and screening. This would allow for a body of knowledge to be developed that could contribute to the effectiveness of school health nursing practice over time.

Collaborative working is a feature of public health practice (DoH 2001) and the school health nurse is an expert at working in this way. Meeting the health needs of children requires a high level of interagency and interdisciplinary working, collaboration and co-ordination. An important component to enable this to take place is effective communication. The sharing of information particularly in relation to children with special needs and child protection information is seen as vital to the welfare of the child (Polnay 1995). School nurses are in the unique position of interfacing with may organizations to benefit the child and family, from hospital admission through

to discharge and community care. They work across the boundaries of health, social services and education to benefit the needs of the school-aged child and must continue to do so in the new world of public health.

There has been a distinct lack of training opportunities for school health nurses, although this has improved over the last 8 years since the UKCC included them into the specialist community practitioner framework (UKCC 1994). This has resulted in Higher Education Institutes providing school nursing programmes, although Humphries and Tonge (2000) warn of the difficulties some school nurses face in accessing level 3 programmes and call for courses at level 2 to facilitate entry into these first-degree courses. They also comment on the lack of further education available after undertaking specialist practitioner programmes, that allow school health nurses to develop a higher level of expertise in public health. The development of modules with a school health nursing focus at Masters level would correct this deficit.

School nursing also requires a management structure that is supportive and recognizes the potential of school nurses to influence the public health agenda. A leader or manager with appropriate skills and knowledge can act as a change agent, and in doing so facilitate development and collaborative working (Shaw & Bosanquet 1993). With direction, school nursing can work both operationally and strategically in influencing the health of children and moving the profession forward. (See Chapter 16 for further discussion on professional leadership.)

CONCLUSION

The school nurse is an independent practitioner able to assess the health needs of the school child. They are able to act as the link between school, the family, other professionals and the wider community. The role is complex and involves an in-depth knowledge of child and adolescent health and welfare. Contact with school children maximizes the opportunities for school nurses to positively influence the lifestyles of children, adolescents and their families, thereby contributing to the reduction of high-risk behaviour and increasing the possibilities of achieving health gain within local communities.

This chapter has attempted to define the historical perspective and outline the current practice of school nurses. It has identified how school nurses can adapt a child-centred public health approach to their work and articulated the barriers to future development. School nursing has great potential to influence the health of the school child and consequently the future population of the country, however more resources are required, coupled with training opportunities and research to allow this profession to reach its full potential.

SUMMARY

◆ The decline in school nurse numbers over the past decade is set to be reversed to meet current government health objectives.

◆ The school nurse role has evolved into one that is responsible for child-centred health assessment and surveillance, care and treatment, and health promotion.

◆ The school nurse role has been much undervalued, despite successes such as measles and MMR vaccination and antismoking campaigns; this can be remedied by collection and dissemination of evidence of successes.

DISCUSSION POINTS

1. How would you go about profiling a school population? Consider the basic elements that should be included and discuss how you would prioritise needs identified.

2. Consider the 12 criteria for a health promoting school and discuss how you would achieve these in collaboration with school staff.

3. Identify a health need in young people and discuss how you would address this through a health promotion initiative. Consider planning, implementation, monitoring and evaluation of outcome in your answer.

REFERENCES

Bagnall P 1995 School nurse's response to the measles vaccination campaign. Nursing Times 91(40): 38–39

Bagnall P, Dilloway M 1997 In a different light. Department of Health, London

Barlow J, Brown SS, Fletcher J 1987 Systematic review of the school entry medical examination. Health Services Research Unit, Oxford

Bolton P 1994 School entry screening by the school nurse. Health Visitor 67(4): 135–136

British Paediatric Association (BPA) 1995 Health needs of school aged children. BPA, London

Charleston S and Denman S 1997 The school nurse's contribution to health promotion. Health Visitor 70(8): 302–304

Clark J, Buttigeg M, Bodycombe-James M, et al 2000 A review of health visiting and school nursing in Wales. University of Swansea School of Health Care Science, Swansea

Cowley S, Bergen A, Young K, Kavanagh A 1996 Establishing a framework for research: the example of needs assessment. Journal of Clinical Nursing 5: 53–61

Crowe A 2000 Providing a drop-in centre in partnership with young clients. Community Practitioner 73(10): 796–798

Department of Health 1999a Saving lives: our healthier nation. HMSO, London

Department of Health 1999b Making a difference: strengthening the nursing, midwifery and health visiting contribution to health and health care. HMSO, London

Department of Health 2001a Investment and reform for NHS staff – taking forward the NHS plan. HMSO, London

Department of Health 2001b The health visitor and school nurse development programme: school nurse practice development resource pack. Department of Health, London

Department of Education 1907 Education Act. Department of Education, London

Department of Education 1944 Education Act. HMSO, London

Department of Education 1981 Education Act. HMSO, London

Department of Education 1993 Education Act. HMSO, London

DES/DHSS 1983 Assessments and statements of special educational needs. DES Circular 1/83/HC/(83)/3/LAC (83)/2

English National Board 1996 An investigation into the changing educational needs of community nurses with regard to needs assessment and quality of care in the context of the NHS and Community Care Act 1990. Research Highlights Number 23. ENB, London

Fletcher K, Baldwin J 1992 School nurses do it in schools. Amalgamated School Nurses Association, London

Fletcher J, Brown S, Barlow J 1997 Systematic review of reviews of the effectiveness of school health promotion. Health Services Research Unit Oxford, Oxford

Hall D (ed) 1996 Health for all children. Report of the 3rd Joint Working Party on Child Health Surveillance. Oxford University Press, Oxford

Hancock C 1994 Schools for scandal. Health Service Journal (April) p. 21

Health Committee, House of Commons 1997 Health services for children and young people in the community, home and school. The Stationery Office, London

Humphries J, Tonge J 2000 Looking ahead: a forum on the future of school nursing. Community Practitioner 73(12): 881–883

Lightfoot J, Bines W 1996 Meeting the needs of the school aged child. Health Visitor 70(2): 436–437

Mullaly S 2001 Forward. In: Department of Health (2001) The health visitor and school nurse development programme: school nurse practice development resource pack. Department of Health, London

Naidoo J, Wills J 2000 Health promotion: foundations for practice, 2nd edn. Baillière Tindall, Edinburgh

Pearson A, Hart S 1996 School asthma teams make the difference. Practice Nurse May: 66625–66628

Polnay L 1995 Polnay Report: The health needs of school aged children. British Paediatric Association, London

Poulton BC 1998 Roles, responsibilities and conditions of service for nurses working in independent and boarding schools. Unpublished Committee Paper (Nursing Policy), London

Royal College of Nursing School Nurses Forum, cited in Health Committee, House of Commons 1997 Health services for children and young people in the community, home and school. The Stationery Office, London

Shaw J, Bosanquet N 1993 A way to develop nurses and nursing. King's Fund Centre, London

Shepard J, Stuart D 2001 School nurse health interviews: effectiveness and alternatives. Community Practitioner 74(5): 185–189

Snowdon S, Stuart Brown S 1997 Pre-school vision screening: results of a systematic review. NHS Centre for Reviews and Dissemination, Health Service Research Unit, University of Oxford, York

Strehlow M 1987 Nursing in educational settings. Harper and Row, London

United Kingdom Central Council (UKCC) 1994 The future of professional practice – the councils standards for education and practice following registration. UKCC, London

United Nations 1992 Convention on the rights of the child. United Nations, Geneva

Wainwright P, Thomas J, Jones M 1999 School nursing: a review of the literature. Health Promotion Wales, Cardiff

Waley M 1995 Just a reminder … Health Visitor 68(3): 116

Welsh Office 1997 The health of children in Wales. Welsh Office, Cardiff

Welsh Office 1998 Better health, better Wales: strategic framework. Welsh Office, Cardiff

White M 1997 Developing guidelines on catheterisation in schools. Professional Nurse 12(12): 855–858

World Health Organization 1993 The European network of health promoting schools. WHO, Copenhagen

FURTHER READING

Department of Health 2001 The health visitor and school nurse development programme: School nurse practice development resource pack. Department of Health, London

This excellent package provides guidance on the child-centred public health role and new government policies. It summarizes the principles of public health practice extremely well and suggests activities that school nurses could engage in to assist working in new ways.

Naidoo J, Wills J 2000 Health promotion: foundations for practice, 2nd edn. Chapter 9 – Public health work; Chapter 14 – The health promoting school. Baillière Tindall, Edinburgh

This whole book is of relevance to the school nurse, however the two chapters outlined above are of particular relevance for those who wish to work towards the health promoting school concept and incorporate public health principles into their work.

Challenges for the future

SECTION CONTENTS

This final section presents opportunities for community nurses to expand their professional roles and illustrates significant developments and innovative nursing practice undertaken in some parts of the United Kingdom. Readers are not only encouraged to explore the concept of 'value for money' in relation to health service provision, but also to consider the political and professional issues associated with providing community nursing services in new and diverse ways. Different perspectives are adopted to consider the consequences of shifts in the development and organization of primary care, public health and community nursing.

Chapter 24 commences with a discussion on alternative ways of working, where the tensions between maintaining nursing values in the face of new technologies are explored. Examples drawn from service developments such as 'triage', 'walk in clinics' and NHS Direct are used to illustrate new and innovative ways of working. Throughout this chapter examples are provided of nurses emerging as prime caregivers, in some parts of the country. Chapter 25 moves on to discuss issues surrounding the use and impact of information technology on health care and community nursing. The significance of access to information, the use of the Internet as virtual health care and the source and quality of information is explored. The chapter concludes with the use of case studies to illustrate the application of theory to practice.

The third chapter discusses significant concepts such as 'value for money' and an alternative way of looking at difficult choices when faced with scarce resources. Community nurses seeking to resolve complex issues related to service provision are challenged to think through and apply the techniques and strategies outlined.

The closing chapter is concerned with the shift from health promotion to the 'modern' public health movement. The author traces the global history of health promotion up to present day practice and outlines opportunities for all nurses working in a community setting, to become actively involved in contributing to the public health agenda. Throughout this chapter, excellent links are made to the evidence base underpinning health promotion and public health, providing the reader with a range of material on which to base practice.

All of the issues covered in this section have implications for the future of community nursing and the reader is challenged to reflect critically on his or her practice in the light of the topic areas explored.

24

Alternative ways of working

M. Jones

KEY ISSUES

- ◆ Alternative ways of working for nurses as a solution to healthcare problems of the 21st century.

- ◆ Tension between medicine and nursing as traditional working practices are called into question.

- ◆ Benefits for patients as alternatives are found to meet demand and maximize use of resources.

- ◆ Maintenance of 'nursing values' as we progress into a health system dominated by new technologies.

- ◆ The emergence of nursing as prime care-giver within the NHS.

- ◆ Alternatives and the NHS Plan.

INTRODUCTION

The relationship between doctors and nurses has never been straightforward. The differences of power, perspective, education, pay, status, class and – perhaps above all – gender have led to tribal warfare as often as peaceful co-existence. Creative collaboration is rare. Nurses' readiness to be slighted and doctors' reluctance to be challenged create an undercurrent of tension. This may be masked in practice settings by the pressing need to get the work done, but it is there all the same. (Salvage 2000, p. 24)

The editor of the *Nursing Times Journal* so introduced her pioneering endeavour – jointly publishing an issue alongside the *British Medical Journal* – designed to raise the level of debate on the state of play in medicine and nursing in the early 21st century. As Salvage points out, undercurrents steeped in decades of tradition and accepted role demarcation simmer under the surface, but today as never before new ways of working – alternatives to those accepted unchallenged by doctors and nurses of previous times – are increasingly being examined, discussed, piloted and implemented in an attempt to ready the NHS for the greatest acts of modernization since its inception a half century ago. The realization is that by whatever means, we do 'need to get the work done' and changes will happen. This chapter seeks to examine the ramifications of these changes. Are new ways of working simply desperate attempts to manage an overburdening demand on our health services, a means of dealing with human resource issues, or in fact an honest attempt to provide the best possible care in a modernizing NHS?

THE NHS PLAN

The Government is first to admit that – despite many achievements – 'the NHS has failed to keep pace with changes in our society' (DoH 2000a, p. 2). The NHS Plan for England is blunt in its readiness to acknowledge 'there are unacceptable variations around the country. What patients receive depends too much on where they live and the NHS has yet to fulfil the aspiration to provide a truly national service' and 'constraints on funding mean that staff often work under great pressure and lack the time and resources they need to offer the best possible service (DoH 2000a, p. 2).

The NHS is faced with not only having to deal with an increasing demand from, on the one hand an ever more sophisticated consumer, and on the other increasingly marginalized members of society, but also the need for more staff to be available at a time when the workforce is ageing and a career in the health service is not the most attractive option. In an attempt to deal with this somewhat daunting duality, alternative ways of working are being examined and implemented so as to improve access to, and efficiency in, healthcare delivery, whilst making the best use of personnel and making their work more interesting and attractive.

CNO 'TOP 10'

All four UK countries have an NHS plan, however the English version is probably the most ambitious, and certainly the one that focuses most on developments for nursing. Considering changes planned, the Chief Nurse for England developed Health Secretary Milburn's desire for a health service that 'liberates nurses not limits them' (espoused at the RCN Congress a year earlier (Beecham 2000)), by identifying 10 key roles (DoH 2000, pp. 83–84):

◆ to order diagnostic investigations such as pathology tests and X-rays
◆ to make and receive referrals direct, say, to a therapist or a pain consultant
◆ to admit and discharge patients for specified conditions and within agreed protocols

◆ to manage patient caseloads, say for diabetes or rheumatology
◆ to run clinics, say, for ophthalmology or dermatology
◆ to prescribe medicines and treatments
◆ to carry out a wide range of resuscitation procedures including defibrillation
◆ to perform minor surgery and outpatient procedures
◆ to triage patients using the latest IT to the most appropriate health professional
◆ to take a lead in the way in which local health services are organized and in the way that they are run.

The Plan admits that all of these nursing roles are already undertaken somewhere in the country, but the emphasis is on these skills becoming part and parcel of common, widespread practice. For many nurses – such as those working as nurse practitioners – the proposals will be far from radical, but for others, achieving them will present a significant but hopefully exciting challenge. Other professionals – notably doctors – also divide similarly. Those used to working with nurses running their own clinics, managing caseloads, and asking doctors to intervene when they see fit, will not be particularly concerned about these new ways of working. But for a good deal more, these proposed new ways of working will represent nothing more than a junior profession reaching for a foothold in their territory and carving out parts of the medical role to increasingly become the prime care provider.

CASE STUDIES OF THE ALTERNATIVE

With these concepts in mind – the need for the NHS to respond to a changing demand, a need for efficient use of resources, and a need to make working for the healthcare system an attractive choice, we can move to consider examples of alternative ways of working which attempt to address all three. In doing so we examine the ramifications of these developments for both nurses and doctors, and in doing so, ask whether nursing actually gains as it embraces these alternatives, or whether the profession is just being used as a relatively easy means to plug the gaps, and as Castledine theorizes, make the nursing workforce into mini-doctors (Castledine 2000). The final, and of course foremost, question which needs to be addressed is whether these alternatives are actually any good for the patient. With these points in mind let us consider further the following innovations in service delivery:

◆ NHS Direct
◆ NHS Walk-in Centres
◆ Nurse-led Primary Medical Services (PMS).

NHS DIRECT

The telephone triage and consultation service – NHS Direct, together with its 'eyes and hands' partner – the Walk-in Centre, are fundamentally intended to address the two issues of demand and access. There is incontrovertible evidence which everyone appreciates without a string of referencing, that demand for GP and accident and emergency (A/E) services is growing exponentially, the result sometimes of there being a wait of several days for a GP appointment, and of many hours to be seen in the emergency environment.

HISTORY AND DEVELOPMENT

Considering the telephone service first, there is a long history of success in providing a centre into which anxious individuals can call and speak to an experienced nurse for advice and support, with potential outcomes ranging from self-care advice through to visiting a GP, or using the emergency services. Toronto's Medical Information Center based within the city's Sick Children's Hospital opened in the late 1970s, with Australia and Sweden having developed successful services in addition to the project here in the UK (Edmonds 1997, Fifield 1996, Glasper et al 2000, Lattimer et al 1998, Markland & Bengtsson 1989, Timpka & Arborelius 1994). In the UK, Health Secretary Milburn first announced proposals for

the introduction of 'medical helplines' following a recommendation in the Chief Medical Officer's report of 1996 (Glasper et al 2000). This translated into the concept of NHS Direct, born out of the White Paper 'The New NHS: Modern, Dependable' (DoH 1997).

Between March 1998 – when NHS Direct was piloted in three call centres in Preston, Milton Keynes and Newcastle – and March 2000, the service handled 1.8 million calls, with a projected call volume for 2000–2001 of 3–4 million calls (DoH 2000b). So far as the objective of managing demand for healthcare services is concerned, the NHS Direct prospectus believes 'this scale of expansion reflects the importance NHS Direct will play in the future provision of NHS Services. This call volume is required to meet the needs of GPs, pharmacists, staff in A/E and NHS Walk-in Centres providing integrated out-of-hours care' (DoH 2000b, p. 5). Basically this means the service is expected to effectively triage callers, assisting them to look after themselves, and where absolutely necessary use the appropriate face-to-face service, whether this be an urgent or routine GP appointment, or a visit to an A/E department or community pharmacist.

IS NHS DIRECT WORKING?

But is NHS Direct meeting this objective? A snapshot survey of 350 consecutive calls from the three pilot sites during one week of September 1998 gleaned 719 (71%) responses from a total of 1050 calls. Ninety-five percent found the service 'quite helpful' and 85% stated that they had followed the nurse advice (O'Cathain et al 2000). More robust data covering the totality of NHS Direct service provision bears out the satisfaction index with the same 95% of callers being satisfied or very satisfied with the service (Medical Care Research Unit, University of Sheffield (MCRUUS) 2000). As for impact on other areas of the NHS, the data are not so conclusive, with little association being found between the introduction of NHS Direct and the increase in demand for A/E or 999 services (MCRUUS 2000). However, MCRUUS did find a correlation with slowing down of the increasing demand for GP out-of-hours services and there does seem to be evidence that people are directed to use A/E and other services appropriately (DoH 2000b). The 2002 National Audit Office review confirmed this general picture, indicating a 90%+ satisfaction score amongst callers. This is considered a success for NHS Direct as it has more than achieved its target of 60% awareness of the service in the general population by March 2002. In addition to the main triage function, NHS Direct has come to the fore in dealing with specialist 'one off' issues such as the introduction of the meningitis C vaccination programme, the MMR controversy, and latterly taking 5000 calls concerning the organ retention scandal (Ward 2001). No doubt NHS Direct does assist people to care for themselves and use the NHS appropriately, but it is still an additional service rather than a replacement or alternative.

WHAT'S IN IT FOR NURSING?

So far as nurses are concerned, NHS Direct does seem to be an attractive proposition. In spite of estimates ranging up to 15 000 nurses needed to run NHS Direct from its 22 call centres (Ashmore et al 2001), there has been little difficulty in employing the 1000 whole-time equivalent individuals actually working within the service. With 60% of these working part-time and many being unable to work elsewhere because of injury, it obviously fits the lifestyle of modern nurses (Clark 2000, Ward 2001). Also, in spite of concern that NHS Direct would 'cream off' nurses from other parts of the NHS, this hasn't happened to any great extent, the reality being that only two NHS trusts have lost more than two staff, with the worst example being Leeds Teaching Hospitals NHS Trust losing 13 out of a total of 5,000 nursing staff (Scott 2000). Overall NHS Direct employs 0.4% of the total whole time equivalent NHS nursing workforce, and 20% of its nurses came from outside the NHS (NAO 2002). If anything, the big question is whether NHS Direct will find it so easy to source appropriately qualified staff as the current nursing workforce ages. Glasper et al (2000) point out that whilst the nursing pool today contains a wealth of experience and expertise, future nurses graduating from more narrow

focus Project 2000 courses will not have the breadth of knowledge needed to be an effective provider of care, through the necessarily generalist NHS Direct. The contra argument to this is that NHS Direct requires more specialist nurses. For instance, the National Service Framework for Mental Health identifies NHS Direct as a new point of access to appropriate mental health services (Ashmore et al 2001), yet even though calls concerning mental health issues make up only 4% of calls, they create more stress in general nurses, especially those new to the service, and take twice as long to process (McMillan 2000). NHS Direct is addressing this issue through the introduction of mental health advisers in each provider site, and generally there is a move toward rotating NHS Direct nurses through other posts in the mainstream health service (Pearce 2001).

What of the question of whether this alternative way of working is a proper development of nursing skills? It could be seen as an attempt to create a hybrid telephonist to push people around an overburdened system, but there is evidence to suggest that nurses working in the system find their past experience invaluable even when they are working with computerized decision support. The national support system developed by AXA aims to ensure consistency of advice and minimize any danger to callers. This 'NHS nurse clinical assessment system' can be seen as directive in its use of an algorithmic approach to sorting problems, but expert nurses are still needed to ensure the right questions are asked and the correct information put into the system. In spite of a reliance on IT systems and managing the care process just through talking and listening, the patient/client relationship and nature of interaction does have the same sequence and characteristics as a 'normal' patient contact (Moore 2001). As Clark (2000) observes, the real challenge for nurses working with such systems is to strike a balance between responding to the healthcare imperatives of the 21st century, using its technology, and retaining the core values of nursing and attention to the constant of basic human need. Tempting as it might be to use 'lower-grade' nurses working to rigid algorithms just to save cash, this would be the undoing of NHS Direct as the ability for an experienced nurse to think around a problem and tease relevant details from a caller, would be lost. This is a significant point which, according to the National Audit Office, must be given serious attention if the service is to guarantee swift caller contact with a nurse when this is required (NAO 2002).

ALTERNATIVE THREATS

NHS Direct finds itself firmly in the firing line for a whole range of perennial doctor vs nurse controversies (Glasper et al 2000)

This chapter began by suggesting that alternative ways of working which bring nurses to the fore, might not sit well with others – in particular doctors. True enough, even though they have complained for years about the need for more appropriate application of their complex skills of diagnosis and management, derived from years in medical school, consolidated in hard times on the wards and as a registrar, GPs were quick to line up and castigate NHS Direct as an ill-thought out, potentially dangerous government wheeze which would do nothing but increase the number of patients attending their surgeries (Burley 1999, Glasper et al 2000, Kenny 2000).

After 3 years of operation the criticism continued, and even eminent TV personality/fertility expert Professor Lord Winston joined the fray condemning NHS Direct as dangerous, based on just two cases (Kenny 2000). In one, a 60-year-old man experiencing nausea and vomiting was advised on self-care. He subsequently died from a ruptured aortic aneurysm. In the other case, the mother of a 7-week-old baby with a fever was advised to call back in an hour if the self-management advice was not working. This she did and the child was admitted to hospital only to die of septicaemia. In fact, research from Sheffield University shows that from 106 396 calls they examined only these two critical incidents were identified – 0.002% of the total, and as Kenny (2000) points out, if we were to survey the whole diagnostic process of the NHS we would find numerous similar mistakes made by GPs and registrars. Nobody suggests that because doctors make errors of judgement, then all medical consultations must be unsafe!

The Consumer Association fanned this fire of criticism by reporting the results of a 'mystery patient' exercise in which the consistency of advice was questionable (Health Which? 2001). This led to critical 'banner headlines' in the *Times* and *Guardian*, stoked by the medical profession, yet a good part of the report was actually positive, praising the improved access to the 24-hour service provided and lauding its principles around confidentiality.

Nevertheless, by early 2001 the medical profession moved into a position of truce and their press even saw reports of the positive benefits NHS Direct has brought to practices (e.g. Durham 2001). This change of heart lay in no small part to those running NHS Direct services both nationally and locally, appreciating that a teamwork approach with GPs was the only sensible way forward. Many GPs have a financial stake in out-of-hours co-operatives, something which could possibly cloud their judgement when faced with the potential of their being replaced as gatekeepers to the NHS by a nurse on a phone line. From the early days of NHS Direct, as part of the tender exercise for second wave bids in May 1998, a consortia of London healthcare trusts and health authorities working with the HARMONI co-operative, showed that collaboration between the accepted model and the new, could work (Burley 1999) and more partnership approaches were developed, thus easing the climate of tension and conflict between the hitherto opposing sides (Reynolds 2000). With NHS Direct having met its target to integrate providers of GP out-of-hours services for 10 million people by March 2002 (NAO 2002), the future of integrated services and collaborative effort is looking good.

NHS WALK-IN CENTRES

'These centres will offer a service to the public, when the public need it and where the public need it'

As he issued these words at the launch of the Walk-in Centre (WIC) project on 16 July 1999 (BBC Online 1999, pp. 1–2), Health Secretary Frank

Dobson knew only too well he was courting controversy. The statement implied that existing services didn't always provide the accessibility required. Even though he went on to emphasize the centres were not intended to replace general practice, rather 'they supplement and complement it' (Beecham 1999, p. 12), Dobson had stirred up once again the unease within the medical profession which had accompanied the inception of NHS Direct. In spite of the Department of Health seeking to ensure that GPs with practices close to the initial 19 WIC sites were on board with the proposals and had 'given their blessing to the project' (BBC Online 1999, p. 2), the British Medical Association (BMA) chairman Ian Bogle had already engendered suspicion among colleagues, at the organization's annual conference just prior to the launch. Bogle suggested the plans would simply 'pander to public demand for 24 hour access to the NHS' and asked 'will they relieve pressure on an understaffed and under resourced service?' (BBC Online 1999, p. 3).

SAME WAR, DIFFERENT BATTLE

Again, we see the introduction of an alternative way of working intended to relieve demand on general practice simply raising criticism from that profession. Again the key elements for dissent are there – an alternative access point to NHS services, to the traditional 'gate keeper GP' (see later in the chapter for more discussion of this issue), and a nurse-led and dominated service deciding who needs to see a doctor and when. The rationale for setting up WICs was also pretty similar. The Government knew people were fed up waiting for GP appointments and that many turned to A/E services when their GP was inaccessible, leading to problems there. Also, GPs themselves had been describing how overworked and understaffed their part of the health service really was. What GPs did not want though, was an alternative to their domination of the market. A discussion paper jointly published by the Royal College of General Practitioners (RCGP) and the NHS Alliance stated that 'for those patients who are away from home or who work during the opening hours of their surgery,

access to urgent facilities is of value. However, there are long-standing "temporary resident" and "immediately necessary treatment" schemes in general practice; out-of-hours co-operatives and deputising services; and accident and emergency. Offering yet another option for immediate access seems unnecessary' (1999, p. 1).

ON WITH REFORM

In a speech in Solihul addressing the concerns of the medical profession, Frank Dobson pledged to 'raise the pace of NHS reform rather than slow it down in response to BMA fears' (BBC Online 1999, p. 3).

The Health Secretary did not exactly say it, but the implication was that if GPs were able to have offered all these services in a way in which the public could understand, and use, there wouldn't be a problem. As they hadn't, WICs were the answer he had come up with. It is important to note that no resources were being diverted away from general practice – the £30 million which would eventually be spent on setting up 36 WICs throughout England was all new money – just that GPs felt it should be spent on them, rather than, as John Chisholm (the leader of BMA GPs) put it, 'shift investment of money from the urgent and serious to the relatively trivial' (BBC Online 1999, p. 3). (See Chapter 26 for further discussion on decision-making with reference to the use of scarce resources.)

DO WALK-IN CENTRES MEET NEED?

The answer depends on one's perceptions of 'serious' and 'trivial'. If 'serious' was perceived to be complex conditions requiring medical intervention, and 'relatively trivial' were less complex problems which could easily be handled by nurses in a WIC, then Chisholm had a point. But for someone suffering from a 'relatively trivial' problem the WIC could be ideal – as Dobson reckoned. Taking a look at the range of conditions the average WIC is intended to deal with, does seem to suggest it is a useful facility (DoH 2001):

◆ coughs, colds and flu-like symptoms
◆ information on staying healthy/local services

- minor cuts and wounds – care, dressings
- skin complaints – rashes, sunburn, headlice, nappy rash
- muscle and joint injuries – strains and sprains
- stomach ache, indigestion, constipation, vomiting and diarrhoea
- women's health problems, e.g. thrush, menstrual advice
- hayfever, bites and stings.

As it turns out, nurses working in WICs have been quick to expand this list and develop additional services in respect of their individual skills and demands on the centre. For example the Birmingham WIC ran an outreach programme with ethnic minority women's groups and now provides a cervical cytology screening programme for Somali women who found it difficult to use local GP services, and this WIC and the majority of others have moved into sexual health advice and the provision of emergency postcoital contraception (Peake 2001). This potential for innovation and role development has made WICs an attractive place for nurses to work. A background in A/E or primary care nursing seems to be a common factor, and for similar reasons to those given for NHS Direct above, nurses have been keen to move into the WIC environment.

JUSTIFIED CRITICISM?

Not surprisingly, given the track record of NHS Direct, criticisms of WICs followed a similar course. The main GP criticisms were that WICs would reduce continuity of care, erode the doctor–patient relationship and dilute the 'values of general practice in the United Kingdom' and that 'Overall the effect of Walk-In Centres on access will be minimal, while the potential for degradation of general practice – the internationally acknowledged gem at the centre of the NHS – is significant' (RCGP/NHS Alliance 1999, pp. 1–2). One does not need to be an expert in semantics or to look deeply into these statements, to see where the doctors were coming from! Having said this, the warnings of the medical profession struck home with patient groups who, whilst welcoming

the convenience WICs would offer, reiterated the possible danger to patients because of poor communication between the WIC and GPs (BBC Online 1999, p. 1). The accessibility of records was seen as a crucial factor and Mike Stone, general manager of the Patient's Association, raised the fear of mistakes due to inaccessibility of GP records by nurses in WICs.

These are indeed valid points, and true seamless care for patients at whatever point of the healthcare system they choose to access it, will not be a reality until we achieve the goal of a true electronic patient record. The NHS Plan (DoH 2000a, Ch 10) acknowledges this, together with the additional benefit of patients being able to see their own record via smart card access. These are truly alternative ways of working which will liberate both patients and clients as all would have access to contemporaneous information, so reducing the input of criticisms levied around poor communication. Of course a patient-held paper system could be introduced right now if there was the will to do it.

Evaluation, or lack of it, in WICs is again a source for concern. The Consumers' Association used a similar method to their tactics with NHS Direct and introduced a series of 'mystery patients' making 24 visits to eight of the centres in operation during 2001 (Jones 2001). The report in Which? (2001) criticized the WICs for inconsistent advice and failure to provide a full assessment for some patients. The Department of Health acknowledged some of these failings and has subsequently embarked upon a programme to extend the AXA decision support software system from NHS Direct to WICs. This will not only facilitate communication between the two services – including referral of a caller to the WIC if a face-to-face consultation was considered beneficial – but nurses within the centres will have a standard reference point upon which to base their triage and assessment decisions.

As with NHS Direct, the introduction of WICs as an alternative way of working, has brought nurses into the frontline of controversy, as traditional systems which have been in place since the inception of the NHS, are challenged. GPs have been threatened and reacted accordingly, yet again where co-operation has been encouraged, leading medical commentators have highlighted the positive benefits for themselves and their patients (e.g. Everington in Beecham 1999).

NURSE-LED PERSONAL MEDICAL SERVICES (PMS)

The modernization of the health service in line with the NHS Plan is throwing up alternative ways of working which challenge the very firm status quo of the NHS as it has existed for over 50 years. A key element to that status quo is the medical practitioner as the dominant healthcare provider, and in the context of primary care, the GP as focal point and gatekeeper to the system. According to the Royal College of General Practitioners (RCGP), 'Along with dentists, pharmacists and opticians, general practitioners form the primary care level of the NHS and as such are the "front line" of the health service' (RCGP 1999). Even in the midst of the rapid change facing the NHS at the turn of the century, GP academics still see the 'enduring stereotype in this era as a GP' (Dowell & Neal 2000). A great deal of importance is placed on the relationship between patient and GP – see the BMA comments re introduction of Walk-In Centres above – with only general practice having the 'obligation of care 24 hours a day, and offering continuity in the context of the family and the community' (RCGP 2001). With over 95% of the population registered with a GP and around 1800 patients vying for the care he or she can provide (RCGP 1999) as part of the 300 million consultations made per year (Office of Health Economics 1997) it is hard not to recognize the notion of 'family doctor' as the prime focus of primary care provision.

If these assertions are unpicked however, and we ask why this is so, an obvious answer is that it has always been done that way. Even without the purchasing aspect associated with fund holding, access to secondary care services – even for something as minimal as having an X-ray of a suspected fracture performed – has been as a result of referral from a GP, provided of course one

wanted this done 'on the NHS'. Similarly, high rates of registration with GPs do not necessarily represent a considered response from a public keen to select the best provider for their needs, rather that without such registration it is nigh on impossible to access state-funded health services. GPs have also benefited from a range of ring-fenced skills and rights such as the ability to prescribe drugs for example. Yet even the most ardent supporter of the medical practitioner as the natural team leader and centre of care provision in primary care, cannot turn a blind eye to the 40 000 or so community nurses employed by Primary Care Trusts (PCTs) nor the exponential increase in numbers of practice nurses from a little over 1500 in 1980 to some 17 500 today (Jones 1996).

THE GP AS HUB

It is all well and good postulating that the 'right person' to deliver primary care to any given person might not necessarily be the GP, especially as roles traditionally reserved for them – prescribing for instance – are being shared with others, but an examination of the organizational systems in place leads us to appreciate that the established model of GP as team leader/centre of provision is quite difficult to move away from. The place of GP as independent contractor 'selling' his services to the NHS and earning a living through a series of payments based on a number of patients on his list, and what he does or does not do for them, does little to motivate entrepreneurial spirit, or for the GP to play his part in a team which might take away a little of his profit margin. This is no fault of doctors, rather the organizational – including financing – system of primary care, which has grown up in a way so as to recompense the GP for services rendered, as the one and only gatekeeper. With its emphasis on purchasing care to the best value, Thatcher's fundholding scheme only served to entrench these values.

As Wilson (2000) points out, it was not until the NHS Community Care Act (DoH 1989) attempted to integrate primary health and social care services that the extent to which professionals view the same problem from different perspectives was really appreciated. Each professional group uses its own language and vocabulary and is routed in tradition, ideology and philosophy, which sets it apart from others. With a population which has differing health needs, according to individual needs and the community concerned, it is easy to see how such a disparity would militate against the best provision with professionals working to their own treatment paradigm (Dorwick 1997) and a lack of cohesion within the team made worse by organizational systems which were never intended to support joint working in the first place.

CHANGING THE RULES – PRIMARY CARE ACT PILOT SITES

The organizational development which gave the opportunity for the GP-dominated primary care provider model to be seriously challenged, was the experimental changes made to legislation, deregulating the provision of personal medical services – the so called 'Primary Care Act Pilots Sites (PCAPS) (DoH 1997). PCAPS were designed to allow primary care professionals to put forward new and innovative alternatives to the GP-centred model. In some of the models, GP groups simply re-jigged their existing services and highlighted the importance of their attached nursing staff, others were more radical, with nurses taking over the administrative and leadership role in the practice and employing GPs to take up referrals from the nursing team (Vanclay 1998). PCAPS allowed for the side-stepping of existing regulations and procedural barriers and marked the moment when the GP monopoly in the provision of personal medical services was brought to an end and true interdisciplinary approaches to primary care delivery really began to be considered.

NURSE-LED PMS

Moving on from PCAPS projects, Health Secretary Dobson announced another development encouraging health professionals to take a different approach to delivering primary care

services – the Personal Medical Services (PMS) pilots. Perhaps the most significant development in these PMS initiatives was the decision by nine nurses to lead the delivery of PMS care from 1 April 1998. The so-called 'nurse-led PMS pilots' demonstrated a radical shift in primary care dynamics with some of them even employing a GP on a salaried basis. A review of the sites by the King's Fund (Lewis 2001) 2 years into their operation found all of them had experienced resistance in their neighbourhood ranging from antagonism from GPs in the area, through to hospital consultants not accepting nurse-originated referrals, and even nurses seeing their PMS colleagues as rather strange. The report highlighted the dramatic effects of supplanting a medical model led service with one based on nursing ethic and systems which quite often was more appropriate to addressing the needs of underserved practice and locality populations. Nevertheless, the nurse-led PMS sites indicate that as they built up their services and demonstrated their ability to do a good job, a good deal of the initial reticence concerning their operation began to subside. (See Chapter 5 for further discussion on cultural issues relating to the quality of care.)

PMS BENEFITS?

Returning to the original issues of meeting need in alternative ways, best use of resources, and providing attractive new options for nurses, how have nurse-led PMS projects faired? PMS has generally been described as giving 'GPs, nurses, and their teams freedom to decide how to organise themselves and their resources so as to meet local needs, and provide an opportunity to take advantage of the particular skills of each member of the team' (pricare 2001, p. 5) and commentators such as Lewis and Jones (Jones 1999, Lewis 2001) have identified their ability to provide an appropriate alternative for some patient groups, this being particularly relevant for inner cities with relatively large deprived and homeless populations. These authors maintain the established model of an NHS, organizationally geared to the traditional model of general practice, is open to challenge and the adoption of alternative systems.

This is not just for political reasons associated with the diminution of the GP powerbase, but because a mixed market of primary care delivery will offer many insights into the feasibility of addressing need and utilizing resources in ways which were never even considered, and Primary Care Trusts (PCTs) should find nurse-led PMS invaluable as they accept responsibility for the configuration of primary care in the future (Jones 1999, p. 49).

AND NURSING?

These developments have not been without personal costs for the nurses involved. A punishing workload and a highly politicized environment, with resistance, or blockages, from many quarters, appear to have been the norm. Certainly the NHS juggernaut will not turn on a sixpence. Nor should the 'forces of conservatism' be underestimated. Nurse leads have faced professional and bureaucratic obstacles that have proved quite unyielding; to the extent that the pilots have been successful, this has been despite the 'system' and not because of it. However, this is not to say that, having been the brainchild of Ministers, the nine leads have been abandoned to their fates. As one nurse lead commented wryly: 'never have nine nurses had such access to Ministers' (Lewis 2001).

CONCLUSION

There is no doubt our Government is 'hell bent' on modernizing the NHS and will do all in its power to ensure that, at the end of the day, the resource we have will bring maximum benefit to the most people. We can debate the pros and cons of such a utilitarian principle elsewhere, but for the purposes of this chapter, it is plain to see that novel, alternative ways of working, have seen the light of day as a result of the commitment to making the NHS as accessible and efficient as possible through the best use of both human and physical resources. If this means addressing some of the 'sacred cows' such as medical dominance of the system and the GP as hub of primary care, then so

be it. But let us not be fooled into thinking that if the NHS had a bountiful supply of cash and people flooding in to work as doctors and nurses, it would still be like that. As the saying goes, necessity is the mother of invention, and holding out the hand of friendship to nursing in the form of a revitalized identity, in the healthcare system, is something in which the Government really had little choice.

Having said this, when a Health Secretary writes a leader in a nursing journal to the effect that 'NHS Direct is an important element of the modernisation of healthcare. It is a powerful symbol of the new NHS, and is an example of the exciting opportunities for nurses which the new NHS offers. The success of NHS Direct is a credit to the skills and vision of the nurses who staff it' (Dobson 1999), this is not just the guff of politics. This Health Secretary and his successor have seen the true value in 'liberating' nursing, and no doubt appreciated the risk in upsetting the apple cart of the medical profession as they introduced pretty radical nurse-led service models such as NHS Direct and Walk-in Centres. In a way, these initiatives have been a 'gift' for those who have argued the benefits of putting the nurse at the centre of the healthcare delivery system, and by and large nurses have risen to the challenge. This is perhaps not so evident with the PMS pilots.

Throughout this chapter, the role of medics in general terms has been considered, while that of GPs has been explored in more detail. Certainly alternative ways of working have been considered in terms of giving GPs 'a run for their money'. But, when entering the field of GP payment systems and contractual obligations we get into a whole new ball game. Bevan realized at the very inception of the NHS, that if GPs were not on board the whole thing would fail. From those times right up until just a couple of years ago, GPs held an independent practitioner contract with the Secretary of State and made a living according to a rigidly set and calculated formula. PMS has changed all of that. It has been tough enough for some GPs to accept more control over their work from the Primary Care Trust/Scottish Primary Care Group/Local Health Group and taking away the rules, whilst at the same time putting in more performance management, makes for an uneasy situation. Bring along the concept of a GP being salaried to a PMS provider team run by a nurse and we are talking radical. The almost unthinkable novelty of this situation has brought the battle alluded to by Salvage right at the beginning of this chapter back into sharp focus, although this time around it is not just doctors who are jumpy, but as can be seen from Lewis' analysis for the King's Fund, nurses themselves are questioning the viability of such a proposition.

No doubt the day of true interdisciplinary PMS will arrive with neither medicine nor nursing claiming the lead, but until then all we can see from the evidence to date is that nurses who have attempted to pioneer in this arena, have a much tougher ride than colleagues in the telephone and walk-in services. Perhaps these nursing pioneers and their influence on the traditional healthcare system, will lead us into a new world of primary care in which power bases and traditional ways of doing things are once and for all abandoned in favour of an approach which best meets the need of the people needing care, rather than those of the professionals seeking to provide it.

Alternative ways of working are good news in principle, but we need to check they meet need in appropriate ways and make the best use of our resources (see Chapter 26 for further discussion of the economic perspective). Being selfish in conclusion – but this is a nursing textbook – we need to be sure these alternatives are good for nurses and that nursing isn't being liberated today only to be reined back in tomorrow. Our medical colleagues know this lesson only too well.

SUMMARY

◆ Alternative ways of working for nurses include NHS Direct, NHS Walk-in Centres and nurse-led Primary Medical Services.

◆ Although these services have created some tensions between medicine and nursing, tangible benefits have been seen by patients.

◆ Nursing is emerging as prime care-giver in the modern NHS.

DISCUSSION POINTS

1. Are exciting developments for nursing happening because our skills are recognized at last, or because we are the last ditch solution for a struggling government?

2. Does innovation in nursing always have to lead to conflict with medicine, and if not how can we prevent this?

3. What makes the alternative ways of working described above attractive propositions for both nurses and patients?

REFERENCES

Ashmore R, Hemingway S, Lees J 2001 Assessing therapeutic intervention used by NHS Direct nurse advisers. British Journal of Nursing 10(10): 662–664
BBC Online 1999 Walk-in centres could be a danger. BBC News: Health (online). July 16th, pp. 1–4. BBC, London
Beecham L 1999 GPs must get involved in walk-in centres. British Medical Journal 319: 2
Beecham L 2000 UK health secretary wants to liberate nurses' talents. British Medical Journal 320: 1025
Burley D 1999 Educational provision for nurses operating in 'NHS Direct'. Journal of Community Nursing 13(10): 4–5
Castledine G 2000 Reinforcing the medical stereotypes of nursing. British Journal of Nursing 9(15): 1026
Clark J 2000 Old wine in new bottles: Delivering nursing care in the 21st century. Journal of Nursing Scholarship First Quarter: 11–15
Department of Health 1989 Caring for people: community care in the next decade and beyond. HMSO, London
Department of Health 1997 The new NHS: modern, dependable. The Stationery Office, London
Department of Health 2000a The NHS plan. A plan for investment. A plan for reform. The Stationery Office, Norwich
Department of Health 2000b NHS Direct. A new gateway to healthcare. The Stationery Office, Norwich
Department of Health 2001 NHS walk-in centres. Department of Health, London (www.doh.gov.uk/nhswalkincentres/info.htm)
Dobson F 1999 A direct hit. Nursing Times 95(33): 32
Dorwick C 1997 Rethinking the doctor patient relationship in general practice. Health and Social Care in the Community 5(1): 11–14
Dowell T, Neal R 2000. Vision and change in primary care. In: Tovey P (ed.) Contemporary primary care – The challenges of change. Open University Press, Buckingham
Durham N 2001 NHS Direct pilots cut day visits by a fifth. GP March 16: 16
Edmonds E 1997 Telephone triage: 5 years' experience. Accident and Emergency Nursing 5: 8–13

Fifield M 1996 Telephone triage: protocols for an unacknowledged practice. Australian Journal of Advanced Nursing 13(2): 5–9

Glasper EA, Lattimer VA, Thompson F, Wray D 2000 NHS Direct: examining the challenges for nursing practice. British Journal of Nursing 9(17): 1173–1181

Health Which? 2000 NHS Direct investigated. Health Which? August: 12–16

Jones D 1999 Nurse led PMS pilots. In: Lewis R, Gillam S (eds) Transforming primary care. King's Fund, London

Jones J 2001 NHS walk-in centres fail to assess patients properly. British Medical Journal 322: 70

Jones M 1996 Accountability in practice. A guide to professional responsibility for nurses in general practice. Quay Books, Dinton

Kenny C 2000 Jury still out on the safety of NHS Direct. Nursing Times 96(50): 13

Lattimer V, George S, Thompson F et al 1998 Safety and effectiveness of nurse telephone consultation in out of hours primary care: randomized controlled trial. British Medical Journal 317: 1054–1059

Lewis R 2001 Nurse-led primary care – putting policy into practice. Learning from the first wave nurse-led PMS pilots. King's Fund, London

Markland B, Bengtsson C 1989 Medical advice by telephone at Swedish health centres. Who calls and what are the problems? Family Practitioner 6(1): 42–46

McMillan I 2000 Dial 'M' for mental health. Mental Health Practice 3(9): 6

Medical Care Research Unit, University of Leicester 2000 Evaluation of NHS Direct first wave sites. Second interim report to the Department of Health. Medical Care Research Unit, University of Leicester, Leicester

Moore R 2001 A framework for telephone nursing. Nursing Times 97(16): 36–37

National Audit Office 2002 NHS Direct in England. Report by the Comptroller and Auditor General. HC505 Session 2001–2002: 25 January 2002. NAO, London

O'Cathain A, Munro JF, Nicholl P, Knowles E 2000 How helpful is NHS Direct? Postal survey of callers. British Medical Journal 320: 1035

Office of Health Economics 1997 10th compendium of health statistics. OHE, London

Peake G 2001 Personal communication between Gerri Peake, manager Birmingham walk-in centre, and author.

Pearce L 2001 Walk-in wonderland. Nursing Standard 15(18): 22–23

pricare 2001 Simple guide to PMS. (in association with Doctor, RCN, napc). Pricare, London

Reynolds M 2000 The quiet revolution. Nursing Standard 14(40): 18

Royal College of General Practitioners 1999 General practice in the UK. Information Sheet no.4. RCGP, London

Royal College of General Practitioners, NHS Alliance 1999 Walk-in centres. RCGP, London (www.rcgp.org.uk/rcgp/corporate/discussion/nhswic14.asp)

Royal College of General Practitioners 2001 Access to general practice based primary care. A position statement for consultation. RCGP, London

Salvage J 2000 Who wears the trousers? Nursing Times 96(15): 24

Scott G 2000 First port of call. Nursing Standard 14(40): 13–14

Timpka T, Arborelius E 1994 The primary care nurses' dilemma: a study of knowledge use and need during telephone consultation. In: Smith J (ed.) Research and its application. Blackwell Scientific Publications, London

Vanclay L 1998 Team working in primary care. Nursing Standard 12(20): 37–38

Ward S 2001 Dial M for…medical advice. Health Service Journal May 24: 26

Which? 2001 Survey of NHS walk-in centres. Which? January: 7–9

Wilson AE 2000 The changing nature of primary care teams and interprofessional relationships. In: Tovey P (ed.) Contemporary primary care – The challenges of change. Open University Press, Buckingham

FURTHER READING

Department of Health 2002 Liberating the talents. Helping Primary Care Trusts and nurses to deliver the NHS Plan. DoH, London

Gabe J, Kellemer D, Williams G (eds) Challenging medicine. Routledge, London

Gillam S, Abbott S, Banks-Smith J 2001 Can primary care groups and trusts improve health? British Medical Journal 323: 89–92

Moon G, North N 2000 Policy and place: general medical practice in the UK. Macmillan, Basingstoke

KEY ISSUES

◆ Information technology and nursing.

◆ Resources for community nursing.

◆ The Internet and the practitioner/patient relationship.

◆ Health and digital inequalities.

25

The challenge of information technology

M. Hardey

INTRODUCTION

This chapter is about the opportunities and challenges of information and communication technologies (ICTs) for community nursing, as well as health and social care in the UK. The chapter opens with an examination of the new virtual world of the Internet. It then moves on to consider problems of unequal public access to Internet resources. Drawing attention to the virtual, it explores some of the more significant health resources that are available to practitioners and the public. The role of newsgroups and home pages is also discussed. This leads to questioning the nature of identity and the choices open to contemporary society. These themes will be drawn together in the conclusion, which will suggest that the new space of the Internet is transforming how we think about health and how care should be delivered.

The nursing profession has not faired well in the introduction of new technology into the public services. The short history of the implementation of information technology into government services is marked by large cost over-runs, late delivery and poor usability. Few professions are more aware of the 1980s myth of the 'paperless office' than nursing, who since computers appeared on the wards or in the community office have been struggling with ever-increasing demands for documentation.

HISTORY AND DEVELOPMENT

Information technologies have been central to the modernization of the NHS since the first tentative introduction of general management with the Griffiths Report (1983). Since the 1980s, computational technology has been transformed by the production of increasingly fast microchips, graphically based software and a fall in real costs. This has driven the development of what is known as the new Information and Communications Technologies (ICTs). The expansion of the ICTs sector has been rapid, for example an estimated 623 web sites were on the Internet in 1993 and in only six years this grew to 5.4 million.[1] (Relevant website addresses are given at the end of the chapter.) The Internet is by far the most visible of ICTs and is rarely out of the news, including the World Wide Web, e-mail, chat room and other ways in which people can interact with others, or identify and view, information. It is the global and unmediated nature of the Internet which has frequently captured the interest of the news media with stories that have included a Webcast of a woman giving birth, an attempt to sell human kidneys on an auction site and the promotion and sale of potentially dangerous treatments to consumers. Health is commonly cited as the second most visited category in the Internet. Such are the expectations about the potential of ICTs that policy documents are confident that the Internet will be a major public resource that will connect users to health professionals and social care organizations. For example, the Department of Health (2000) information technology strategy claims that public access to health and social services should be fully available electronically by 2005.

In the 1970s information technology led to the founding of a new medical specialty labeled 'telemedicine'. The word derives from the Greek 'tele' meaning '*at a distance*' and the present word 'medicine' which itself derives from the Latin 'mederi' meaning '*healing*'. Reflecting a more 'social' orientation the label 'telecare' is often used by projects that are seeking to, for example, monitor an individual's health in their own home. Policy emphasis on enabling people with chronic health problems to stay in the community has led to a number of projects that have included provision of home alarm telephones and monitoring bodily functions.[2] The technology exists to provide interactive home consultations, detailed patient monitoring and the surveillance of lifestyle

(e.g. use of the kitchen, social contact, etc.). However cost-effectiveness of large-scale implementation is questionable given other health and social care priorities (Wootton 1998). (See Chapter 26 for more detailed discussion of health economics.) The related specialty 'nursing (or medical) informatics' developed out of computer informatics which, as the title suggests, is focused on the creation and delivery of computer-mediated information (Graves & Corcoran 1989, Simpson 1992). This includes many information technology specialists who have been responsible for creating and maintaining computer systems in hospitals and elsewhere. There is, for example, a nursing specialist group within the British Computer Society. However the specialties reflect institutional and professional boundaries and so less effort has been expended in nursing informatics (which is dominated by the United States) than in other areas.

The introduction of computers is often taken for granted as a good thing. This may not always be the case. A glance at journals such as *Information Technology and Nursing* will reveal articles about the problems and opportunities of implementing and using computers in practice. The emphasis is on 'technology' and this masks the way the implementation and use of information technology is profoundly social. In the 1980s the 'Florence' project attempted to build a ward-based computer records system with the collaboration of nurses who would be the users (see Bjerknes & Bratteteig (1987) for a description of Florence). It became apparent that information used by nurses on wards is complex and the processes and material may be hidden to observers (Robinson et al 1996; see also Hardey et al 2000). Computerization therefore is far more than simply replicating written material in line with a vision of a 'paperless' ward. However, relatively little information technology is currently used in the UK to integrate the delivery of community care or even to promote collaboration between health and social care professionals (Hardey et al 2000).

CONSIDERING THE VIRTUAL

It is worthwhile taking a geographical analogy when considering the nature of the Internet, which we can think of as a new virtual space. This reflects a metaphor common in the United States of the 'electronic frontier' that captures the sense of a new space waiting to be occupied and moulded by people as they move into it. Within this 'landscape' there are different territories, which have more or less distinct boundaries. For example, a space devoted to email has a distinct architecture and pattern of use compared to a personal home page. The latter is one of the ways that anyone can establish their own 'home' on the Internet by designing a space around their interests and experiences. Issues surrounding home pages, which users have established as a resource for people who share their health problems, are worth exploring. Sitting at a computer at home or work, means entering a space that is occupied by a vast collection of libraries where it is possible to read literary classics, or the most recent issue of your favourite clinical journal. Virtual spaces are both local and global in that I can enter the virtual world while sitting at the computer in my spare bedroom and read a paper published in Australia, or interact with people from other parts of the globe, in a chat room. Note that on the one hand I am alone and isolated in my room but at the same time I am communicating with others and participating in what has been described as an 'electronic community'. The Internet seems to promise the advantages of privacy, cultural richness, altruism and infinite possibilities for sociability. It is also a space where users are disembodied.

The virtual landscape is so vast and made up of so many different features that it might be useful to outline the main resources that are commonly claimed to be useful to practitioners.

Electronic libraries

Most readers will be familiar with electronic libraries, which are increasingly becoming efficient ways to identify new innovations in practice and are central to research.

Electronic journals

Some journals exist independently of libraries and essentially consist of digital copies of print journals (e.g. *Journal of Advanced Nursing*). Other journals only exist on the Internet and are sometimes referred to as 'e-journals' (e.g. *Sociology On-line*). Utilizing the power of ICTs, many journals make past copies instantly available and in some cases resources that are not available in print copies (e.g. *BMJ*, *Nursing Standard On-Line*).

Electronic resources

Medline, CINAHL and other resources enable users to search and retrieve health information. In addition the Cochrane Centre and the NHS national electronic library provide a series of routes to information targeted at specific health professions and for example give access to evidence-based research material.

Newsgroups (USENET)

Discussion groups devoted to nursing issues are usually moderated (i.e. controlled by one or more people who ensure that the topics discussed are appropriate). Users can search the messages from others and leave their own contributions. Many newsgroups have a global membership so a question posted to one about, for example, discharge planning, might receive responses from users in Australia or India.

Chat rooms

Unlike newsgroups communication is synchronous, so users can have real-time interactions between spatially separated participants who can read each other's contributions instantaneously.

Communities online

There are a growing number of neighbourhoods where people have developed a community on the Internet. In the UK these may be part of regeneration schemes aimed at poorer communities and represent a potentially important source of information about the history, concerns and opportunities that exists in an area where individuals live and work.

Distance learning

Potentially using any number of technological resources the Open University and other education institutes offer courses that are partially based on self-directed learning supported by the Internet. There are also a number of attempts to create 'virtual universities' where whole courses are delivered on-line (e.g.[3]). The NHS Information Authority Education and Training strategy is investing in information technology as a means to prepare nurses for future practice. Indeed the reader of this chapter may be part of this program.

Government data and policies

As part of the 'e-government' initiative, it is anticipated that not only will the policy documents now posted on government sites be available but that also all government services, both local and national, should be available electronically by 2005 (DoH 2000 Section 2, Paragraph 2–3). Most readers will be familiar with the NHS Website that has links to other resources including health authorities.

Professional organizations

Bodies such as the UKCC and the ENB maintain Websites and some provide on-line support to members.

HEALTH AND DIGITAL INEQUALITIES

The association between poverty, morbidity and mortality is generally accepted and has been manifest in attempts to improve the nation's health since the Black Report (Townsend & Davison 1982) if not earlier (see Hardey 1998, Ch. 5 for a discussion of this). A new inequality has been identified at the beginning of the 21st century, which has been described as the 'digital divide'. Ownership of home computers is highest in the United States but growing rapidly in Europe and the UK. Computers were present in nearly one in six UK households in 1986 and by 2000 this had grown to one household in three (Office of National Statistics 2001, p. 118). While the UK is well placed among the bigger EU countries in the ownership of information technology it lags behind Scandinavian nations. The Internet is also available in many places of work, most schools, colleges and universities, libraries, Internet cafes, Internet-based public phones, public Internet access points in many cities and other places. Relatively few nurses have easy access to a networked computer at work and may be dependent on their own home machine, or those available in educational institutions (Anthony 2000). A survey of community nurses undertaken in Aberdeen reported that just under half had access to the Internet at home or work (Lawton et al 2001). However, some areas of nursing such as mental health may have less access at work than others (Anthony 1998). (See Chapter 5 for a discussion on the link between quality assurance and access to research-based evidence of clinical effectiveness.)

It has been estimated that there are 11 100 new Internet users per day in the UK (NOP 1999). Another survey undertaken in July 2000 found that 45% of all adults had accessed the Internet (Office of National Statistics 2001). Such generic figures can disguise inequalities of access. For example, men are more likely to use the Internet than women and while nearly all people under the age of 24 years have used the Internet it has been used by only 6% of those aged 75 and over. Ownership of a computer and home access to the Internet is also not common in poorer communities. However, analysis of the postcodes of new Internet users has indicated that the relative income of new UK Internet users is decreasing (Foley 1999). The digital divide is usually conceived in terms of economic inequalities rather than gender or ethnic differences, for which there are fewer sources of reliable data. While a household may have a computer with Internet access this does not mean that all household members will use it equally. To make matters more difficult we should recognize the convergence of digital technologies. The Wrap mobile phone, handheld computer and digital radio and television all potentially provide access to the Internet. Digital television was introduced in the UK in 1996 and can be received through a conventional aerial, cable or a satellite dish. Unlike the analogue system that it will replace, it is a potentially interactive technology that will enable people to access a limited number of Internet services through their televisions. Despite the potential equalizing impact of digital television there is a continuing divide along social class lines that has implications for the broader issues of social exclusions. It should be remembered for example that some communities are likely to experience disproportionately higher levels of disability and premature death. For example, South Asian men in the UK experience up to half as much greater risk from heart disease than white men (Balarajan 1996). Government policy promotes the Internet as a means to provide access to healthcare information and services, which increase the quality and efficiency of care. There is potential here for the information rich to take advantage of opportunities that are not available to the information poor, who are consequently further disadvantaged.

Lack of access to ICTs has potentially serious consequences for individuals, communities and countries, if we accept that we live in what government policy documents refer to as the 'knowledge economy'. A number of initiatives have therefore been developed as part of broader schemes to provide skills and education as well as improved employment opportunities to people who live in poor neighbourhoods. Various projects around the UK (and Europe) have built on existing community associations and voluntary organizations to provide the resources to enable people to design and maintain their own on-line communities. Through involvement in such projects people not only gain important information technology skills but are also able to highlight the opportunities and problems associated with their neighbourhood. For example Artmedia, based in Batley grew out of community arts and now has an established Internet site developed by local people. Their site includes African-Caribbean women telling their family histories, a digital gallery and the local multiple sclerosis support group who explain their experiences and give information about where support can be found. In contrast to this urban community there are also a number of projects that are based in rural areas. WREN telecottage, for example, is based in Warwickshire. Following information technology training provided by WREN, a number of people have set up

local businesses and others have moved into working in the information technology industry from home (see CIRA for links to community sites and research on them).[4]

Although the focus of this chapter is on the UK it is important to remember that the Internet is not distributed equally across the globe. The United States continues to dominate it whether this is measured by the population of users, or in terms of content within Web pages. Spatial analysis of computers that 'host' (i.e. store and provide access to the content of Web resources) or users of the Internet, generates a map that echoes earlier geographies where resources were disproportionately owned by colonial powers (Dodge 1999). Many African and South American countries have few links to the Internet while other countries including China, Saudi Arabia, Iran, Algeria and the United Arab Emirates not only restrict public access to the Internet but also filter all traffic that flows into the country to prevent users accessing what is thought to be undesirable content.

VIRTUAL HEALTH CARE

Any brief review of virtual health care will highlight NHS Direct Online[5] as it is the most visible example of a state gateway that provides health information in the UK. It is designed to complement the nurse-led NHS Direct telephone-support service. It has a disease focus, although there is some advice about healthy living, and has a limited amount of information that is not presented in the English language. In addition there are some audio/video presentations about self-treatment. The BBC Web site[6] which contains Online Health and Fitness provides a less disease-based information service and through dynamic links to radio and television programmes, has a degree of interactivity lacking in NHS Direct. For example, a media-led national 'stop smoking' campaign run in 2000 included radio, television and Internet advice with support groups for smokers being organized through the BBC site. The United States, where the e-health market is estimated to be worth $205 billion dollars by 2003, leads the way in commercial health Web resources. This reflects the estimated 24.8 million Americans who use the Internet to find information about health and, in a system dominated by health insurance, to seek medical care (Reents 1999). There are an increasing number of private health portals in the UK. Boots and Granada Media have developed the Wellbeing[7] site, which is associated with a digital health television channel and intended to provide information and to advance and sell products and services to users. Reflecting the importance of the health market, other sites like that owned by Lloyds Pharmacy, are seeking to exploit the commercial potential of the Internet. Other organizations, such as NetDoctor,[8] have attempted to replicate broadcast media by generating revenue from sponsorship and advertising. There are also a growing number of UK sites that are oriented to complementary and alternative therapies. These range from organizations that promote and sell products directly to consumers and to individual therapists who have developed their own Web page to advertise their services. At a global level there are a vast number of Internet pages devoted to health and well-being.

Many voluntary organizations have their own space on the Internet. Their use of the Internet reflects the priorities of the organization and is used by some primarily to campaign and by others to provide information and support to users. For example, the Mind Web site contains descriptions of various mental health problems, available treatments and the obligations of health and social services to clients. Not constrained by government policy or commercial considerations the voluntary sector can be more adventurous in the content and form of their Web resources. The National Schizophrenia Fellowship, for example, provides chat rooms where users can interact with each other.

The form and content of sites outside of NHS Direct are more diverse and include a greater degree of social care information but the presentation is predominately in a form congruent with an English-speaking middle class audience. There is therefore something of a paradox at the heart of what is currently available in the UK to users of health and social services in that it fails to reflect the needs of a culturally diverse society. (See Chapter 24 for more detailed discussion of NHS Direct.)

HEALTH POLICY AND THE 'EXPERT PATIENT'

Since the 1980s there has been a drive for health and social services to become more consumer conscious. The resulting rhetoric is constructed around notions of empowerment, rights and partnership and expressed in terminology that includes 'consumers', 'responsibility', 'service users', 'client' and 'providers'. Indeed, social workers now refer to service users or simply users rather than the now dated and paternalistic label, client or case. However, 'patient' remains common currency in nursing and medicine despite being characteristic of a doctor/patient relationship where the patient is in a position of 'technical incompetence' (Parsons 1951, p. 440). This reflects the root of the NHS, which was established on the basis of making the service universal and largely free at point of use, hence, encouraging dependence on health professionals. The NHS National Plan includes an 'expert patient' program that proposes to provide 'patient-friendly' versions of all guidelines published by the National Institute for Clinical Practice (NICE). In addition, 'patients will be helped to navigate the maze of health information through the development of NHS Direct online, Digital TV and NHS Direct information points in key public spaces' (DoH 2000, para. 10.2). However, these changes do not necessarily signal a transformation of relationships or provision of services.

Much of the early utopian writing about the Internet celebrated it as an open and ungoverned space. However, concerns about the potential impact of misleading or incorrect medical information has led to a number of attempts to 'kite mark' sites according to a set of medical protocols. Moreover, many organizations that occupy this new space remain bound by legal and other constrains traditionally associated with their work in the material world. Such constraints may not be apparent to users. Sites including those sponsored by the BBC and Granada include chat rooms where users can exchange views and advice about health matters. However, users' postings are reviewed and are removed if they contain any derogatory comments about pharmaceutical products, medical centres and so forth. Also attempts to make patient records available to practitioners on-line have run into difficulty with the Data Protection Act. Concerns about the lack of clear clinical evidence for the use of most complementary and alternative approaches to health, mean that they are not listed in the content of sites for example in NHS Direct. There is a tension here between pluralistic approaches to health and health knowledge and a biomedical one that rests on the gold standard of the ramdomized-controlled trail.

INSIDE THE INTERNET: NEWSGROUPS

In the 1980s in the United States, electronic notice boards, such as a bulletin board system (BBS) became the forerunner of the vast number of newsgroups that can be found on the Internet, and were used by people who had HIV/AIDS to exchange ideas and experiences. Today most health and social problems have newsgroups where people can read messages posted by other members and contribute their own experiences and ask questions. Newsgroups and chat rooms are particular structures within the landscape of the Internet. Unlike physical spaces these virtual spaces usually contain none of the furniture or other features that shape the interactions that take place (e.g. we behave differently in the bedroom from in the consulting room). Moreover, users are disembodied and therefore loose the 'silent language' of gesture, body position, facial expression and so forth, that set the stage for spoken communication (Goffman 1969). We should note that some chat rooms have attempted to build a three-dimensional representation of space and provided users with avatars (cartoon-like models, which users can speak through, move around, gesture, etc.). At this point it is also important to remember that in the spaces provided by newsgroups, chat rooms and other areas of the Internet individuals are essentially anonymous.

The extract below is taken from a UK-based health newsgroup. Note that the final posting alludes to the problem of the identity of users and shows how one individual has attempted to address this problem. It is also interesting that the second posting comes from a medical researcher based in a large teaching hospital (real names have been change to protect the anonymity of the users).

Case Study 25.1

Subject: Decompression accident

I had a decompression accident while diving some years ago. I have been experiencing head pain and dizziness since. My symptoms are getting worse. My neurologist told me a long time ago that there was nothing to do. I want to give it one more try. I would like to know the name of the top neurologist in London, or in the UK, which might be helpful for my condition.
Thanks,
Paul

Re: Decompression accident

Try looking through this site, it's quite informative and someone may be able to answer questions for you before you see a neurologist.
http://www.vnh.org/FSHandbook.html
It may not be a top neurologist you need, but someone with some interest in this area. Perhaps if you phoned around and asked at different centres to save your GP some leg work, and post to various neurological newsgroups and notice boards.
Are you sure the problem is because of the accident and not something else? Decompression accidents are nasty because they do, do lasting damage very quickly.
Good luck.

Re: Decompression accident

Try a good cranial osteopath.
I know a good one in Sandy Bedfordshire.

Re: Decompression accident

Can get the info on Doctors for you. What part of London? North or South?
Etc.

I have been and probably still am suffering from mental and general health problems due to medications. I decided to create a safe environment unlike some of the newsgroups.

I set up my own website as therapy to help others and myself at the same time. General health, mental health, drugs and medications, misdiagnoses are all dealt with if you leave your message on my message board (So others in the same position as yourself can be helped.) I can then forward you with the info you need.

Anonymity and disembodiment can be both advantageous and dangerous. This reflects broader patterns in contemporary society where space has lost some of the power it had to shape behaviour. In a small town or village the ways people behaved and looked could be observed and remembered by others who knew them. It was not easy to remain anonymous and many spaces exerted a moral pressure to conform to expected behavioural norms. However, people now live in cities with populations of over a million and many individuals are highly geographically mobile. This has led to various explanations of community or cosmopolitan life (for examples see Bauman 1995, Giddens 1994). Many of the spaces we occupy may also lack a sense of locality. Visit any modern shopping centre and the architecture, shops and facilities could be interchangeable with similar centres elsewhere. This disembodying of place means that people can hide behind anonymity and may feel less responsible for the consequences of their behaviour.

In virtual spaces users can feel liberated from the expectations and demands of their everyday social roles. Unencumbered by the corporeal body, locality and biography individuals can form 'second selves' and forge new relationships, which in itself can be therapeutic (Turkle 1995). For example, a paraplegic confined to the home can explore the electronic landscape and participate in Internet communities without any fear of the stigma that may threaten them in the real world. Moreover, the inhibitions, embarrassment, and risks associated with disclosing difficult or potentially stigmatizing experiences or behaviours may disappear in a space where no one knows your 'real' identity. Research that has examined newsgroups devoted to providing on-line support has noted how important anonymity is to users (Burrows et al 2000). The apparent fragility of such identities does not prevent the emergence of genuine reciprocity and support. Self-help through the Internet therefore provides a new way for people to seek reassurance and to protect themselves from a sense of insecurity or isolation. Sharing experiences with others that share common health problems and experiences may also act as a 'buffer' from a sometimes confusing and harsh real world (Cohen & Wills 1985). A study of a newsgroup for people with diabetes revealed that it offered a 'secure space' where information could 'be assimilated and reflexively shaped to inform lifestyle choices' (Loader et al 2002, p. 12). This suggests that it is the social interaction and information from others with diabetes rather than the quality of clinical advice that is important to users.

INSIDE THE INTERNET: HOME PAGES

For the purposes of this chapter home pages are defined as a space on the Internet that has been designed by an individual to give information about him/herself, family and other things that they feel to be important. This may also include accounts of illness, a diary, autobiography and links to other Web sites. The text below has been taken from a UK Web site in order to illustrate the nature of the material such home pages contain. Note that it is not possible to reproduce the lay out and full design of the site. The phrases underlined contain hyperlinks to other parts of the page or other places on the Internet.[9]

Case Study 25.2

Chronic fatigue syndrome & environmental illness Richard's pages

This section of my site is devoted to Chronic Fatigue Syndrome (also known as Chronic Fatigue and Immune Dysfunction Syndrome or Myalgic Encephalomyelitis) and Environmental Illness. A few preliminary points:

◆ I am a patient, not a health professional, and do not claim expertise: nothing on my site is intended to replace the advice of your health professional. I have, however, been very careful about the material I have prepared for this site and the documents I have posted here have first been checked by doctors.

◆ I have included links to sites that looked worthwhile to me, but have not read everything on those sites – so the opinions expressed on those sites may not be my own.

◆ Most people with CFS or EI do not get as severely affected as me.

◆ Take a look at my homepage – please make my day and sign my Guestbook.

Contents

◆ Links to CFS and Environmental Illness sites.

◆ Living With CFS – a collection of pieces I've written from time to time about living with CFS (some humorous) and some writing that has inspired me when I needed it.

◆ Writing – stories and poetry arising from my illness (and some not arising directly from it).

◆ Notice Board – if anyone wants to put up a notice to do with CFS or Environmental Illness here, they are welcome. Just email me.

◆ Sign Guestbook | View Guestbook.

◆ Email me (Note: as I am battling exhaustion every day, I may take a while to reply.)

Highlights

Just so you don't miss them, here are some pages that I think are worth a look, if you are interested.

◆ CFS and Me – a brief account of my illness.
◆ Being Me – a piece about what it's like to live with CFS.

The above extract indicates the depth of understanding a person can achieve about their illness. It also shows how experiences of illness and health care are interwoven with biography and lifestyle. Such accounts of illness are similar to the more familiar narratives that have formed part of research on lay understandings of health. We can see how changes in the body and emotional states are understood in a way that is different from the biomedical model (Frank 1995, Radley 1999).

Like many other contemporary conditions a diagnosis of chronic fatigue syndrome (CFS) is not universally accepted or easy to treat. It is sometimes associated with psychosocial dysfunction and

medical treatment may be seen as stigmatizing by some patients. In the face of medical orthodoxy the Internet provides access to other forms of expertise. This may take the form of consultations with medical authorities in other parts of the globe; advice from a network of lay experts and information from libraries and other resources as noted earlier. It is also possible for home page authors to move from the provision of information to the delivery of products or advice through their Web pages (Hardey 2001).

DOUBT, CHOICE AND LIFESTYLE

In 1999 Anthony Giddens gave the annual Reith Lectures which were broadcast and debated on the Internet (they remain on the Web and you can read them for yourself).[10] In these lectures he brought together some of the themes of his earlier work and drew on the work of others, including Beck (1992), who were trying to understand contemporary society. To briefly summarize the issues that are relevant here, it is argued that the pace and scope of change is unique to contemporary life. Doubt, unpredictability and uncertainty therefore characterize social and economic life. Reflect on your own experiences of family life or your work and you can probably see that compared with previous generations, life is less predicable (for example, think about the number of courses you have taken or up-date classes you have attended). A further change has been highlighted by Beck, which involves our relationship with the environment. He argues that in the past people were concerned about things like rain or drought that appear to happen naturally. Today, few aspects of the natural environment have not been affected by humans and we are now concerned about our impact on nature (e.g. pollution, global warming). Moreover, we can no longer fall back on traditional certainties to help us make choices in an uncertain world. For example, when medical science gained widespread acceptance as a way to understand disease, medical experts were trusted to provide answers to health problems and the role of the doctor was accorded considerable social prestige. Scientific knowledge is now questioned; parents, for example, no longer just assume that medical advice to have their child inoculated with the combined measles, mumps and rubella vaccination (MMR) is the right thing to do.

As Giddens and others have noted, we are confronted with a vast array of choices and feel that we may constantly be at risk of making the wrong ones. In what he calls a 'reflexivity of the self' Giddens argues there is a constant need to access information so that we can make assessments on which to base our choices. This permeates all aspects of our lives and is often taken for granted. There is a diversity of information available on the Internet and this is accompanied by an ever-increasing number of specialized television channels and magazines that offer all kinds of visions of potential lifestyles. (For example, the BBC series 'Changing Rooms' offers an instant DIY lifestyle change in participants' homes.) This flood of information gives a momentum to the reflexivity of the self so that 'lifestyle choice is increasingly important in the constitution of self identity and daily activity' (Giddens 1994, p. 5). We should recognize that resources always shape choices and that the choices made by some people may limit those open to others. Buying organic beans, for example that have been imported from Africa in your local supermarket, may limit the choices available to people who once grew their own crops on the land now used for export crops. Giddens brings together his conceptualization of risk, reflexivity and the planning of lifestyles to suggest that many people may experience a sense of insecurity. Briefly what he calls 'ontological insecurity' may arise when an individual feels detached from his/her past and surrounded by uncertainties and risks. People may become locked in a state of constant scrutiny that may challenge a coherent sense of self-identity and the ability to make everyday choices.

CONCLUSION

A quick literature search using Medline for articles related to asthma revealed over 50 000 citations.

A similar search using an Internet search engine, pointed to over 185 000 Web sites. Fifteen years ago it was suggested that if a clinician read two medical articles a day he or she would be 55 centuries behind that 1 year's production of medical papers (Haynes et al 1986). There is a lot of information available to practitioners and consumers of health care. This marks a break with the past when medical information was largely confined to a hierarchy of professionals headed by doctors. This may transform the nature of the relationship between health professional and patient or client (Hardey 1999). However, doctors sometimes negatively refer to patients who attempt to introduce information they have found on the Internet into consultation, as 'netters'. Grounds for such labels are found in the traditional stance of medicine to protect the public and in this case it is implied that they need 'protection' from the mass of unmediated information now available to them. Perhaps nurses who practice patient-centred care may be more able to benefit from and promote the negotiation of care with these new expert patients.

SUMMARY

- The virtual space of the Internet provides an anonymous space where people can take on new identities and transcend 'real' world problems such as disability or illness.

- Information may be written by anyone and therefore the quality of clinical advice may be open to question.

- The Internet is both global and local. This challenges local (i.e. national) regulations and practices and makes patients aware of diagnosis and treatments that may not be available in the UK.

- Nurses remain relatively poorly supported with information technology.

- The digital divide may further disadvantage poorer communities.

- Patients provide their own electronic advice networks and may create their own resources to tell their story and explain their approach to health and illness.

DISCUSSION POINTS

1. In what ways might the Internet be a dangerous place that undermines patients' confidence in practitioners and overloads them with information of questionable veracity?

2. How could the health divide be closed or exacerbated by the Internet?

3. In what ways do 'Online Communities' represent an important resource for practitioners to become involved in community life and to promote the health of an area?

4. Consider the statement that people reinforce their sense of 'illness' by becoming immersed in a virtual world of sickness?

REFERENCES

Anthony D 1998 A qualitative study of computer networks in the British National Health Service Nursing Standard Online 12(43): www.nursing-standard.co.uk/vol12-43/ol-art.htm

Anthony D 2000 Are nurses excluded from the web? In: Bryant J (ed) Current perspectives in health care computing. British Computing Society 4: 10–18

Balarajan R 1996 Ethnicity and variations in mortality from coronary heart disease. Health Trends 28: 45–51

Bauman Z 1995 Life in fragments: essay in post-modern morality. Blackwell, Oxford

Beck U 1992 Risk society. Towards a new modernity. Sage, London

Bjerkins G, Bratteteig T 1987 Florence in Wonderland: systems development with nurses. In: Bjerkins G, Kyng M (eds) Computers and democracy: A Scandinavian challenge. Avebury, Norway

Burrows R, Nettleton S 2000 Reflexive modernisation and the emergence of wire self-help. In: Renninger KA, Shumar W (eds) Building virtual communities: learning and change in cyberspace. Cambridge University Press, New York

Burrows R, Nettleton S, Pleace N, Loader B, Muncer S 2000 Virtual community care? Social policy and the emergence of computer mediated social support. Information Communication and Society 3(1): 23–31

Charles C, Gafin A, Whelan T 1997 Shared decision-making in the medical encounter: what does it mean? (Or it takes two to tango). Social Science and Medicine 44(5): 681–692

Cohen S, Wills T 1985 Stress, social support and the buffering hypothesis. Psychological Bulletin 98: 310–357

Department of Health 2000 The NHS plan: a plan for investment, a plan for reform. The stationary office, London

Department of Health 2000 Information for social care. HMSO, London

Dery M 1993 Flame wars: The discourse of cyberculture. Duke, Durham, NC

Dodge M 1999 The geographies of cyberspace. CSA Working Paper 8: www.casa.ucl.ac.uk/cyberspace.pdf

Foley P 1999 Whose Net? Characteristics of Internet users in the UK. Department of Trade and Industry, London

Frank AW 1995 The wounded storyteller: Body, illness, and ethics. Chicago University Press, Chicago

Giddens A 1994 Beyond left and right: The future of radical politics. Polity Press, Cambridge

Glastonbury B 2001 Calling the tune in social care information. NTHS 13(3/4): 1–10

Goffman E 1969 The presentation of self in everyday life. Penguin, Harmondsworth

Graves J, Corocran S 1989 The study of nursing informatics. Image: The Journal of Nursing Scholarship 21: 227–231

Griffiths R 1983 NHS management inquiry: Report to the Secretary of State for Social Services. Department of Health, London

Hardey M 1998 The social context of health. Open University Press, Buckingham

Hardey M 1999 Doctor in the house: The Internet and as a source of lay health knowledge and the challenge to expertise. Sociology of Health and Illness 21(6): 820–835

Hardey M 2001 The transformation of patients into consumers and producers of health information. Communication, Information and Society 6(4): 1–21

Hardey M, Payne S, Coleman P 2000 Scraps: Hidden information and its influence on the delivery of care. Journal of Advanced Nursing 32(1): 208–214

Hardey M, Payne S, Hawker S, Kerr C, Powell J 2001 Professional territories and the fragmentation of elderly care. Journal of the Royal Society for the Promotion of Health 121(3): 159–164

Haynes RB, McKibbon KA, Fitgerald D, et al 1986 How to keep up with the medical literature: Why try to keep up and how to get started. Annuals of Internal Medicine 105: 149–153

Lawton S, Montgomery L, Farmer J 2001 Survey and workshop initiative on community nurses' knowledge of the Internet. Computers in Nursing 19(3): 118–121

Loader BD, Muncer S, Burrows R, Pleace N, Nettleton S 2002 Medicine on the line? Computer mediated social support and advice for people with diabetes. International Journal of Social Welfare 11: 1–13

National Opinion Polls 1999 Internet User Profile Study, NOP Research Group. June

Office of National Statistics 2001 Britain 2001. The Stationery Office, London

Parsons T 1951 (1991) The social system. Routledge, London

Radley A 1999 The aesthetics of illness: narrative, horror and the sublime. Sociology of Health and Illness 21(6): 778–796

Reents S 1999 Impacts of the Internet on the doctor–patient relationship. The rise of the Internet consumer. Cyber Dialogue http://www.cyberdialogue.com

Robinson K, Robinson H, Davies H 1996 Towards a social constructionist analysis of nursing informatics. Health Informatics 2: 179–187

Simpson R 1992 Informatics: Nursing's newest specialty. Nursing Management 23: 26

Taylor C 1999 The E*Volution of Healthcare, E*Offering Working paper. E* Trade Group, Menlo Park, California

Townsend P, Davision N 1982 (1992) The Black Report in inequalities in health. Penguin, Harmondsworth

Turkel S 1995 Life on the screen: Identity in the age of the Internet. Simon and Schuster, New York

Wootton R 1998 Telemedicine in the National Health Service. Journal of the Royal Society of Medicine 91: 614–621

FURTHER READING

Hardey M 1999 Doctor in the house: The Internet as a source of lay health knowledge and the challenge to expertise. Sociology of Health and Illness 21(6): 820–835

One of the first studies of the role of the Internet and the changing nature of lay knowledge. An abridged version can be found in Davey B, Gray A, Seal C (eds) 2002 Health and disease: A reader, 3rd edition. Open University Press.

Hardey M 2004 e-health: The Internet and the transformation of health. Routledge, London

Takes up some of the issues noted here in more depth and more theoretically.

He@lth Information on the Internet

This is the journal published by the Royal Society of Medicine which is available on-line. It provides news of the latest resources that may be of interest to practitioners as well as articles written by some of the experts in the field.

Webb S, Burt E (eds) 2003 Information and communication technology in the welfare services. Jessica Kingsley, London

An edited collection of papers that bring together health and social care. Some chapters draw on research while others are more theoretical. A useful source of up-to-date research, highlighting important issues related to the integration of care.

Welsh S, Anagnostelis B, Cook A 2001 Finding and using health and medical information on the Internet. Aslib, London

One of the better guides to using the Internet. There is a UK bias, which means that 'local' resources are well represented. As in other cases there is an irony in that the publisher fails to use the Internet to offer on-line support or updating for Web material that changes rapidly.

WEBSITE ADDRESSES

1. http://www.netcraft.com/survey/Reports/1999/graphs.html
2. http://www.vivatec.co.uk
3. http://www.vu.org/
4. http://www.cira.org.uk
5. http://www.nhsdirect.nhs.uk
6. http://www.bbc.co.uk/health
7. http://www.wellbeing.com
8. http://www.netdoctor.co.uk
9. http://www.geocities.com/Athens/Parthenon/7015/cfs-ei/index.html
10. http://www.lse.ac.uk/Giddens/reith_99/

26

Value for money

D. Cohen

KEY ISSUES

◆ Principles of economics.

◆ Resource scarcity.

◆ Efficiency.

◆ Objectives of community care policy.

◆ Cost–benefit analysis.

◆ Cost–effectiveness analysis.

◆ Cost–utility analysis.

INTRODUCTION

This chapter explains why considerations of value for money are important when comparing community care with other forms of care and in determining how the resources devoted to community care could best be deployed. Its framework is that of economics and it provides an alternative way of looking at the sometimes difficult choices which resource scarcity makes necessary. A brief description of the techniques of economic appraisal is given together with examples, but the chapter's main aim is to show how application of the thinking behind economic appraisal can be of value even when the techniques are not rigorously applied. Community nurses should be able to apply this thinking to the problems and issues they face.

VALUE FOR MONEY: THE NEED TO ASK THE RIGHT QUESTIONS

Although government documents may give the impression that recent shifts toward community care are motivated solely by a concern for the well-being of patients, many commentators have accused Government of promoting community care as a means of saving money (see for example, Harrison et al 1990). This begs the question 'is community care cheaper than other forms of care?'

Anyone who has not been exposed to the principles of economics would probably regard this as an important question which economists ought to be addressing. They might be surprised to hear that few economists would regard it as a key economic question at all. The reason – as will be explained in this chapter – is simply that economics is not 'about' money and most certainly not about saving money. It is about achieving value for money which concerns the relationship between what is achieved and the cost of achieving it.

Nevertheless, the cost of community care is clearly of interest to Government, policy makers and those who deliver services. Unfortunately, costing community care is not a straightforward exercise and depends on whose perspective is taken and which costs are included (for a discussion of the difficulties of costing community care see Knapp 1993). From the perspective of the National Health Service, community care is almost certainly cheaper because many costs are borne by local authority social services and by social security. From the perspective of the public sector as a whole, community care may be cheaper because many costs are borne by patients and their relatives and much care is provided by unpaid informal carers. From the perspective of society as a whole, the answer is unclear.

Whether or not community care is cheaper than institutional care, though, is largely irrelevant for purposes of evaluation because saving money is not the primary objective of community care policies. A better question, and one which would recognize the health and welfare objectives of policy as well as Government's natural concern to control public expenditure, would be 'does community care offer better value for money?' The remainder of this chapter will demonstrate how economics provides an approach which allows value for money issues to be addressed.

THE GROWING ACCEPTANCE OF THE THINKING OF HEALTH ECONOMICS

The basic tenet of health economics is that resources for health creation are scarce relative to the demands made on them. This means that resource allocation choices are inescapable. Given scarcity, a decision to fund any particular programme or activity means that resources will be diverted from other potentially beneficial uses, i.e. every decision involves trading-off benefits gained against potential benefits forgone. Economics is concerned with comparing these trade-offs.

Until recently, this economic view was largely shunned by health professionals who tended to argue that their duty is to provide the most effective health care possible. Considerations of costs are not only anathema to their whole way of thinking, but taking cost into consideration in decision-making would compromise their ethical principles (see for example, Loewy 1980). While there are no doubt many who still hold this view, such rigid opposition to the economic perspective is becoming less commonplace. One reason for this is the fact that the gap between the health needs that *could* be met in a perfect world of infinite resources and the health needs that *are* being met in the real world of finite resources, is growing. This became evident in the UK when the purchaser and provider functions of the NHS were separated in 1991. Purchasers were given budgets, instructed to assess the needs of the populations they served and told to purchase healthcare services to meet those needs from within the budgets. It became immediately obvious that the budgets could not possibly purchase enough health care to meet all health needs fully, immediately and in the most patient-friendly way. Some form of prioritizing – or to use an uglier term 'rationing' – appeared to be necessary.

Soon after the introduction of this 'internal market' in the NHS, a conference organized by the British Medical Association, the Kings Fund and the Patients' Association carried a motion 'This house believes that rationing in health care is inevitable'. It is unlikely that such a motion would have even been debated, let alone carried, had it been considered at a similar conference 10 years earlier.

There are many other examples of the growing acceptance of the need to make hard resource allocation choices. The National Institute for Clinical Excellence was recently set up to examine the evidence on various healthcare interventions and recommend which should or should not be available on the NHS. It was made clear from the start that these recommendations would be based on evidence of cost effectiveness as well as clinical effectiveness, implying that beneficial treatments could be rejected if shown to provide poor value for money. Indeed bodies which fund healthcare research are increasingly demanding as a condition of funding that researchers address cost–effectiveness issues in addition to those of safety and efficacy.

Of course, the need to make resource allocation choices can be lessened by increasing the overall level of funding. At the conference mentioned above, Christine Hancock, then secretary of the Royal College of Nursing said 'If doctors and nurses are seduced by the idea of rationing they give politicians the perfect excuse not to increase resources' (quoted in Smith 1983). Mark Jones in Chapter 24, for example, adopts a very different perspective to complex resource allocation.

Accepting the idea of rationing, however, does not mean having to accept that current funding levels are adequate. Indeed, by any international comparison the UK NHS is badly underfunded. In 1998, the UK spent £970 per person on health care compared to £1423 in France, £1670 in Germany and £2521 in the United States. In terms of health spending as a percentage of gross domestic product, the UK was 23rd out of 29 OECD countries (OHE 2001). While there are always dangers in comparing spending patterns in different countries with different healthcare systems and different patterns of health needs, these figures at least suggest that the UK could greatly increase its spending on health care.

But additional spending cannot make resource allocation choices go away. If the 'need' for health care is perceived in terms of 'capacity to benefit from treatment' (including prevention) then it is clear that need is growing at a faster rate than any realistic growth in funding. Apart from the obviously higher needs of an ageing population, healthcare technology is advancing at a rapid and increasing pace. New pharmaceuticals, diagnostic procedures, equipment and surgical techniques among many other advances, mean that some

patients who were previously untreatable can now benefit from treatment. Very-low-birthweight babies, for example, did not have a need for treatment until the technology of neonatal intensive care units was developed. Today they have a need. New advances are also allowing people who could previously be treated to now receive better treatment, i.e. their need (capacity to benefit) has increased as a consequence of advances in medical knowledge and technology.

Constantly increasing funding is therefore required just to prevent the gap between met need and total need, from widening further still. So long as society has other needs as well (for education, defence, law and order, not to mention private consumption) closing the health needs gap completely cannot be done.

PRINCIPLES

For present purposes health economics may be regarded as a discipline whose way of thinking is more important than its range of techniques. As stated above, the main principle is that of resource scarcity; 'In the beginning, middle and end was, is and will be scarcity of resources' (Mooney 1992).

MONEY VERSUS RESOURCES

In common usage the terms 'money' and 'resources' are often used interchangeably. In economics, they have quite different meanings. Resources contribute to the production of healthier people either directly (e.g. nurses, doctors, drugs, dressings, equipment) or indirectly (e.g. administration). Money gives a command over resources, but will not make people healthier unless used to pay for resources. Some resources such as volunteer workers or informal carers do not receive money payment. Most healthcare resources do. Thus more resources normally means more money expenditure and vice versa.

The distinction is important, though, as often the scarcity problem relates to a resource rather than to cash. A Community Trust which is having difficulties retaining and recruiting community nurses will be constrained in the service they can offer by a shortage of nurses regardless of the size of their budget.

OPPORTUNITY COSTS

Because of scarcity, devoting resources to X means sacrificing the benefits that could have been produced in Y. Economists regard the cost of X in terms of the benefits sacrificed from Y, and use the term opportunity cost to emphasize this notion of opportunity forgone.

Opportunity costs are not necessarily the same as money costs. Moving a nurse from A to B may mean no change in the nursing wages bill, but if the move to B means sacrificing the benefit she used to achieve in A, then an opportunity cost is incurred. By the economic way of thinking, cost always means opportunity cost and is one of the features which distinguish economic appraisal from financial appraisal.

EFFICIENCY AS A CRITERION FOR CHOICE

Scarcity means that we cannot do everything we would like to do and resource allocation choices are inescapable. Economists have long argued that when making choices, the criteria being used should be stated explicitly. The economist's preferred criterion is *efficiency* which is about maximizing the benefit to available resources – but efficiency is never presented as the be all and end all of resource allocation. Inefficient allocations can be defended on political, public relations, ethical, equity or other grounds, but inefficiency carries a price since (by definition) inefficient allocations mean less total benefit than could have been achieved.

THE COST–BENEFIT APPROACH

All healthcare activities involve the use of resources which are expected to produce benefits but at the same time incur opportunity costs. The process of comparing gains (benefits) with sacrifices (costs)

is called the cost–benefit approach. Its decision rule says to do only those things where the value of the gain exceeds the value of the sacrifice. Failing the cost–benefit test does not mean that the potential benefits of a programme are not worth some amount of cash, but that the cost of pursuing them in terms of other benefits, which will have to be forgone, cannot be justified.

It is also important to stress that the cost–benefit approach is advocated as an aid to decision-making and never as a substitute for it. Failing the cost–benefit test does not mean that something must not be pursued since, as stated above, efficiency is not the only noble social objective. Cost–benefit analysis cannot therefore be the be all and end all of decision-making.

Two examples of the use of the cost–benefit approach are given below. The first demonstrates how the use of cost–benefit 'thinking' i.e. a crude application of the cost–benefit framework, helped deal with a problem that required resolution. Although the exercise was conducted by economists, this provides a good example of how community nurses – with a bit of formal training – could apply economic thinking to a local problem. The second example illustrates a more formal application of the technique of cost–benefit analysis in appraising a new community nursing initiative.

APPLYING THE COST–BENEFIT APPROACH: CARS FOR COMMUNITY NURSES

In 1983, Lothian Health Board began to question why community nurses and health visitors who apparently once provided a satisfactory service by walking, cycling or using public transport to visit their patients, were increasingly regarding a car as a virtual necessity for the job. The question was generated by a concern that a large and growing proportion of the community nursing budget was being spent on transport rather than directly on patient care. Did the current expenditure on transport represent good value for money? For a variety of reasons an answer was needed quickly and a full and costly economic appraisal was not practical. It was decided nonetheless to examine the issue using the cost–benefit framework.

The first problem encountered was the reluctance of the community nurses and health visitors to participate. They shared the commonly held belief that economics is about economizing and therefore assumed that the objective of the study was to save money by taking their cars away. They argued that the study was inappropriate and unnecessary because they 'needed' their cars. The following passage illustrates how translating such commonly heard statements into economic language can help frame the issue in a way more consistent with economic thinking.

Economic appraisal is based on the idea that there are always alternative uses for resources and that there are always choices to be made. When one hears it argued that in some particular circumstance there is no choice – Nurse Jones must have use of a car – then it is implied that Nurse Jones currently provides a service which benefits patients in the community. If she did not have the use of a car and had to rely on other forms of transport, she could not possibly do as much. The resulting loss of benefit to the community would be so great relative to the savings in transport costs as to be not worth considering. Put another way, there is unlikely to be any other use to which the freed resources could be put which could compensate for the loss of the benefit resulting from withdrawal of Nurse Jones' car. (Cohen & Yule 1984)

Stated this way the questions that needed addressing were:

◆ How much money would be saved by providing nurses with alternative transport?
◆ How much additional travel time would this imply, i.e. how much less time would be available to care for patients?
◆ What would be the loss of benefit associated with less time with patients?
◆ What benefits could be produced by using the saved money to expand other services?

It was decided that crown car users with the lowest annual mileage and private car users with the lowest miles per visit ratios would be included in the study. Seven district nurses and eight health visitors were identified. On the basis of their knowledge of the local geography, etc., and in consultation with the nurses and health visitors concerned, nursing officers were asked to identify the most appropriate alternative form of transport and estimate the implications for extra travel time.

Benefit loss was estimated by converting the extra travel time into numbers of home visits forgone, but as explained below, loss of services can be a misleading proxy for loss of health benefits. Although crude, the results indicated that 1.38 district nurse home visits or 1.06 health visitor home visits would be lost for every £1 saved.

The issue of 'what is a visit worth?' was addressed by asking a wide range of other service providers to describe what they could achieve if they were given additional funding. Their answers, scaled to reflect the extra benefit per pound, could then be compared with the perceived benefit attached to the home visits which would be forgone by removing car user status from the identified community nurses and health visitors.

It is, of course, not possible to state objectively whether the benefits from the present level of expenditure on transport exceed the benefits forgone elsewhere. This requires a value judgement. The advantage of applying the economic framework is that the trade-offs are clearly identified, thus ensuring that judgements are made about the right things.

In this case, the appraisal bore out the initial feelings expressed by the nurses. No other use for the savings from reduced expenditure on transport could be found that was judged to be of greater value than the loss of benefit to community patients which reduced transport expenditure would cause. Now, though, instead of the uninformed statement that community nurses 'must have cars', we see an investigation using economic principles, albeit on a crude basis, which indicated that the benefits derived from current expenditure on transport exceeded the opportunity costs. This implies that the present level of provision of cars for nurses was in fact good value for money.

APPLYING COST–BENEFIT ANALYSIS: PRESCRIBING EXERCISE

In a formal cost–benefit analysis (CBA) all costs – defined as resources with alternative uses, i.e. which incur opportunity costs – and all benefits – defined as everything of value which results from an activity – are identified, measured and then valued in money terms (Drummond et al 1997). While benefits such as resource savings are easy to value in money terms, improvements in health and well-being are not. Nevertheless, health gains clearly *are* of value independently of any resource savings, or increases in productivity which they may bring about. Moreover, they are normally the principle reason why any programme or activity is advocated in the first place. Their importance cannot be overemphasized. (See Chapter 7 for further discussion on health promotion strategies related to health gain.) However, because of the obvious difficulties of placing money values on intangible health benefits, fully comprehensive CBAs are few and far between (OHE 1998). While it is important not to lose sight of the importance of intangible health benefits, there is one situation where they can legitimately be ignored. This is illustrated in the following example.

On the basis of evidence that exercise could reduce the number of falls incurred by elderly people, Robertson et al (2001) examined the costs and benefits of district nurses prescribing individual home exercise programmes to people aged 75 and over, in New Zealand. While the addition of this activity to the community nurses' workload would clearly incur opportunity costs, these were expected to be offset, at least in part, by reductions in the costs of treating injuries due to falls.

This study found no statistically significant reduction in falls by those aged 75–79 as compared with a control group. For those in the study aged 80+, however, a highly significant reduction in falls was shown. For the programme as a whole, the direct cost per fall prevented was $NZ1803 which fell to $NZ155 when the savings from avoided injuries were included ($NZ1 = £0.30 at the time of the study). For the subsample aged 80+, however, the cost saving from avoided falls exceeded the cost of the intervention. This produced a negative cost per fall prevented of −$NZ576.

With respect to this specific age group, there was no need to value the health benefits of avoided falls (avoided pain, etc.) since the resource savings brought about by the intervention more than offset its cost. The health gains from avoided falls

are in addition to this and any attempt to value them is now unnecessary since adding them to the analysis could only reinforce the conclusion that had already been reached.

Unfortunately, the number of cases where resource savings exceed resource costs are few and far between. Even with prevention programmes, the total cost of reducing preventable illness and injury is normally higher than the cost of dealing with them without prevention (Cohen & Henderson 1988). This, of course, does not mean that economics is opposed to prevention. It only would be if the sole objective of prevention were to save resources. If, more realistically, the objective of prevention is to achieve health gains – in this case via reductions in preventable morbidity – then economic appraisal can identify which prevention programmes do so most efficiently and how these compare with treatment or other means of producing health.

DIFFERENT OBJECTIVES, DIFFERENT TECHNIQUES OF APPRAISAL

The above discussion of prevention raises the important issue of 'objectives'. Cost–benefit analysis is based on the pursuit of efficiency which implies that the objective of the policy or programme in question is 'to maximize total benefit'.

Often, however, healthcare interventions have very specific objectives which are taken as given, i.e. are assumed to be worth pursuing. For example, if a government decides to introduce a national breast screening programme it may express the objective of the programme in terms of detecting as many presymptomatic cancers as possible, i.e. that early detection reduces mortality provided that treatment is available. In such cases, the question of whether or not to pursue the objective is assumed to be answered and the relevant question becomes one of *how* to pursue it.

In the case of the home exercise prescription intervention discussed above, a decision may have been taken (on whatever grounds) to commit resources to reducing falls in the elderly. If so, then the task becomes solely one of finding the best way of doing so. From an economic perspective 'best' would be perceived as that method which produces the greatest reduction in falls for any given expenditure, or that method which minimizes the cost of achieving any given reduction in falls. This is known as *technical efficiency* as opposed to *allocative efficiency* (should resources be allocated to pursing the objective?) which is a cost–benefit question. Technical efficiency is a cost–effectiveness question and is addressed through cost–effectiveness analysis (CEA). Here, comparisons are made of alternative ways of pursuing a given objective.

Two examples of CEA in the area of community health care are presented below. The first relates back to the prescribing of exercise to prevent falls to illustrate how CEA can deal with the sample for which the intervention did not produce a net saving of resources. The second highlights the difficulties of determining the basis on which to make the cost–effectiveness comparison.

COST–EFFECTIVENESS ANALYSIS 1: PRESCRIBING EXERCISE

In the district nurse home exercise study discussed above, CBA showed that for the subsample aged 85+, the intervention produced net savings and therefore clearly passed the cost–benefit test. For the sample as a whole, however, the net cost of the intervention was positive, meaning that a cost–benefit conclusion could not be drawn without taking account of the value attached to the intangible health benefits. While this is no easy task, there are several methods which economists employ to do just that (see for example discussion of the willingness-to-pay method in Drummond et al 1997).

A simpler way of addressing the issue, though, is to reach a cost–effectiveness conclusion by assuming that the objective to reduce falls had already been accepted as worth pursuing. CEA will identify the most technically efficient way of doing so.

The authors did this by comparing the intervention in question (which cost $NZ1803 per fall prevented, or $NZ155 per fall prevented when resource savings are included) with an American multifactorial intervention ($NZ6141 per fall prevented) and an Australian home assessment and modification programme ($NZ5602 per fall prevented). District nurse prescription of individual home exercise programmes was thus shown to be more cost effective than these other alternatives.

COST–EFFECTIVENESS ANALYSIS 2: EFFECTIVE AT DOING WHAT?

In 1983 the UK Government made £6 million available to support a policy objective of maintaining elderly people with severe or moderate organic disorders at home rather than in long-term institutional care. One of the innovative projects it funded was a Family Support Unit (FSU) in South Tees which offered respite care, day care, evening care and special occasional residential care to support the carers of elderly mentally infirm people. A study was undertaken to compare the cost effectiveness of community care including an FSU with conventional community care (Donaldson & Gregson 1989).

Unlike the above example, where the single objective of the intervention was to prevent falls, the objectives of the FSU were multiple and far less specific. It was thus much more difficult to identify a single unit of effectiveness (a condition of CEA) against which the alternatives could be compared. Given that the stated objective of the policy was to maintain older people at home, the authors of this study chose 'time in the community' (measured as number of at-home days between assessment and either admission to long-term care or death) as the unit of effectiveness. Note that this takes no account of the quality of life of older people, or of any other health effects of the policy, including those to informal carers who arguably are the principal beneficiaries of the respite care and other services provided by the FSU. Of particular interest here might be the question of whether or not a family or carer would be willing to provide long-term care without some level of support.

The study showed patients in the FSU group having a mean of 664 days in the community compared to 492 days for the controls. The cost of community care with FSU was £6.60 per patient day compared to £2.30 without. The total extra cost of community care to the FSU group – including the cost of the extra days spent in the community – was £3200 per patient. This however, meant 172 fewer days in hospital (664 − 492) which would have cost £7912.

Is community care with an FSU more cost effective than community care without? Given the way effectiveness was measured the answer is clearly yes. However, since effectiveness was only measured (quite correctly in these circumstances) as days spent in the community, the authors hedged their conclusion by stating that the FSU is more cost effective only '… if it is assumed that clients and their carers find time spent at home in the community at least as desirable as long term hospital care' (p. 205). If the health status of the two groups had been monitored and compared in terms of cost per unit of health (see below), then the study could have shown whether community care with FSU is a more cost–effective way of pursuing a health objective than community care without.

BROADENING THE OBJECTIVE

A major limitation with cost–effectiveness analysis is that it can only compare alternative ways of pursuing the same objective, i.e. alternative ways of producing the same unit of effectiveness. In the above examples the analyses identified the most cost–effective way to prevent falls and the most cost–effective way of keeping elderly patients in the community. The information from the studies could not be combined to determine if exercise prescription is more cost effective than FSUs. Indeed such a question makes no sense since the two programmes, although both in the area of care of the elderly in the community, seek to do different things.

It is possible, however, to reduce this limitation by broadening the objective and thus broadening the unit of effectiveness to one produced by a variety of different programmes. For example, although it may have a more immediate objective in terms of early detection, a breast cancer

screening programme can also be seen as having an ultimate objective of saving lives. If alternative ways of screening for breast cancer are assessed in terms of cost per year of life saved, then the CEA can not only identify the most cost–effective way of screening for breast cancer but this result can be compared with that from any other life-saving programme which has been assessed in similar terms. Unlike the example above, here we can determine whether breast screening is more cost effective than (say) heart transplantation.

Two major problems, however, still remain. Firstly, a large number of healthcare interventions – including both home exercise prescription and community FSUs – are not specifically about saving lives and therefore cannot be included in the comparisons. Secondly, comparisons of cost per life year saved assume that an extra year of life bedridden and in pain is of equal value to an extra year of life in perfect health. Both problems can be overcome by broadening the objective further still, to the production of 'health' defined to include both time (how long) and quality (how good) dimensions.

Economists have advanced this concept in recent years by arguing that in principle, all effective healthcare interventions – whether caring or curing, treatment or prevention – either make people live longer or improve the quality of their lives, over what otherwise would be the case. In other words all effective interventions produce a common output in the form of quality-adjusted life years (QALYs). If the unit of effectiveness is measured in QALY terms then an exercise prescription programme, provision of FSU, breast cancer screening and heart transplant can all be compared in terms of cost/QALY.

It should be noted that many different measures of health status are currently used in (non-economic) healthcare research (for a good review see Bowling 1997 and Chapter 8 of this volume). Some of these yield multidimensional health *profiles*, others unidimensional health *measures*. It is inevitably easier to present dimension by dimension profiles than to attempt to combine the dimensions into an overall score since this involves attaching weights (values or 'utilities') to the different attributes of health. Does a reduction in pain represent a greater or lesser health gain than an improvement in mobility? Despite this difficulty, only single index health measures can provide the sought after universal unit of effectiveness. The term QALY is increasingly being used as a generic term to describe a number of different single-index utility-weighted measures being developed.

A cost–effectiveness analysis which uses QALYs as the unit of effectiveness is called a cost–utility analysis (CUA). Cost–utility analyses are the most recent form of economic evaluation in health care but are rapidly gaining in popularity as the methodology improves (OHE 1998). At the time of writing, few full cost–utility analyses in the area of community nursing have been undertaken, although attempts to develop the methodology in this area are being made (see for example, Vick 1996).

CONCLUSION

The messages from this chapter are simple. Scarcity means that decisions on the appropriate level of resource devoted to community care and the way in which those resources are deployed both require value-for-money information. Value for money, however, cannot be assessed without clear reference to the broad objectives of policy or the narrower objectives of specific interventions. Too often these objective are either poorly defined or misleading. (See Chapter 4 for a different discussion on quality and value for money.)

Examining whether or not community care is cheaper than institutional care is not a straightforward task but on its own only provides information which aids decision-making if the stated objective of policy is to save money. If objectives are more health orientated, then other questions need to be asked.

Economics provides a framework based on sound principles which allow issues of value for money to be addressed in a scientific way, while emphasizing that the values attached to the various benefits of care can never be determined objectively. Since the value-for-money definition makes value judgements, economic appraisal can never be a substitute for decision-making.

Examining issues using the economic way of thinking, or more formally applying the techniques of economic appraisal, can, however greatly aid such decision-making.

SUMMARY

◆ The starting point of economics is the fact that resources for health care are scarce relative to the demands made on them. This means that there are opportunity costs to all uses of resources and thus resource allocation choices (i.e. prioritizing) are inescapable.

◆ One key criterion for choice is *efficiency* which seeks to identify those choices which maximize the total benefit possible from available resources.

◆ Three main techniques of economic evaluation – cost–effectiveness, cost–utility and cost–benefit analyses – can help to assess the efficiency of community health nursing.

DISCUSSION POINTS

1. How would you respond to someone who stated that the health of your patients must be 'beyond considerations of cost'?

2. What arguments could you use in support of a request for funding for some new equipment which you know will greatly benefit your patients?

3. Why should you be sceptical about the claim that a measure of the success of the NHS is the fact that it is treating more patients than ever before?

4. From a nurse's perspective what are the key issues of community care requiring economic appraisal and why?

REFERENCES

Bowling A 1997 Measuring health: a review of quality of life measurement scales, 2nd edn. Open University Press, Buckingham
Cohen D, Henderson J 1988 Health prevention and economics. Oxford University Press, Oxford
Cohen D, Yule B 1984 The case for community cars. Nursing Time: Community Outlook May 9: 173

Donaldson C, Gregson B 1989 Prolonging life at home: what is the cost? Community Medicine 2(3): 200–209

Drummond M, O'Brien B, Stoddart G, Torrance G 1997 Methods for the economic evaluation of health care programmes, 2nd edn. Oxford University press, Oxford

Harrison S, Hunter DJ, Pollit C 1990 The dynamics of British health policy. Unwin Hyman, London

Knapp M 1993 The costing process: background theory. In: Netten A, Beecham J (eds) Costing community care: theory and practice. Ashgate Publishing, Aldershot

Loewy EL 1980 Letter. New England Journal of Medicine 302: 6970

Mooney GH 1992 Economics, medicine and health care, 2nd edn. Wheatsheaf, Brighton

Office of Health Economics 1998 Trends in Economic Evaluation. Office of Health Economics, London

Office of Health Economics 2001 Compendium of health statistics. Office of Health Economics, London

Robertson MC, Devlin N, Gardner M, Campbell AJ 2001 Effectiveness and economic evaluation of a nurse delivered home exercise programme to prevent falls. British Medical Journal 322: 1–6

Smith R 1983 Editorial. British Medical Journal 306: 737

Vick S 1996 Caring for ventilated patients in the community: a pilot study examining costs, quality of life and preferences. Health and Social Care in the Community 4(6): 330–337

FURTHER READING

Donaldson C, Gerard K 1993 Economics of health care financing. Macmillan, London

Mooney GH 1992 Economics, medicine and health care, 2nd edn. Wheatsheaf, Brighton

These two publications explain the principles of health economics more fully.

Drummond M, O'Brien B, Stoddart G, Torrance G 1997 Methods for the economic evaluation of health care programmes, 2nd edn. Oxford University Press, Oxford

Jefferson T, Demicheli V, Mugford M 2001 Elementary economic evaluation in healthcare, 2nd edn. BMJ Publishing, London

These two publications explain the techniques of economic evaluation in health care.

Netten A, Beecham J (eds) 1993 Costing community care: theory and practice. Ashgate Publishing, Aldershot

This discusses problems and methods for costing community care programmes.

27

Promoting public health: implications for community nurses

G. Macdonald

KEY ISSUES

◆ Health promotion has developed rapidly as a discipline and practice over a relatively short period.

◆ The Ottawa Charter is often viewed as the 'founding' base for health promotion developments.

◆ 'Settings' for health provide a useful way of developing health promotion practice.

◆ Health promotion is 'breaking free' from the narrow medical model of health and embracing a broader social model.

◆ Health promotion is trying to establish an evidence base of effectiveness based on appropriate research methodologies and best practice case studies.

◆ Community-based nurses are well placed to take advantage of policy and practice changes related to the 'new' public health.

INTRODUCTION

The history and development of health promotion over the last 30 years has been a contentious one, both within the UK and across the globe. From the Lalonde Report in 1974 (Lalonde 1974) to the Mexico Ministerial Statement in 2000 (Health Promotion International), the discipline has been subjected to critical discourse, scrutiny and scepticism in equal amounts. Much of this concern has centred on the role of health promotion in preventing ill health, and/or promoting positive health. It has particularly focused on the effectiveness of health promotion interventions, and whether health promotion should subscribe to a biomedical model or social model of health. Some further discussion has concerned itself with the role health promotion might have in shaping health policy generally, and public health policy more specifically. However there has been, and continues to be, considerable debate on what *appears* to be less important issues, such as terminology, role delineation and training for health promotion practice, but, *in fact*, figures largely in practitioners' everyday views and attitudes towards the subject.

This is not altogether surprising. Health promotion, in relation to other more established disciplines such as psychology or medicine, is still in its infancy. It might, as Kuhn (1970) has suggested, still be searching for its academic credentials and trying to establish its base paradigm. Indeed many still question its right to call itself a 'discipline' at all (Macdonald & Bunton 1992). Nevertheless the debate that has been fermenting and evolving internationally, and has subsequently been adopted and adapted by individual nation states, has served to inform the rapid development of health promotion as a 'discipline' and practice. Today health promotion is studied and practised in most developed countries in the world (Haglund & Macdonald 2000, Mittelmark et al 2000) and has an increasing interest from many developing countries in Latin and South America, South East Asia and Africa (Westphal 2000). As we face the dawn of a new century, health promotion has become, truly, a global endeavour.

However the dynamic and discourse surrounding health promotion continues, as indeed it should with all emerging subjects or fields of study, and this chapter attempts to highlight some of the issues central to this debate. It will trace, albeit very briefly, the history of contemporary ideas surrounding the emergence of health promotion as a concept, as a discipline and as a movement, but it will concentrate much more on teasing out arguments concerned with four current tensions. Firstly, it will discuss the breaking free of health promotion, from the biomedical straight jacket, into the more comfortable attire of the social model of health. Secondly, it will explore an issue that springs from this, namely the tension between the logical positivists and the phenomenologists, in relation to health promotion research. Thirdly, it will trace the move towards evidence-based health promotion (ebhp) and the problems that move has highlighted; and lastly it will consider the continuing tension surrounding terminology, nomenclatures and the associated skills base needed to practice health promotion and public health. The final section of the chapter will devote itself to the implications these four issues have for nurses working at the community level.

FROM OTTAWA TO MEXICO CITY; GLOBE-TROTTING WITH HEALTH PROMOTION

The global development of health promotion since Lalonde is one characterized by a series of international symposia, punctuated by novel initiatives designed to reflect the key themes of the symposia. The principal proponent of these symposia and

initiatives has been the World Health Organization (WHO) and more particularly its European Office (WHO Euro). The Health For All (HFA) programme, which emanated from this office, was the catalyst for the rapid development of ideas and interventions within the public health field across the globe (WHO Euro 1977). It set in train a series of ideas (WHO Euro 1984) and conferences, such as Ottawa, and programmes, such as Healthy Cities, that have fanned initiatives and policy in many member countries ever since.

The conference in Alma Ata in 1978 was the first to capitalize on HFA and produced a 'Declaration' which articulated a set of values supporting the development of human health globally. It particularly recognized *the* central place of primary health care (PHC) as the mechanism for promoting human health, and declared that the principle of 'people participation' would make health resources more relevant to, and supportive of, community health. The Alma Ata Declaration (WHO 1978) reflected the values and goals of the HFA programme, but it was the 38 specific targets within HFA that really engaged member countries, and helped shape public health policy development in those states and would, through its adoption, 'ensure' health for all by the year 2000.

These targets were based on the *four field concept of health*, first espoused by Lalonde when he was the Minister for Health in the Canadian Government in 1974. His report, to that Government, recognized that the multifactorial causes of (ill)health, could be subsumed under four broad categories or fields; namely human biology, environment, human behaviour and healthcare organization. The Canadian Government, as a result of this report, began to shift policy priorities in health towards a broader concern for structural determinants of (ill)health, and laid the foundation for the modern health promotion era. This Canadian health policy innovation, coupled with WHO (Euro) conceptual developments (WHO Euro 1984) brought leading academics, practitioners and policy makers in health promotion, to Ottawa in 1986.

The Ottawa Conference and the subsequent Charter that concluded the debate at that conference laid down the founding principles of modern health promotion and the new public health. The 38 countries that sent representatives to that conference produced a simple but effective Charter that provided impetus and direction for a new public health movement. Its five core themes of 'strengthening community action'; 'developing personal skills'; 'creating supportive environments'; 'reorienting health services'; and 'building health public policy' are still used today to support policy and programme initiatives in member countries of WHO (WHO 1986). Health promoters and public health practitioners were urged to adopt strategies and practice locally, nationally and internationally, that encouraged the development of these themes through 'advocacy', 'mediation' and 'enabling'. The Charter was seen as fundamental to the contemporary debate which focused on the way society is organized and resources are distributed. These advocated structural changes can be related to the different concepts of community. Health promotion views 'community' as a setting or form of social system, that has the potential to act as a resource for health development (Macdonald & Davies 1998). This differs from the more passive interpretation of community, favoured, *inter alia*, by the media that sees the community as a population to be targeted for selfish and/or subjective reasons, and one that is not able to generate co-operative action or reaction. The German concept of *gemeinschaft* (an able and co-operative community) contrasted to *gesellschaft* (a disparate, non co-operative community, or more simply *'only* society') summarizes this tension admirably. The community is central to current health promotion thinking and practice, as witnessed in other chapters in this book.

The Ottawa conference was followed up with a series of symposia, across the globe, that focused on various aspects of the Charter but added subordinate conceptual strands to satisfy the growing complexities within health promotion 'disciplinary' developments. For example the first conference following Ottawa, in Adelaide in 1988, focused on issues relating to healthy public policy, but had a clear subordinate strand on women's health and the role the 'new' public health could play in prioritizing that as an issue.

The conference in Sundsvall in Sweden in 1991, concentrated much more on the notion of sustainability for health through the creation of supportive environments for health, one of the core themes of Ottawa. It focused on critical aspects of the environment such as transport, housing and the workplace and usefully included case studies from across the world to illustrate how 'Ottawa' could work (Haglund et al 1992). For the first time participants from the developing world were encouraged to attend, and the provision of scholarships and bursaries facilitated this. The involvement of participants from developing countries was further developed with the fourth international conference in health promotion in Jakarta, Indonesia in 1997. This symposium adopted the strap line of 'new players for a new era' (WHO 1997) and positively promoted the participation of a global audience sponsored, controversially, through private commercial funds. Its main theme, building still further on Ottawa, was the twin concepts of (community) participation and partnership. It produced a declaration which emphasized the need for increased investment in health, a variation on the reorienting of health services, and the idea of 'settings' as the 'organisational base of the infrastructure required for health promotion' (Editorial, *Health Promotion International* 1997). This idea of a settings approach to health promotion is picked up below.

The most recent conference took place in Mexico City in 2000. 'Bridging the Equity Gap' the theme of the meeting, again took Ottawa forward by addressing a key issue in all public health policy and practice. Over 90 countries sent participants, including Ministers of Health, or ministerial delegations. All delegates and Ministers were invited to endorse the 'Mexico Ministerial Statement for the Promotion of Health; from ideas to action' (Health Promotion International, WHO 2000). The statement reworked Ottawa's call for 'healthy public policy' and added points on the value of research which advances knowledge, and sufficient resources to implement countrywide programmes with supporting evaluation methodologies. It called for improved networks which promote health at national and international levels.

Clearly the Ottawa Charter still has utility value but the thinking in health promotion and the 'new' public health has moved on to incorporate new, similarly broad, concepts like sustainability and health, partnership, community participation, and appropriate evaluation methodologies to improve the evidence of effectiveness base. These additional elements to the international health promotion endeavour reinforce the multidisciplinarity of the subject or field of study. Thematic concepts selectively borrowed from other more established disciplines, will strengthen, through the application of their ideas and practice, the focus on 'community' as a setting for health development, and indeed promote a more general 'settings' approach.

SETTINGS FOR HEALTH PROMOTION

Over the last ten years or so, one of the central ideas emerging from the global conference circuit outlined above was the notion of 'settings'-based health promotion. It was, and still is, a recognition of the significance of *context* in the promotion of public health. It was one attempt to reduce the over-reliance on individualized forms of health promotion (Whitelaw et al 2001) and again took much of its cue from the WHO (Euro) Office. WHO planned, developed and implemented a number of programmes in the late 1980s and 1990s that reflected a settings approach.

Kickbusch (1987) justified this on the grounds that health is generated, shaped and developed in those places where we live and love (the family or home), where we learn (the school or university), where we work (the workplace), where we access health care (the hospital or primary care centre) and the community environment (the city, town or countryside). As a result, a number of programmes, reflecting this philosophy, were implemented by WHO and its European Collaborating Centres. The first and most widespread was the 'Healthy Cities' programme which highlighted a number of indicators a city should develop to be considered 'healthy'. These generally related to a city plan for health, a designated co-ordinator, and a raft of policies on the environment and antipollution measures and such like. It ultimately involved the signing of an agreement with WHO, to pursue a health-promoting agenda. Well over a hundred cities signed up to the programme at the *fin de siecle* (Tsouros 1995). The 'European Health

Promoting Schools' programme soon followed, with similar proposals and prerequisites for schools to enable them to join the project (WHO 1993). This approach to health education in schools, has spilt over into current education policy in the UK with the Healthy Schools initiative (DfEE 1997).

Other programmes, such as Health Promoting Hospitals (WHO 1991) complemented these settings and added further currency to the settings approach. This approach to health promotion was adopted by one national health-promotion agency in the UK (HEBS 1994), as the most effective way of planning programmes, and is currently profiled in both England's Our Healthier Nation strategy (DoH 1999) and in Wales' Better Health Better Wales strategy (NAfW 1998). This use of settings as a means of delivering health-promotion interventions, whilst increasingly popular, has not been without its critics (Poland et al 2000, Whitelaw et al 2001). They argue that there is the 'potential for the homogenisation of practice, where sharply contrasting activities are inelegantly brought under a single setting banner' and when it comes to matching the settings approach to circumstances 'one size fits all'. In other words, as far as practitioners are concerned, trying to adopt the unidimensional concept of a settings approach to health promotion with little understanding of the organization in which the activity takes place, makes for failure and disillusionment. Public health and health promotion specialists have to contextualize their approach not only through a good understanding of the setting, but also the place of the setting within a community or society. Settings-based approaches, like individualistic approaches, need to recognize the significance of *context*.

FOUR TENSIONS IN CURRENT HEALTH PROMOTION DISCOURSE

STRUCTURAL/LIFESTYLE

The move towards a 'settings' approach, has in part been caused by a growing disillusionment with the focus on individual health and illness.

Much early work in health promotion utilized the so called biomedical model of health and tended to view individuals in isolation from their surroundings, environment and social context. In many ways it fostered the now much criticized 'victim blaming' approach to health promotion that blamed the targeted individuals for their own bad health if they didn't adopt new forms of health behaviour and lifestyle. The poster campaign promoted by the then Health Education Council in the late 1970s, which profiled a naked, smoking and heavily pregnant women with a strap line that read 'Do you want a cigarette more than you want a baby?', epitomized this approach. It did little to put the woman and her predicament within any social context, but simply appealed to her already overwhelmed conscience. The pervading wisdom at that time was that if only individuals had the knowledge about what was thought to cause ill health they would then be in a position to do something about it. An image was canvassed that saw individuals as 'victims of their own ignorance' (Davison et al 1992). Many of the interventions were therefore aimed at individuals using essentially a biomedical approach which tended to divorce individual health status from environmental and/or structural relationships.

Lalonde opened up thinking in this area with the *four fields concept*. Here individual health and well-being were viewed within a much broader context. Whilst biological and behavioural factors undoubtedly play a role in determining health status, Lalonde argued that the broader factors such as the environment and healthcare organization had perhaps a more profound impact on individual, and indeed community, health. These structural factors soon became the focus for research and emerging results in the 1980s and 1990s appeared to suggest that health status was indeed the result of a complex combination of the individual risk factors coupled with broader social and structural determinants. Researchers and academics working in this area produced a wealth of data that correlated poor health with the social determinants of morbidity and premature mortality. The pioneering work by Marmot and colleagues (1984), supported by many others including Wilkinson (1996), Davey-Smith et al (1997) and eventually WHO (WHO (Euro) 1998), led to the emergence of social epidemiology as a legitimate field of study and research. These researchers have indicated very strong associations between a variety of social indicators, such as (un)employment, poverty, social class, ethnicity and income and health status. The research has spawned seminal edited readers such as Marmot and Wilkinson's the 'Social Determinants of Health' (1999) and Berkman and Kawachi's 'Social Epidemiology' (2000) and helped reshape approaches to traditional epidemiology (Tannahill 2002).

Whilst much research and health promotion practice continues at the level of the individual, there is a growing movement towards broader conceptual analyses. Some even suggest that it is a combination of social systems, that is the systems that promote work, promote competition, promote transport, etc. that militate against health (Harrison 1999, Macdonald 2000). Systems research focuses on the evidence surrounding the effect of sustained stress on individuals struggling in a society that has no 'system for health', merely systems that promulgate economic development. Sometimes these two goals are incompatible. Most recently social scientists and other researchers have begun to look at the effect social cohesion has on communities and individual health (Mustard 1996, Stansfeld 1999). By concentrating on certain social indicators that can be measured such as social networking or social capital, early results seem to indicate a relationship between social cohesion and health. However, more research is needed in this vital area if health promoters want to develop interventions based on sound evidence.

RESEARCH METHODS

In much the same way that early health promotion programmes were influenced by a narrow biomedical view of health and disease, early research methodologies employed in health promotion and public health were seduced by the logical positivist approach to research. Prospective controlled experimental studies epitomize logical positivist approaches to research and evaluation, and they have been reviewed through the establishment of the Cochrane Collaboration. This collaboration is committed to the systematic review of research evidence on the effects of health care and has given rise to over 40 Collaborative Review Groups focusing on different aspects of health care and disease prevention. The methodology employed for reviewing interventions relies very heavily on data collected through experimental, randomized controlled trials (RCTs). Here, the evaluation is carried out by comparing the effects of an intervention on a group of people receiving the intervention (or dose) – the case group – with a group of people who do not – the control group – but the selection of membership of either group is random. The data are collected under strict 'laboratory experimental' conditions and the results may determine the efficacy of a particular intervention.

This particular kind of approach to evaluative research is valuable for clinicians wishing to determine the most effective clinical intervention, dose or drug, but it doesn't lend itself so well to public health and/or health promotion interventions. In health promotion the concern is not so much with the *efficacy* of a particular intervention, for example a comparison of one school-based health programme compared with another. Efficacy relates to effectiveness *under ideal conditions* – the laboratory experiment. Clearly carrying out research within schools brings a contamination to the research method. Health promoter researchers in this scenario may try to control for real life situations, that is differing teaching styles, pupil background, school curriculum policy, etc., but they cannot control for all variables in a real world situation. Health promotion is more concerned therefore with *effectiveness*, that is, in a sense, real world *efficacy*. Further, some of the questions health promoters and public health specialists may want answered cannot be determined by experimental design. It might be that answers are needed to questions such as 'what values does a community have that might drive health needs?' or 'how do we involve people more in helping to set priorities for public health?' This concern for the limitations of the RCT, and indeed other forms of experimental design, has led to calls for the employment of other types of research

methods (Macdonald et al 1996, Williams & Popay 1994).

The research methods problem for health promotion is all the more acute since it can be seen as lying at the interface between the medical and social sciences (Oakley 1998). Many in health promotion subscribe to the ideas in contemporary social science that promote qualitative or phenomenological approaches to research. They suggest that experimental studies have little or no place in health promotion research since, they argue, health promotion has, at its core, a brief for ensuring respect for individual autonomy, acknowledgement of subjective belief and values, and public participation in research. This contrasts with the logical positivist, quantitative position in the biomedical sciences, which might see no place at all for small, nonrandomized sample selection, researcher (interpretative) bias and nongeneralizability.

However, in the last few years this apparent hostility between quantitative and qualitative research methods has been ameliorated through the development of multimethod evaluative research and forms of triangulation (Tones & Tilford 2001). Indeed some have argued that social science has always played a part in promoting and utilizing positivist approaches and that this tension is somewhat illusionary (Oakley 1998). The current policy need for researchers and practitioners to address inequalities in health, promote public participation in healthcare policy, and to provide value for money services that produce the most effective 'returns' means that a combination of research methods will be necessary if these fundamental issues are to be answered effectively.

THE SEARCH FOR EVIDENCE IN HEALTH PROMOTION

The concern with adopting and/or adapting the appropriate research method to evaluate health promotion interventions has developed, more recently, into a discussion on the use (and abuse) of evidence to support effectiveness. Evidence-based health promotion (ebhp) has in many ways mimicked the more established evidence-based medicine (ebm). However, because of the problems surrounding the adoption of positivist methodology to research in health promotion, the definition and understanding of what is meant by evidence has been questioned (Speller et al 1997). It may be the case that a properly conducted RCT offers the best form of evidence, but what if it is badly planned and carried out? Other nonexperimental types of research, if well conducted, can offer more valuable evidence than poorly implemented RCTs. This means that some form of quality assurance needs to be applied to research methodologies to produce justifiable evidence (Macdonald 1997). Any review of published research studies should include an assessment of the quality of the design and not just an analysis of the results, but in practice, this is rarely the case.

Ebhp may, therefore, be more prepared to accept evidence from nonexperimental studies and certainly the Health Promotion Review Group of the Cochrane Collaboration intends to develop new review criteria for this purpose. Unlike ebm, ebhp is as much concerned with the processes involved in the planning, implementation and delivery of interventions as it is in the outcome (Tones & Tilford 2001). Often this interest in process evaluation can only be demonstrated through qualitative research designs. Qualitative research designs help to illuminate *why* and *how* a particular programme has or has not achieved its objectives, not simply *whether*. Only by gaining a better understanding of these aspects can programmes be improved for greater effectiveness in the future (Macdonald et al 1996). Health promotion is rarely able to demonstrate a cause and effect continuum in the same way that ebm aspires or needs to. Too many practical problems exist within dynamic, ever-changing communities and environments, that make it impossible to control for all the different variables. Therefore any evidence that does emerge has to be treated with some caution. Even the association between smoking and lung cancer, though strong and statistically significant, is still only an association. There may be a causal link there in epidemiological terms but strictly speaking in this strongest of all associations we cannot say that if you smoke you will get lung cancer.

In other areas of health promotion and public health the associations are often much weaker, and if we include process as well as outcome data, the relationship between cause and effect is much more tentative. It is therefore necessary to consider evidence in a different way. It should be thought of in the same way that juries are instructed to consider evidence within a courtroom trial. They are asked to weigh up the evidence and make a decision based on the 'balance of probabilities' or resting on a conviction which is 'beyond reasonable doubt'. This could be called the judicious use of evidence (Tones 1997), and would be a useful mechanism if employed in ebhp (Macdonald 2000).

Health promoters need to weigh up best evidence to support and justify an intervention, but they need also to consider what theoretical evidence there is to inform a method or approach to a programme. There needs to be a kind of symbiotic relationship between theory and practice, where theory informs practice, which in turn informs and develops theory. The old adage that there is nothing so practical as a good theory is very true in public health and health promotion. By combining a sound theoretical base with a mixture of process and outcome indicators, and assessing the results judiciously, health promoters can begin to get better at making use of best evidence.

TERMINOLOGY AND MEANING

The relatively rapid development of health promotion over a 20-year period has, almost inevitably, caused confusion with terms associated with the discipline, and their meaning. In the 1970s and early 1980s health education was more or less the accepted standard term. Indeed there are those who still profess that it is an appropriate term for most health promotion today (Tones & Tilford 1994) although most recently they have accepted health promotion as a broader more relevant term (Tones & Tilford 2001).

Health education, as a concept and practice, borrows heavily from education and pedagogical philosophy. It is concerned primarily with communication and teaching. One definition that encompasses these two elements is a modification of

WHO's position and illustrated in Tones and Tilford's book (2001). It states that health education 'is any intentional activity that is designed to achieve health … related learning … effective health education may, thus, produce changes in knowledge and understanding or ways of thinking; it may influence or clarify values; it may bring about some shift in attitude or belief; it may facilitate the acquisition of skills; it may even effect changes in behaviour and lifestyle'.

This definition, which reflects the 'personal skills development' strand of the Ottawa Charter, concentrates clearly on the 'one to one' and 'one to group' scenarios, where good communication and teaching inform the learning outcomes. However this more narrow view of the promotion of health has resonances in the biomedical model of health, briefly touched on above. Just as the medical model of health views the body as a machine, isolated from its social environment, so the educational model for health sees teaching and learning in a value-free social structure. This link is all the stronger, if the teaching within the health education model errs on the side of *persuasion*, as opposed to teaching for knowledge's own sake. Generally health education within any healthcare setting is more about persuasion, that is, persuading clients and patients to modify their behaviour or lifestyle for some health gain goal in the future. It doesn't simply allow for the provision of education about health in a neutral, value-free way, which then lets the client decide on a course of action. This approach is often referred to as the 'preventive model of health education' (Downie et al 1996). It is centrally concerned with persuading the client or patient to adopt a lifestyle that prevents health problems in the first place (primary prevention) or prevents problems from getting worse (secondary prevention), or is about rehabilitating patients into some form of health following a critical ill health episode (tertiary prevention).

In the 1980s, WHO and others began to question the validity and acceptability of a model that promoted health in a political and structural vacuum. HFA 2000, and the subsequent set of targets, clearly demonstrated that promoting the public health was much broader than simply providing knowledge. Ottawa gave voice to this broader view and the concept of health promotion was refined and defined in the Charter and other subsequent declarations and documents. Health promotion is seen as 'any measure or planned activity that seeks to improve health, or prevent disease'. In this sense it incorporates the preventive health education model, but allows for a much broader approach that could, indeed should, include legislative, fiscal and policy initiatives that facilitate the promotion of public health. In other words it is as much concerned with the structures which militate against health at local, national and international levels, as it is with education for health at the individual or community level (Macdonald & Davies 1998).

It might be then, that health promotion is very largely related to public health, particularly the so-called 'new public health'. Some may argue that there is virtually no distinction between the two. It is true that health promotion does represent new ways of addressing contemporary health and social care needs and problems; it does offer a means for intellectual development that challenges the 'old' order in terms of healthcare provision and healthy public policy; and it does offer novel participative and empowering ways of working for professionals and clients alike. It is therefore reasonable to view health promotion as a *product* of public health, but a product which has offered a new and intellectually challenging aspect to the 'new' public health (Kickbusch 1999, Macdonald & Bunton 2002).

Interestingly, over the last few years, certainly at least in the UK, there has been a discernible shift in terminology, particularly in government policy, towards the use of the term public health. If health promotion was utilized in 'Health of the Nation' (DoH 1992) and the target setting agenda that followed on from that, more recent policies and government documents such as 'Our Healthier Nation' (DoH 1999), and the NHS Plan (DoH 2000), have referred to policy development and practitioner support in this area as 'public health'. A recent policy document on workforce planning and developments (DoH 2000) actively encouraged the promotion of multidisciplinary training and new roles for public health specialists at local and national levels, with little or no reference to health promotion as a specialism.

The picture is further complicated by the plethora of terms now commonly used within public health and health promotion literature. For example, 'health development', 'health gain', 'health improvement', are all variations on the results expected from health promotion. 'Population health', 'people-centred health promotion' and community/settings-based health promotion give an indication of the bias or slant of a particular public health initiative or programme. Terms such as 'health investment' focus on viewing health as a positive investment opportunity which offers returns, both social and economic, in the same way as one might view economic investment as an opportunity for commercial return. 'Health literacy' has crept into the health promotion literature most recently and is used, as a concept, to help assess people's ability to read, understand and act on health education messages. Health Impact Assessment, on the other hand, is more concerned with attempting to measure the impact on health of any major policy initiative at local or national level. All these terms serve to add to the confusion surrounding health promotion meanings. A useful glossary that includes many of these concepts can be found in *Health Promotion International* (Nutbeam 1998).

CONCLUSION

There is little doubt that all nurses have a critical role to play in helping to promote the public health. Recent government policy White Papers such as 'The NHS Plan' and 'Our Healthier Nation – Saving Lives in England' and 'Improving Health In Wales' reiterate the important role nurses can play in both preventing disease and more positively, promoting health. This is particularly the case for nurses working at the community level.

Nurses working in primary health care and community settings more generally have a particularly crucial role to play. Within the context of an expanded role for primary care, these community-based nurses will help in the development and implementation of primary care strategies with

their emphasis on public health, and more radically, in the pioneering programmes associated with Sure Start and Children and Youth Partnership interventions. They will implement what is essentially health education programmes, with the emphasis on primary prevention (as outlined above), or they will begin to play a more ambitious role in promoting health through a version of the social model of health, again, as discussed above.

Within a more narrow health education context this could mean, for example, further developing the support given to parents by health visitors in the form of information and health advice and perhaps tailoring specific health plans to family needs. Or it could mean, for practice nurses, the employment of techniques designed to get patients to give up smoking through the current Government's strategy for smoking prevention and cessation. For school nurses it allows, *inter alia*, for the development of school-based counselling services, and for occupational health nurses, workforce screening would be an option. District nurses could be encouraged to develop secondary and tertiary prevention strategies to prevent further morbidity in the elderly. Community psychiatric nurses could and must play a pivotal role in reversing the overwhelming emphasis on treatment of mental health problems towards an approach that values prevention, and more particularly mental health promotion (Tudor 1996). Similarly those trained in learning disability nursing need to be aware of what role they can play in helping to improve, for example, the sexual health of their patients, which remains a neglected health education area.

There is a wealth of examples given in the 'Saving Lives' White Paper and some of them touch on a more expanded health promotion role for community nurses. For example health visitors could be encouraged to initiate and develop outreach programmes based on their experience with Sure Start, or school nurses could take a more active role in supporting the healthy schools initiative. Midwives could target socially disadvantaged groups such as single parents or minority ethnic groups and set up pregnancy clubs, and occupational health nurses could promote the concept and practice of a health-promoting workplace. Community mental health nurses can join organizations such as 'Mind' or 'Mentality' to help lobby for improved provision and swing the pendulum towards prevention and health promotion. Learning disability nurses need to help other practitioners and policy makers become more aware of the dearth of health promotion provision and research in this area. It is still too often viewed as something of a 'Cinderella service', struggling to cope with clinical support let alone providing health promotion strategies for people with learning difficulties.

Both these approaches, the health education preventive model and the broader health promotion approach, lend themselves nicely to community nurse-led interventions. However nurses need to be aware of the wider implications of the Ottawa Charter and its sequelae if they wish to support the spirit of contemporary health promotion practice. Ottawa emphasized the need to both reorient health services towards primary health care, and to strengthen community action. Community nurses could take a prime lead in lobbying for these changes. Whilst it may be true that resources are slowly being put into primary health care (to some extent at the expense of acute care) this process is all too slow. Furthermore, the vast majority of research monies made available for healthcare research go into hospital-based care and treatment and relatively little is allocated to community care and health promotion (Carter & Thomas 1999). In addition community-based nurses have first hand experience of the communities in which they work and could be invaluable in terms of supporting community participation and involvement, in the planning, implementation and, indeed, evaluation of community-led services. The Sustainable Health Action Research Programme (SHARP; NafW 2000) in Wales is an example of work that could easily accommodate community-based nurses.

However Ottawa calls for more than this. It asks all professionals in health, social and educational services to take on extra roles as mediators, between funders of services and the public, as facilitators in making things happen, but most importantly as advocates on the part of communities both socially excluded and included. Nurses can enact a very influential role here by banding together, within professional groups or through

geographical location, and lobby for change on behalf of 'their patients'. They can lobby for representation on primary care trusts or local health groups; they can research critical public health issues and publish results in order to encourage change. This expanded role for nurses is crucial if health promotion and public health are to become the 'new' focus for healthcare delivery in the future. Of course it will require new knowledge and skills and the White Paper 'Saving Lives' (DoH 1999) recognizes this. It suggests a new professional to lead in this new public health arena, the 'specialist' in public health, who would be trained in the skills necessary for the proper delivery of this function. The Government intends to lift 'the glass ceiling' within public health that denies nonmedically qualified specialists the option of becoming Directors of Public Health. In the future this will be open to medical specialists in public health and nonmedical specialists and nurses. Community-based nurses are particularly well placed to take advantage of the training opportunities now on offer in this emerging specialism.

Community-level nurses are in a key position to develop and deliver health promotion or the new public health agenda, in line with current government policy. With the acquisition of new knowledge and skills and the determination to extend the role beyond the individual, community nurses could be pivotal in helping to reduce health inequalities across the country and promote health gain at the individual and population levels.

SUMMARY

◆ Health promotion continues to develop and establish itself as a field of study and practice.

◆ The WHO has taken a strong lead in establishing the conceptual base to health promotion interventions, teaching and research.

◆ Health promotion may be seen as the delivery mechanism for the 'new' public health and certainly, with recent policy initiatives, there is scope and support for the development of the role of community nurses (and others) to capitalize on new training and positions associated with the 'new' public health agenda.

◆ New, imaginative, but rigorous forms of evaluation and effectiveness studies need to be developed to establish a more secure evidence base.

DISCUSSION POINTS

1. Do you consider health promotion to be a legitimate discipline or field of study? Can you justify your answer?

2. Are health promotion and public health one and the same?

3. What are the strengths and weaknesses of the Ottawa Charter?

4. What are the problems associated with measuring the effectiveness of health promotion interventions?

5. What different or expanded role could community-based nurses play in promoting health in the locality of current practice?

REFERENCES

Berkman L, Kawachi I 2000 Social epidemiology. Oxford University Press, Oxford

Carter Y, Thomas C (eds) 1999 Research opportunities in primary care. Radcliffe Medical Press, Oxford

Davey-Smith G, Hart C, Blane D, Gillis C, Hawthorne V 1997 Lifetime socio-economic position and mortality; prospective observational study. British Medical Journal 314: 547–552

Davison C, Frankel S, Davey-Smith G 1992 The limits of lifestyle; reassessing fatalism in the popular culture of illness prevention. Social Science and Medicine 34(60): 675–685

Department for Education and Employment 1997 Building excellence in schools together. HMSO, London

Department of Health 1992 Health of the nation. HMSO, London

Department of Health 1999 Saving lives; our healthier nation. HMSO, London

Department of Health 2000 The NHS plan. HMSO, London

Downie RS, Tannahill C, Tannahill A 1996 Health promotion; models and values. Oxford University Press, Oxford

Haglund B, Macdonald G 2000 A global internet survey of health promotion training. European Journal of Public Health 10(4): 316–318

Haglund B, Pettersson B, Finer D, Tilgren P (eds) 1992 Creating supportive environments for health; report from the 3rd International Conference on health promotion; Sundsvall, 1991. WHO, Copenhagen

Harrison D 1999 Social system intervention. In: Perkins E, Simnett I, Wright L (eds) Evidence based health promotion. Wiley, Chichester

Health Education Board for Scotland 1994 Health education and health promotion; from priorities to programmes. No 1 WHO Regional Office for Europe, Health Promotion Country Series. HEBS/WHO, Edinburgh

Kickbusch I 1987 Think health; what makes a difference? Health Promotion International 12(4): 265–272

Kickbusch I 1999 Global public health; revisiting healthy public policy at the global level. Health Promotion International 14(4): 285–288

Kuhn T 1970 The structure of scientific revolutions. University of Chicago Press, Chicago, IL

Lalonde M 1974 A new perspective on the health of the Canadians. Government of Canada, Ottawa

Macdonald G 1997 Quality indicators and health promotion effectiveness. Promotion and Education 4.2: 5–8

Macdonald G 2000 A new evidence framework for health promotion practice. Health Education Journal 59: 3–11

Macdonald G, Bunton R 1992 Disciplines or disciplines. In: Bunton R, Macdonald G (eds) Health promotion; disciplines and diversity. Routledge, London

Macdonald G, Bunton R 2002 Disciplines and developments. In: Bunton R, Macdonald G (eds) Health promotion; disciplines, diversity and developments. Roultedge, London

Macdonald G, Davies JK 1998 Reflection and vision; proving and improving the promotion of health. In: Davies JK, Macdonald G (eds) Quality, evidence and effectiveness in health promotion; striving for certainties. Routledge, London

Macdonald G, Veen C, Tones K 1996 Evidence for success in health promotion; suggestions for improvement. Health Education Research 11: 367–376

Marmot M, Wilkinson RG (eds) 1999 Social determinants of health. Oxford University Press, Oxford

Marmot MG, Shipley MJ, Rose G 1984 Inequalities in death – specific explanations of a general pattern. Lancet i: 1003–1006

Mexico Ministerial Statement for the Promotion of Health 2000 From ideas to action. Health Promotion International 15(4): 275–276

Mittelmark MB, Kvernevik AM, Kannas L, Davies JK 2000 Health promotion curricula; cross national comparisons of essential reading. Promotion and Education VII: 27–32

Mustard JF 1996 Health and social capital. In: Blane D, Brunner E, Wilkinson R (eds) Health and social organisation. Routledge, London

National Assembly for Wales 1998 Better health – better Wales. National Assembly for Wales, Cardiff

National Assembly for Wales 2000 The sustainable health action research programme. National Assembly for Wales, Cardiff

Nutbeam D 1998 Health promotion glossary. Health Promotion International 13(4): 349–364

Oakley A 1998 Experimentation in social science; the case of health promotion. Social Sciences in Health 4(2): 73–89

Poland B, Green L, Rootman I (eds) 2000 Settings for health promotion. Sage, Thousand Oaks

Speller V, Learnmouth A, Harrison D 1997 The search for evidence of effectiveness in health promotion. British Medical Journal 315: 361–363

Stansfeld S 1999 Social support and social cohesion. In: Marmot M, Wilkinson R (eds) Social determinants of health. Oxford University Press, Oxford

Tannahill A 2002 Epidemiology and health promotion; a common understanding. In: Bunton R, Macdonald G (eds) Health promotion; disciplines, diversity and developments. Routledge, London

Tones K 1997 Beyond the randomised control trial; a case for judicial review. Health Education Research 12(2): i–iv

Tones K, Tilford S 1994 Health education; effectiveness and efficiency. Stanley Thornes, Cheltenham

Tones K, Tilford S 2001 Health promotion; effectiveness, efficiency and equity. Nelson Thornes, Cheltenham

Tsouros A 1995 The WHO healthy cities project; state-of-the-art and future plans. Health Promotion International 10: 133–141

Tudor K 1996 Mental health promotion. Routledge, London

Westphal M 2000 Mobilisation of Latin America to promote health. Promotion and Education VII(4): 2–3

Whitelaw S, Baxendale A, Bryce C, MacHardy L, Young I, Whitney E 2001 'Settings' based health promotion; a review. Health Promotion International 16(4): 339–353

Wilkinson RG 1996 Unhealthy societies; the afflictions of inequality. Routledge, London

Williams G, Popay J 1994 Researching the people's health; dilemmas and opportunities for social scientists. In: Popay J, Williams G (eds) Researching the people's health. Routledge, London

World Heath Organization 1977 Health for all by the year 2000. WHO, Geneva

World Health Organization 1978 Report on the International Conference on Primary Health Care Alma Ata. WHO, Geneva

World Health Organization 1984 Health promotion; a discussion document on the concepts and principles. WHO Regional Office for Europe, Copenhagen

World Health Organization 1986 Ottawa Charter for health promotion, an international conference on health promotion. WHO, Copenhagen

World Health Organization 1988 Healthy public policy; report on the Adelaide Conference. WHO, Copenhagen

World Health Organization 1991 The Budapest declaration on health promoting hospitals. WHO European Regional Office, Copenhagen

World Health Organization 1993 The European network of health promoting schools; a joint WHO (Europe) and the Commission of the European Communities and Council of Europe Project. Commission of European Communities and Council of Europe, Brussels

World Health Organization 1995 Building a healthy city; a practitioners guide. WHO, Geneva

World Health Organization 1997 The Jakarta Declaration on leading health promotion into the 21st century. Health Promotion International 12: 261–264

World Health Organization 1998 Social determinants of health. The solid facts. WHO Regional Office for Europe, Copenhagen

World Health Organization 2000 Mexico ministerial statement for the promotion of health; from ideas to action. Health Promotion International 15.4: 275–276

FURTHER READING

It is difficult to highlight a few texts that capture the essence of health promotion, and are at a level which makes demands on the reader; the list below, does I think, achieve both.

Bunton R, Macdonald G (eds) 2002 Health promotion; disciplines, diversity and developments. Routledge, London

This book provides an introduction to health promotion as a discipline; it has over a dozen chapters devoted to demonstrating the contribution other disciplines, such as psychology, sociology, education, ethics and genetics, have made to the development of health promotion theory and practice. It is a second revised edition, based on a successful first edition first published in 1992.

Perkins E, Simnett I, Wright L (eds) 1999 Evidence based health promotion. John Wiley and Son, Chichester

A collection of contributing chapters designed to discuss and critique the various approaches to evidence and how practitioners might learn from them. It attempts to help practitioners assess evidence and base interventions on imperfect evidence.

Poland B, Green L, Rootman I 2000 Settings for health promotion. Sage, Thousand Oaks

A first attempt to analyse the use of 'settings' as the focal point for health promotion interventions. It has a strong Canadian/USA feel to it, but it does provide a comprehensive series of examples and case studies from across the globe to illustrate the strength of a settings approach.

Davies JK, Macdonald G (eds) 1998 Quality, evidence and effectiveness in health promotion; striving for certainties. Routledge, London

This book brings together for the first time, issues to do with quality assurance, research and effectiveness. It is an edited reader with contributions by leading international authorities and divided into three sections. It examines effectiveness studies through different research methodologies; it assesses practice-based quality assurance programmes; and it provides examples of programmes utilizing both concepts.

Tones K, Tilford S 2000 Health promotion; effectiveness, efficiency and equity. Nelson Thornes, Cheltenham

A very comprehensive treatment of health promotion, the book combines a first section dedicated to definitions, indicators of change and research methods, with a second section that looks at settings for health and the use of the mass media. An academic and strong contribution to the understanding of the subject.

Ewles L, Simnett I 1995 Promoting health; a practical guide, 3rd edn. Scutari Press, London

This is a well thought through easy to read guide to planning, implementing and evaluating a health promotion programme or intervention. It is written at a more basic level than the five above but could be a useful starting point.

Index